Transfusion and Transplantation Science

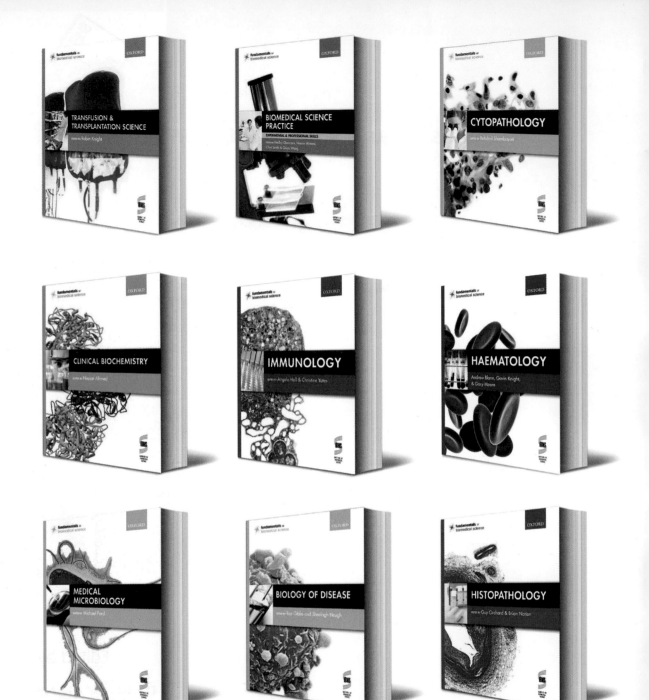

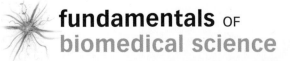

fundamentals OF
biomedical science

Fundamentals of Biomedical Science

Transfusion and Transplantation Science

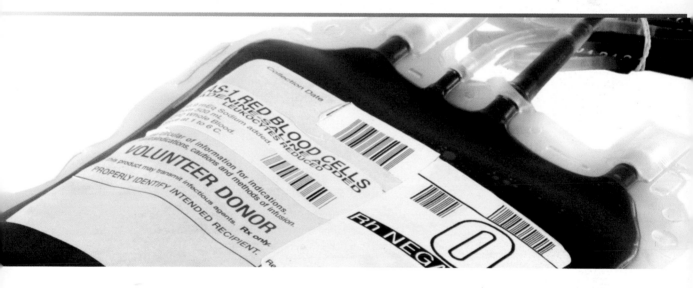

Edited by

Robin Knight
Transfusion Science Consultant

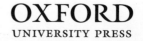

OXFORD

UNIVERSITY PRESS

OXFORD
UNIVERSITY PRESS

Great Clarendon Street, Oxford, OX2 6DP,
United Kingdom

Oxford University Press is a department of the University of Oxford.
It furthers the University's objective of excellence in research, scholarship,
and education by publishing worldwide. Oxford is a registered trade mark of
Oxford University Press in the UK and in certain other countries

Impression: 1

British Library Cataloguing in Publication Data
Data available

Library of Congress Cataloging in Publication Data
Library of Congress Control Number: 201294197
ISBN 978–0–19–953328–2

Printed in Italy on acid-free paper by
L.E.G.O. S.p.A.–Lavis TN

Acknowledgements

Some of the material presented in Chapter 9 draws on material presented in *Human Blood Cells*, May-Jean King (ed.), Imperial College Press, Chapters 9 and 10, 2000 and *Practical Transfusion Medicine* (3rd edition) Michael F Murphy and Derwood H Pamphilon (eds), Blackwell Publishing, Chapter 4, 2008. I am particularly grateful to Mr David Allen (NHSBT, Oxford Centre/University of Oxford), Dr Paul Metcalfe (National Institute for Biological Standards and Control, Potters Bar), Professor Mike Murphy (NHSBT, Oxford Centre) and Dr Willem Ouwehand (NHSBT, Cambridge Centre/University of Cambridge) for their kind permission to use material from the above publications. Some of the material presented in Chapters 1 and 7 draws on that presented in *An Introduction to Blood Transfusion Science and Blood Bank Practice*, Phil Learoyd, Robin Knight, Peter Rogan, and Martin Haynes, British Blood Transfusion Society, 2009; from whom permission has been obtained.

An introduction to the Fundamentals of Biomedical Science series

Biomedical Scientists form the foundation of modern healthcare, from cancer screening to diagnosing HIV, from blood transfusion for surgery to food poisoning and infection control. Without Biomedical Scientists, the diagnosis of disease, the evaluation of the effectiveness of treatment, and research into the causes and cures of disease would not be possible.

However, the path to becoming a Biomedical Scientist is a challenging one: trainees must not only assimilate knowledge from a range of disciplines, but must understand—and demonstrate—how to apply this knowledge in a practical, hands-on environment.

The *Fundamentals of Biomedical Science* series is written to reflect the challenges of biomedical science education and training today. It blends essential basic science with insights into laboratory practice to show how an understanding of the biology of disease is coupled to the analytical approaches that lead to diagnosis.

The series provides coverage of the full range of disciplines to which a Biomedical Scientist may be exposed—from microbiology to cytopathology to transfusion science. Alongside volumes exploring specific biomedical themes and related laboratory diagnosis, an overarching *Biomedical Science Practice* volume provides a grounding in the general professional and experimental skills with which every Biomedical Scientist should be equipped.

Produced in collaboration with the Institute of Biomedical Science, the series:

- understands the complex roles of biomedical scientists in the modern practice of medicine,
- understands the development needs of employers and the Profession,
- places the theoretical aspects of biomedical science in their practical context.

Learning from this series

The *Fundamentals of Biomedical Science* series draws on a range of learning features to help readers master both biomedical science theory, and biomedical science practice.

Case Studies illustrate how the biomedical science theory and practice presented throughout the series relates to situations and experiences that are likely to be encountered routinely in the biomedical science laboratory.

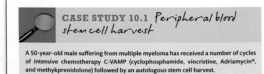

CASE STUDY 10.1 Peripheral blood stem cell harvest

A 50-year-old male suffering from multiple myeloma has received a number of cycles of intensive chemotherapy C-VAMP (cyclophosphamide, vincristine, Adriamycin®, and methykprenidolone) followed by an autologous stem cell harvest.

Additional information to augment the main text appears in **boxes.**

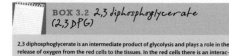

Method boxes walk through the key protocols that the reader is likely to encounter in the laboratory on a regular basis.

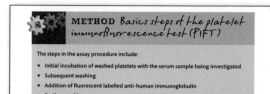

Clinical correlations emphasize at a glance how the material sits in a clinical context.

CLINICAL CORRELATION

The HLA-matching scheme used in the allocation of kidneys in the UK initially takes into account polymorphism at the HLA-A,-B and DRB1 loci:

000   No mismatch at HLA-A, B, or DR

010   One HLA-B mismatch

Key points reinforce the key concepts that the reader should master from having read the material presented, while **Summary** points act as an end-of-chapter checklists for readers to verify that they have remembered correctly the principal themes and ideas presented within each chapter.

Key points

Organ rejection can be minimized by HLA typing, matching, and crossmatching.

Rejection can be categorized as:

Hyperacute, occurring within minutes or hours of the transplant.

Acute, usually occurring within days up to the first three months following transplantation.

Chronic, slow deterioration of graft function, occurring months to years following transplantation.

Key terms provide on-the-page explanations of terms with which the reader may not be familiar; in addition, each title in the series features a **glossary**, in which the key terms featured in that title are collated.

Extravascular lysis
Immune mediated cell removal that takes place outside the circulation in the liver or spleen.

Intravascular lysis
Cells being lysed within the circulation by antibodies that activate the complement pathway, especially anti-A and anti-B.

This mechanism is called **extravascular lysis** as the immune mediate place outside the circulation in the liver of spleen.

Some antibodies, especially anti-A and anti-B can activate the comple complement' as it is sometimes called, that leads directly to the cells b circulation; this is called **intravascular lysis**.

Therefore, antibodies are produced in response to an external antige mary response is slow and IgM antibodies are formed first with the plas ing production to IgG. In a secondary response IgG antibodies are prod with little or no lag phase.

Antibodies by themselves do not cause cell destruction but they acti

Self-check questions throughout each chapter and extended questions at the end of each chapter provide the reader with a ready means of checking that they have understood the material they have just encountered. Answers to these questions are provided in the book's Online Resource Centre; visit www.oxfordtextbooks.co.uk/orc/ knight

components into up to eight paediatric packs. Similarly, adult apheresis platelet donations are split into four paediatric packs. Smaller volumes of methylene blue treated FFP are also available for these patients.

SELF-CHECK 3.8

What are the additional test requirements for blood components intended for neonatal use?

Cross-references help the reader to see biomedical science as a unified discipline, making connections between topics presented within each volume, and across all volumes in the series.

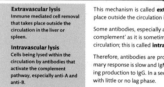

ood components renders the donor lymphocytes non-viable and m potentially developing TA-GVHD. It is recommended that all cel-at risk patients should be irradiated with a minimum of 25 Gray (Gy),

See Chapter 5 for more on irradiated blood components.

nsfusion Services introduced to reduce the incidence of HLA related sion?

Online learning materials

online resource centre

The *Fundamentals of Biomedical Science* series doesn't end with the printed books. Each title in the series is supported by an Online Resource Centre, which features additional materials for students, trainees, and lecturers.

www.oxfordtextbooks.co.uk/orc/fbs

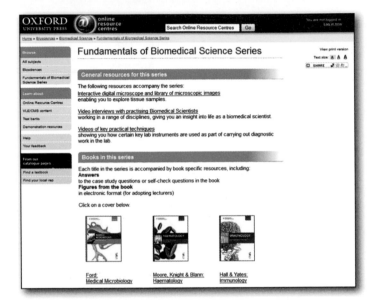

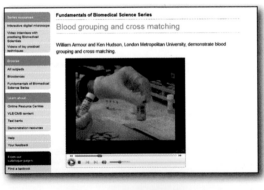

Guides to key experimental skills and methods

Video walk-throughs of key experimental skills to help you master the essential skills that are the foundation of biomedical science practice.

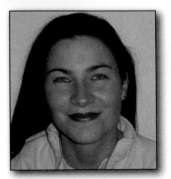

Biomedical science in practice

Interviews with practising Biomedical Scientists working in a range of disciplines, to give you valuable insights into the reality of work in a biomedical science laboratory.

Jane Worthington, Specialist Biomedical Scientist in Microbiology at St Peters Hospital, Chertsey

Digital Microscope

A library of microscopic images for you to investigate using this powerful online microscope, to help you gain a deeper appreciation of cell and tissue morphology.

The Digital Microscope is used under licence from the Open University.

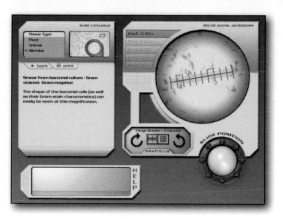

Answers to self-check, case study, and end-of-chapter questions

Answers to questions posed in the book are provided to aid self-assessment.

Lecturer support materials

The Online Resource Centre for each title in the series also features figures from the book in electronic format, for registered adopters to download for use in lecture presentations, and other educational resources.

To register as an adopter visit **www.oxfordtextbooks.co.uk/orc/knight** and follow the on-screen instructions.

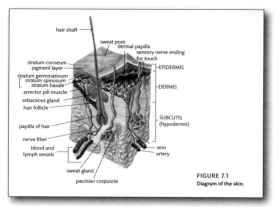

FIGURE 7.1
Diagram of the skin.

Any comments?

We welcome comments and feedback about any aspect of this series.
Just visit **www.oxfordtextbooks.co.uk/orc/feedback** and share your views.

Contributors

John Barker
Gateshead Health NHS Foundation Trust

Colin Brown
NHS Blood and Transplant

Carol Cantwell
St Mary's Hospital Imperial College Healthcare NHS Trust

Bill Chaffe
East Kent Hospitals University NHS Foundation Trust

Tony Davies
NHS Blood & Transplant

Joan Jones
Welsh Blood Service

Robin Knight
Former Head of NHS Blood and Transplant Red Cell
Immunohaematology Division

Richard Lomas
NHS Blood and Transplant

Geoff Lucas
NHS Blood and Transplant

Karen Madgwick
North Middlesex Hospital NHS Trust

Lionel Mohabir
Welsh Blood Service

Malcolm Needs
NHS Blood and Transplant

Robert Walters
North West Wales NHS Trust

Contents

Introduction to Basic Immunology and Techniques

Robin Knight

Learning objectives

After studying this chapter you should be able to:

- Outline the various components of the immune system.
- Outline the functioning of the humoral immune system.
- Describe antibody structure and function.
- Describe antigen–antibody reactions.
- Understand antibody-mediated red cell destruction.
- Understand the detection of red cell antigen–antibody reactions and agglutination.

Introduction

This book essentially covers the laboratory and scientific aspects of the transfusion of human blood and products or components made from blood, and the transplantation of tissues and stem cells, but not the clinical practice of transfusion and transplanting organs. This first chapter reviews the historical background to the science of transfusion and transplantation.

The history of both transfusion and transplantation can be traced back to ancient times, but the real advances have been made within the last 60 years. For many centuries, medicine was founded on the four body humours—blood, phlegm, yellow bile, and black bile, and it was thought that health could be restored by bloodletting, starving, vomiting, or purging. Such practices were still carried out in some places until the end of the nineteenth century.

The circulation of the blood and the function of valves in veins were described by the English physician William Harvey in a book published in 1628. A few years later (1669) another Englishman, Richard Lower, reported his experiments with the transfusion of blood from one dog to another and also between humans. About the same time in Paris, Jean Baptiste Denis also performed some transfusions of humans but after a number of his subjects died the practice was banned in some European countries for the next 150 years.

In 1829, Dr James Blundell, a British obstetrician, first performed a successful human transfusion by taking four ounces of blood from the arm of a dying patient's husband with a syringe and transfusing it into the patient, who recovered. He had conducted a series of well-thought-out experiments using animals, where he showed that as long as the blood was transfused quickly after it had been taken then it would be successful even in resuscitating an animal dying of blood loss.

Many of Blundell's patients were women who were bleeding excessively after childbirth (post-partum haemorrhage) and he devised numerous instruments for the transfusion of blood, many of which we would recognize today. To honour the work of this pioneer the British Blood Transfusion Society still presents an annual James Blundell Award.

In 1849, Dr C Routh, physician to the St Pancras Royal Dispensary in London, reviewed the 44 examples of blood transfusion that had been reported at that time. He concluded that the procedure was one of the safest major operations which may be practised in surgery 'with the rate of mortality of one in three—rather less than that of hernia, or about the same as the average of amputations'.

In 1875, Landois reported that the red cells of one animal species clumped, or *agglutinated* those of another if mixed together. Similar clumping had already been noticed when certain sera had been mixed with bacteria. It was suggested that this was due to antigens on the surface of the bacteria uniting with antibodies in the serum. Therefore, this knowledge of bacterial immunology was applied to the phenomenon of red cell agglutination.

One of the most important discoveries in the history of transfusion was made by the Austrian scientist Karl Landsteiner, who observed the agglutination of human red cells by serum of other humans—a difference within a species, rather than between species. He went on to describe the ABO blood group system in 1901. In 1930 he received the Nobel Prize for Physicians and Medicine and a decade later, together with Dr Weiner, described the *Rh-factor*, now known to be part of the Rh blood group system.

Following the work of Landsteiner, and independently, Moss and Jansky, in describing the ABO groups, the reason why so many early transfusions were fatal was at last understood. The blood of one person can be *incompatible* with that of another, so before a transfusion can be given the donor's blood must be shown to be compatible with that of the potential recipient. Initially this was done by matching the ABO groups, but later more complex tests were devised, the so-called *crossmatch*.

A major contribution to the discovery of further blood groups was 'a new test' described in 1945 by Drs Robin Coombs, Arthur Mourant, and Rob Race: the antiglobulin test. This is still often referred to, erroneously, as the Coombs test. Using this technique IgG, or non-agglutinating antibodies, can be detected on the surface of red cells either as the result of their being coated by antibody *in vivo*, or in an *in vitro* laboratory test.

Since then, more blood groups have been discovered, so that today there are some 30 human erythrocyte antigen (blood group) systems known. The whole arena of histocompatibility (tissue typing) and the human lymphocyte antigen (HLA), human platelet antigen (HPA), and human neutrophil antigen (HNA), systems have been described and their function understood. These, too, are described in greater detail in this book.

The two World Wars of the twentieth century were both times when advances were made in transfusion science and practice. During the First World War it was shown that if blood was collected into an *anticoagulant* to prevent clots from forming, the blood could be stored for a short time before being transfused. By adding dextrose to the sodium citrate anticoagulant, blood could be stored for several days in a refrigerator. Therefore, there was no need to have a donor available at the time blood was needed. The process of storing blood was improved during the Second World War when the first large-scale collection of blood from volunteers was started in the UK under the Emergency Medical Service. From this was born, in 1947, the National Blood Transfusion Service, which has grown to become, in England, by 2006, NHS Blood and Transplant. Scotland, Wales, and Northern Ireland have their own similar services.

There have been two other major developments that enabled advances to be made in transfusion practice. The first is the use of plastic bags for the collection of blood, instead of glass bottles. Dr Carl W Walter was instrumental in this development that has enabled whole blood, as collected from the donor, to be split into its component parts—red cells, plasma, platelets, and white cells. Each of these *blood components* can be stored separately and transfused to patients who require that specific component, for example red cells because they are anaemic.

In the 1940s Dr Edwin Cohn, a Harvard biochemist, developed a method for fractionating plasma into its different proteins, so that specific *blood products* could be produced. These include fibrinogen, gamma globulins, albumin, and various clotting factors. Some of the latter are now made using *recombinant technology*.

Another major advance has been the introduction of *monoclonal antibody technology*. Milstein and his co-workers showed that by fusing an antibody-producing cell with a myeloma cell, a clone of cells could be grown in culture that continued to produce antibody. The supernatant containing the specific antibody can be harvested and used as an antibody reagent. Prior to this, antibodies were obtained from humans or animals, often after deliberate immunization, but the required antibody had to be isolated or unwanted antibodies removed. Monoclonal antibodies, being obtained as a single specificity and in large volumes, do not need to undergo such lengthy treatment. Monoclonal antibodies are now used not just for *in vitro* tests, but also for *in vivo* treatment.

Transplantation has a shorter history, although in Roman times Saints Cosmas and Damian are attributed to have grafted the leg of a recently deceased black Ethiopian to replace the ulcerated leg of a white patient. The major problem of tissue transplantation is that of rejection—the transplanted cells are seen by the recipient's immune system as foreign and mount an 'immune attack' to reject them.

It was the realization that graft rejection was due to incompatibility of antigens on human white cells that lead to the discovery of the HLA system and the *major histocompatibility locus* that has enabled the great advances to be made with transplantation.

Kidney (renal) transplants were first carried out successfully in 1954 and the world's first heart transplant was done in 1967, since which time most organs have been transplanted. Not only can solid organs (e.g. kidneys, heart, lungs) be transplanted, but also bone marrow and stem cells. Stem cell transplantation is a fast growing science, but not without ethical controversy. Some tissues, such as corneas, skin, and bone, can be collected and stored and then transplanted without the problems of rejection associated with more cellular organs. These, too, are covered in this book.

Over the past few years there has been an increase in legislation from the European Union affecting many aspects of our lives, including transfusion and transplantation. Reference will be made to some of these directives in the text and you will learn that this clinical/scientific discipline is now highly regulated by a number of statutory agencies. Details of where you can find the more the important directives and guidelines will be given at the end of the final chapter that deals with quality.

1.1 Basic immunology and techniques

The human immune response will not be considered in detail in this book as it is covered adequately elsewhere. However, the main features that are directly relevant to topics in this book, such as immune cell destruction, are reviewed below.

Humoral immunity
That part of the immune system that is initiated by the recognition of a foreign protein or cell and leads to its removal or destruction through the interaction of a specific antibody.

Cellular immunity
That part of the immune system that is initiated by the recognition of a foreign protein or cell and leads to its removal or destruction by the interaction of complement, or cytokines produced by cytotoxic or killer T cells.

The adaptive immune response is usually divided into **humoral immunity** and **cellular immunity**. Both are initiated by the recognition of a foreign protein or cell and lead to its removal or destruction, either through the interaction of a specific antibody, in the case of humoral immunity, or by the interaction of complement or cytokines produced by cytotoxic or killer T cells, in cellular immunity.

When considering transfusion of blood and blood components, we are concerned mainly with the humoral response to antigens on erythrocytes, platelets, and leucocytes that enter the circulation either by transfusion, with a transplanted organ or during pregnancy, where some of the foetal cells pass into the maternal circulation. In the transplant situation, although antibodies do play a role in graft rejection, the cellular immune response is more important.

The immune system

For an individual to survive in an immunologically hostile world, the cells of its own immune system have to be able to distinguish 'self' from 'non-self' as any foreign cell, virus particle, or protein might cause that individual harm. Once recognized as foreign then it has to be eliminated from the body if possible before it can cause harm. See Figure 1.1.

During foetal and early development B and T lymphocytes learn what is 'self' so that they can then spot what is non-self and potentially harmful. Essentially, B and T cells have HLA receptor molecules that enable each of the millions of lymphocytes to recognize a specific antigen. If anything foreign enters the body then *antigen presenting cells* (APC) isolate the antigen molecules and present them on their cell surface to be recognized by the unique receptors on T or B cells. If seen as non-self then the APC initiates cellular events that lead to the activation of clones of lymphocytes that will in turn deal with the foreign antigen.

Polyclonal antibodies
These are produced by more than one clone of cells.

Monoclonal antibody
Produced from a single clone of cells.

Activated T cells, cytotoxic CD8+ Tc cells, secrete an array of cytokines that can lead to the death of the foreign cells. This is the main immune reaction that causes graft rejection and graft versus host disease. B cells, with the help of CD4+ T helper cells, transform into antibody-secreting plasma cells. More than one plasma cell line is activated, each producing an antibody with a slightly different reactivity against the initiating antigen, although the general specificity is the same. The resulting antibodies are said to be **polyclonal antibodies**—the product of more than one clone of cells. In some disease states and *in vitro*, antibodies can be produced from a single clone—a **monoclonal antibody**.

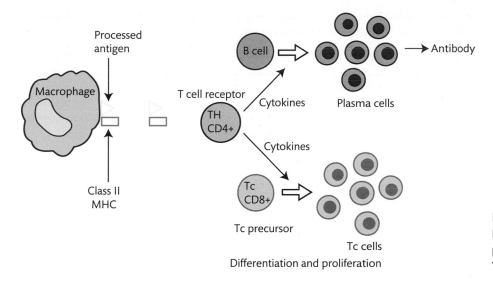

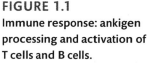

FIGURE 1.1
Immune response: ankigen processing and activation of T cells and B cells.

The clonal expansion that follows initiation takes time and it might be several days, or even weeks, before there is any detectable antibody. At first IgM antibodies are secreted, then the plasma cells 'switch class' and produce IgG molecules. If there is no further exposure to the new antigen then the IgM production peaks and then declines so that IgM antibodies are no longer detectable. However, the IgG antibody production continues and antibodies can be detected many years after the initial exposure, which can, as we shall see, be important when looking for compatible blood for a patient.

Once initiated to a new antigen, some T and B cells become non-secreting memory cells that retain that 'knowledge' and, because of the clonal expansion there will be a large number of primed *memory cells*, so that if there is another contact with that foreign antigen they will be able to respond much quicker than when that antigen was first encountered. Also, the dose of the antigen can be much smaller than that needed for an initial or primary response. Whereas it might take several weeks or months for an antibody to become detectable initially, in a secondary response there is no lag phase as IgG antibody molecules are produced immediately.

It was stated above that for B lymphocytes to be transformed into antibody producing plasma cells the interaction of T helper cells is required. However, some antibodies are produced without T cell involvement. B cells have some antigen receptors that are able to interact directly with sugar-based antigens. A number of polysaccharides, but not polypeptides, especially if they have multiple identical repeats in their molecular structure, can initiate B cells and the proliferation of plasma cells. The antibodies produced are IgM and because of the absence of T helper cell involvement class-switching does not occur and IgM antibodies continue to be produced. Because there are no memory cells produced, antibody production continues only as long as there is continuing exposure to the antigen.

The ABO antibodies are an example of this T-independent immune response. The IgM antibodies are really directed to antigens on bacteria in the gut but they cross-react with the very similar A and B antigens on the red cells. Because these antibodies are produced as a result of exposure to antigens in nature and not as a result of stimulation by foreign red cells entering the circulation, those with blood group activity are often referred to as *naturally acquired* antibodies.

Key points

The immune system recognizes and responds to foreign, or non-self, proteins (antigens) by producing antibodies or cells that interact directly with that protein.

SELF-CHECK 1.1

What are the differences between a primary and secondary immune antibody response?

1.2 Antibody structure

The *humoral immune response* results in the production of specific antibodies that interact with the corresponding, initiating antigen on the target cell, but what is an antibody and how does it bring about cell destruction or removal?

Antibodies are proteins, gamma-globulins, with specific characteristics collectively known as immunoglobulins. An immunoglobulin molecule is composed of two 'heavy' and two 'light' type chains, held together by non-covalent interactions and disulphide bonds. There are five classes of immunoglobulins (Ig) each with their own specific heavy chain:

- IgG-gamma (G or γ)
- IgM mu (M or μ)
- IgA alpha (A or α),
- IgD delta (D or δ)
- IgE epsilon (E or ε)

These heavy chain types differ in the number of amino acid residues and carbohydrate content, giving each class different characteristics and biological activity. The gamma chain has four variations, producing four sub-types of IgG: IgG1, IgG2, IgG3, and IgG4 that results in variations in their biological activity. Most immune IgG blood group antibodies are a mixture of IgG1 and IgG3, and only rarely are they IgG2 or IgG4. There are two classes of IgA: IgA1 and IgA2.

There are two types of light chain, kappa (K or κ) and lambda (L or λ). The light chains of antibody molecules produced by each clone of antibody-producing plasma cells will be the same type. Each IgG immunoglobulin molecule has the two light chains and two γ heavy chains, held together by disulphide bonds between cysteine amino acids and by non-covalent hydrophobic interactions. See Figure 1.2.

An IgG molecule can be broken down by the use of proteolytic enzymes into two Fab fragments, and one Fc fragment. The Fab (fragment antigen binding) is composed of an intact light chain and the amino-terminal end of the γ heavy chain, linked together by interchain disulphide bonding, and acts as the specific antigen binding site.

The Fc (fragment crystalline) is composed of a dimer of the carboxy terminal portions of the two γ heavy chains linked by disulphide bonding. It is associated with some of the IgG

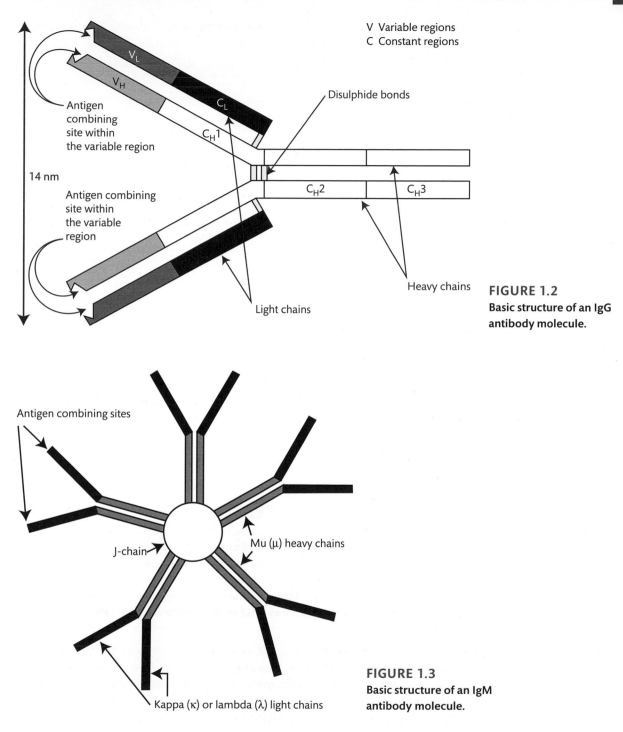

V Variable regions
C Constant regions

FIGURE 1.2
Basic structure of an IgG antibody molecule.

FIGURE 1.3
Basic structure of an IgM antibody molecule.

molecule's biological functions (e.g. complement activation and macrophage binding). The Fc fragment of the IgG molecule contains most of the carbohydrate content.

The IgM molecule is a pentamer, with the five sections, each comprising two light chains and two μ heavy chains, being held together by a J-chain, as shown in Figure 1.3. See Tables 1.1 and 1.2.

TABLE 1.1 Properties of IgG and IgM antibody molecules.

Property	IgG*	IgM
Placental transfer	Yes	No
Complement activation	Yes	Yes
Treatment with dithiothreitol (DTT)	Unaffected	Reduced
Optimal reaction temperature	37°C	4–20°C
Primary immune response involvement	(+)	+++
Secondary immune response involvement	+++	(+)

*See Table 1.2.

TABLE 1.2 Properties of blood group antibody IgG subclasses.

Property	IgG1	IgG2	IgG3	IgG4
Mean percentage of total IgG	~70%	~18%	~8%	~4%
Complement activation (via the classic pathway)	+++	+	+++	−
Placental transfer	++	±	++	+
Macrophage binding	+++	−	+++	−

1.3 Antibody function

The polypeptide chains of immunoglobulin molecules are not straight, linear molecules but are folded and held in place by intrachain disulphide bonds. The specificity of the antibody is determined by the variable regions of the heavy and light chains in the Fab part of the molecule; composed of 110 variable amino acid sequences, and containing the 'hyper-variable' regions where the antigen binding sites are located. With some 500–1,000 heavy chain and over 200 light chain variable region genes, there are more than ten million potential antibody specificities that can be produced by any individual.

The other biological functions of the antibody: complement activation, placental transfer, and the ability to bind to macrophages, are located on the constant regions of the Fc part on the immunoglobulin molecule.

The hinge region (two closely associated triplets of proline amino acids) provides the heavy chain with a degree of flexibility, enabling it to bend. An IgG molecule has a 'T' shape with the antigen binding sites about 14 nm apart, but becomes a 'Y' shape on binding with its antigen. This change in shape also allows the effector functions, associated with the Fc portion, to become activated.

Immunoglobulin M molecules have a diameter of about 30 nm, and as well as being flexible at the hinge regions they can change shape on binding with an antigen by movement of the J-chain. Photomicrographs show them as various 'crab-like' shapes when bound to antigens on a cell surface. IgM antibodies can agglutinate red cells when they are suspended in plasma or saline, by binding to antigens on cells next to one another.

What are the functions of antibody molecules? See Figures 1.4 and 1.5.

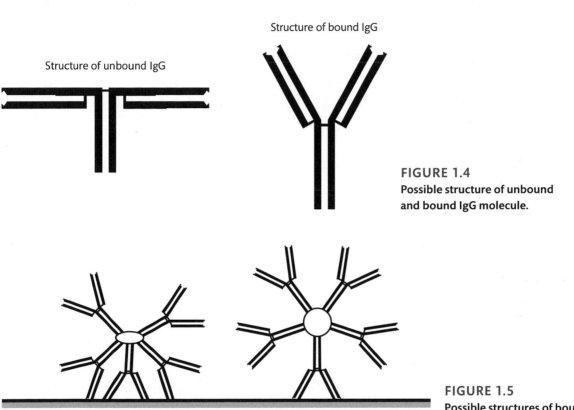

Structure of unbound IgG

Structure of bound IgG

FIGURE 1.4
Possible structure of unbound and bound IgG molecule.

Red cell membrane—antigens

FIGURE 1.5
Possible structures of bound IgM molecules.

1.4 Antigen–antibody reactions

The reaction of an antibody and antigen occurs very quickly. It is a reversible reaction governed by the *Laws of Mass Action* and will eventually come to equilibrium, when the formation of Ag:Ab complexes is at the same rate as the dissociation.

$$Ag + Ab = AgAb$$

The antigen and antibody are held together by relatively weak attracting forces, involving hydrogen, ionic, and hydrophobic bonding as well as van der Waal's forces. As antibodies are produced to a specific antigen by a number of clones of plasma cells the affinity, or association constant, for the antigen will vary within those polyclonal antibodies. Greater differences will be found between antibodies of different specificities. The greater the affinity of an antibody the more likely it is to bind with an antigen. Likewise the greater the amount of antibody that is present for a given amount of antigen, then more antibody will become bound to that cell and the more likely that the antibody-coated or sensitized cells will be recognized and removed *in vivo* or detected in *in vitro* tests.

Key points

Of the five immunoglobulin classes, IgM and IgG antibodies are the most important in transfusion. Antigen binding is a function of the Fab portion, and other effector mechanisms: complement activation, placental transfer, and macrophage binding, are functions of the Fc portion of the molecule.

1.5 **Antibody mediated red cell destruction**

Antibodies do not destroy red cells directly *in vivo*, but initiate their destruction in two ways by:

- The activation of complement
- Macrophage recognition of red cell bound antibody

Complement

The role of complement is essentially to destroy invading cells, such as bacteria, but antibodies to blood cells can also initiate this pathway. The complement system has nine main components, C1–C9, working in a sequential manner; each one, once activated is capable of activating the next in the cascade. The 'classic' complement cascade is activated by the Fc portions of immunoglobulin molecules when bound to a cell surface antigen. Two Fc molecules are required to activate C1. This can be by one IgM antibody molecule or two IgG molecules, very close together on the cell membrane.

The order of the reaction sequence is:

$$C1—C4—C2—C3—C5—C6—C7—C8—C9$$

The final steps of the cascade cause 'channels' to be formed through the cell membrane, allowing water to move into the red cell, resulting in cell lysis or haemolysis of red cells.

The classical complement pathway has three distinct phases:

1. *Activation phase*

The activation of C1 by a red cell antigen–antibody reaction, followed by the activation of C4 and C2 molecules to form the C4b2b complex (C3 convertase).

2. *Amplification phase*

The activation of C3 by C3 convertase', that leads to the binding of C3b to the C4b2b complex and C3b binding to other sites on the cell membrane.

3. *Membrane attack phase*

The activation of C5 by the C4b2b3b complex and the subsequent activation of C6, C7, C8 and C9 leading to cell lysis.

'Activation' phase:

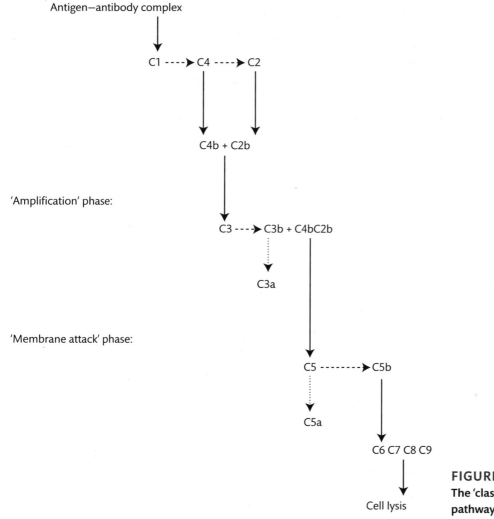

'Amplification' phase:

'Membrane attack' phase:

FIGURE 1.6
The 'classical' complement pathway.

Once activated, complement needs to be carefully regulated so that it does not cause damage to the body itself. There are several regulators that interact with C3b and C4b to inhibit their activity by further splitting the molecules into C3d and C4d, which do not have any effector capabilities. Because of the limited number of complement molecules bound initially to the cell or the action of regulatory mechanisms, the cascade often stops at the C3 (effectively C3b) stage and does not proceed to cell lysis. However, cells coated with C3b can be removed from the circulation by macrophages in the liver but cells with C3d are not recognized and are therefore not removed.

Complement fragments C3a and C5a have properties that are important parts of the overall inflammatory response mechanism. They are chemotactic for neutrophils, attracting them to the site where complement is activated so they can phagocytose cells coated with C3b. The two complement fragments are also anaphylatoxins that bind to basophils in the blood and tissue mast cells, causing them to degranulate and release histamine.

This in turn causes the blood vessels to dilate, allowing more blood containing complement and antibodies to get to the site of inflammation. C5a can also bind to macrophages inducing them to release cytokines such as IL-1 (interlukin) and IL-6 that increase the expression of cell adhesion molecules (CAM) lining the endothelial cells of the blood vessels. Neutrophils attracted to the site then bind to the vessel walls and can be migrated to the inflamed site.

However when considering antigen–antibody reactions of blood cells these are not localized as, for example, a cut to the skin, so therefore the effects of complement and ctyokine activity are not localized, as will be considered later.

Macrophages

As blood cells are not localized but circulating, the effector cells, macrophages, for removing old or damaged blood cells are found mainly in the spleen. As the blood circulates through the spleen IgG antibody coated cells will adhere to IgG receptors (FcR) on the surface of the macrophages that will then engulf the cell, effectively removing it from the circulation. With red cells, the cell is not always engulfed but a part of the membrane is removed allowing the rest of the red cell to break away as a *spherocyte*.

Of the four sub-classes of IgG immunoglobulins; IgG2 and IgG4 seem not to be recognized by these macrophages, whereas IgG1 and IgG3 are. It has been shown that 1,000 IgG1 molecules are required per red cell for it to be sequestered but only 100 molecules of IgG3 are required.

Cells with C3b on their surface are recognized by macrophages in the liver and they, too, are removed from the circulation. However, C3b is quickly broken down *in vivo* to C3d that is not recognized by macrophages, so cells thus coated have a nearly normal life span. The presence of both IgG and complement C3b on the red cell increases the likelihood of the red cells being removed from the circulation, by the 'additive' effect of the removal of complement coated cells in the liver and IgG coated cells in the spleen.

Extravascular lysis
Immune mediated cell removal that takes place outside the circulation in the liver or spleen.

Intravascular lysis
Cells being lysed within the circulation by antibodies that activate the complement pathway, especially anti-A and anti-B.

This mechanism is called **extravascular lysis** as the immune mediated cell removal takes place outside the circulation in the liver of spleen.

Some antibodies, especially anti-A and anti-B can activate the complement pathway, or 'fix complement' as it is sometimes called, that leads directly to the cells being lysed within the circulation; this is called **intravascular lysis**.

Therefore, antibodies are produced in response to an external antigenic stimulus. The primary response is slow and IgM antibodies are formed first with the plasma cells then switching production to IgG. In a secondary response, IgG antibodies are produced from the outset with little or no lag phase.

Antibodies by themselves do not cause cell destruction but they activate the complement cascade that might result in either cell lysis within the circulation or removal by macrophages in the liver of cells coated with C3b. If complement is not activated then cells coated with IgG antibody will be recognized by macrophages in the spleen and removed from the circulation. There are then two types of lysis: intra and extravascular lysis.

SELF-CHECK 1.3

How does complement bring about red cell destruction?

1.6 *In vitro* detection of antigen–antibody reactions

To detect red cell antigen–antibody reactions the cells themselves can be used as markers, as most routine blood bank techniques produce agglutination (antibody-induced clumping). The same technique cannot be used for platelets or granulocyte work and here antibodies are detected by indirect methods such as using flow cytometry. Whatever technique is used it is important to get as much antibody onto the cells as possible as there is a minimum threshold of antibody molecules per cell that will be detectable in routine tests. For the antiglobulin test, for example, this minimum figure is about one hundred antibodies per red cell.

Factors affecting antigen–antibody reactions *in vitro*:

- Antigen–antibody ratio
- Time
- Temperature
- pH
- Ionic strength

  - Increasing the ratio of plasma used in a test to the number of cells will maximize the chances of there being sufficient antibody molecules per cell to be detectable. There are, of course, practicable limits to the volume of plasma that can be used, and other factors such as ionic strength to be taken into account.

  - All reactions need time to come to equilibrium but in most routine techniques it is unlikely that true equilibrium is reached in the incubation times used. Experience has shown what minimum times can be used. In any test the set parameters should not be changed without proper re-evaluation of the technique.

  - Most immune antibodies react better at 37°C than at lower temperatures. But naturally acquired, IgM, T-independent antibodies tend to react better at lower temperatures. As these latter antibodies, with the exception of anti-A/B are not generally clinically significant then most tests are incubated at 37°C.

  - Immune antibodies have a pH optimum around 7.2; therefore tests are performed using buffers to maintain this pH.

  - Lowering the ionic strength of the reactants in a red cell antigen–antibody test from that of physiologically normal saline, 0.45 M, to an equivalent of 0.15 M, increases the rate of antigen uptake of most antibodies. Incubation times in 'normal' ionic conditions are typically 60 minutes but using low ionic strength conditions 15 minutes is sufficient.

Red cell agglutination

When the red cells are joined together by cross-linking of antibody molecules they become agglutinated. Red cell agglutination occurs in two distinct, but inter-related stages, the primary antibody sensitisation stage, and the secondary agglutination stage.

The factors affecting antibody sensitization of red cells have been considered above. In the second stage, the rate of red cell agglutination is determined by the frequency with which the antibody-sensitized red cells collide. Red cells come closer by the action of gravity, which can be increased by centrifugation and by surface tension, or interfacial energy. However, these aggregating forces are balanced by a repelling force associated with an 'ion cloud' around each red cell.

Red cells have an overall net negative charge due to the negative charges on a major constituent of the membrane, the glycoproteins. The negatively charged red cells attract a 'cloud' of positively charged ions from the suspending saline (NaCl) medium. The intensity of the ionic cloud that moves with the red cell decreases with increasing distance from the cell surface. The resulting charge is known as the zeta-potential, and this determines the minimum distance that the red cells are able to approach each other. A number of other forces acting on the red cell membrane, including the movement of water molecules at the membrane surface, are also believed to affect red cell attraction and repulsion.

The repulsive force of the positively charged ion cloud around each cell means that red cells cannot approach close enough to allow an IgG molecule to span the gap between them. An IgM antibody molecule is however, large enough to span this gap and is therefore, capable of causing agglutination of red cells in plasma without any further manipulations. For IgG antibody molecules to agglutinate red cells an alteration in the environment of the red cells is required to enable them to cross-link. Methods employed include the addition of macromolecules, such as albumin; enzyme treatment of the red cells or the use of an anti-human globulin (AHG) reagent. See Figure 1.7.

Red cell agglutination by IgM antibodies

As IgM antibodies can 'span' the gap between red cells they are capable of agglutinating red cells suspended in saline. The first antibodies described in the ABO blood group system were IgM antibodies and until the development of techniques to detect the so-called 'incomplete antibodies' we now know to be IgG, all blood banking techniques used red cells either in their own plasma or suspended in saline. Tests were carried out on glass slides or tiles, or in later years in tubes and more recently in microplates (microtitre plates) that are effectively 96 small tubes in one easy-to-use plastic tray. Because the interaction of IgM antibodies, especially anti-A and anti-B, with their antigens is very quick incubation times can be short or indeed 'immediate'. The *immediate spin technique*, in which the tube containing the reactants is centrifuged without incubation, is widely used when working with ABO antibodies.

In 1990 details of a new test system were published, and this method has subsequently come into widespread use. It uses small microtubes, or columns, containing a gel or bead matrix, to

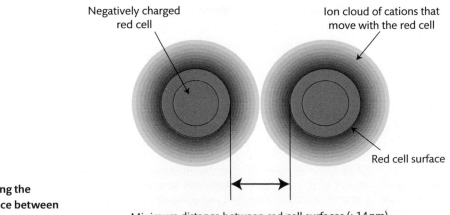

Negatively charged red cell

Ion cloud of cations that move with the red cell

Red cell surface

FIGURE 1.7
Ion cloud affecting the minimum distance between red cells (not to scale).

Minimum distance between red cell surfaces (>14 nm)

which can be added blood grouping or antiglobulin reagents. There are several commercial systems on the market, for example Bio-Rad ID-System, Grifols DG Gel, and Ortho BioVue, each with six or eight columns being presented in a single card. For routine grouping, cards with antisera (e.g. anti-A, anti-B, anti-D) incorporated into the matrix are available. A small volume of a red cell suspension is added to the appropriate column, the card is then centrifuged and red cells that are agglutinated by the antiserum are trapped in the matrix as visible agglutinates.

For reverse ABO grouping, or detecting alloantibodies, a small volume of plasma and the appropriate cells are incubated in the chamber above the microtube that contains a neutral matrix. The card containing the columns is centrifuged after incubation, and any agglutinated cells are trapped within the matrix.

Monoclonal antibodies produced by *in vitro* cell culture for use as grouping or phenotyping reagents are, wherever possible, IgM molecules so that they can be easily used in the laboratory by saline or direct agglutinating techniques, without having to resort to more complex methods that are needed when using IgG reagents.

Red cell agglutination by IgG antibodies

Addition of macromolecules

Macromolecules such as 20% bovine albumin effectively reduce the 'charge density' (the dielectric constant) around the red cells, thereby reducing the net repulsive force between cells. This allows the red cells to approach closer together than is possible in a saline environment, so that IgG antibody molecules can span the gap between red cells, producing cross-linkage and therefore agglutination. It is thought that some macromolecules may also act by binding to the outer surface of the red cell membrane, affecting membrane water and therefore altering interfacial tension. Methods using different macromolecules have variable sensitivity and do not enable all IgG red antibodies to produce agglutination. Although once widely used, especially in the days before monoclonal IgM RhD typing reagents, these techniques are rarely used today.

One exception is the use of Polybrene, (hexadimethrine bromide) which causes red cells to aggregate. In the low ionic Polybrene (LIP) technique, red cells and plasma are incubated for only one minute at room temperature in a very low ionic strength medium so that antibody uptake is very quick. Polybrene is added to 'aggregate' the red cells, then the non-specific aggregation is dispersed leaving antibody mediate agglutination. This rapid technique is not, however, suitable with some antibody specificities (e.g. anti-K) and has a limited, but valuable, use.

Use of enzymes

As the negative charge of a red cell is carried on the glycophorin molecules of the red cell membrane, proteolytic enzymes, such as papain, can be used to remove some of these molecules. This effectively reduces the net negative charge on the red cell membrane, enabling red cells to come closer together, allowing some IgG antibody molecules to agglutinate red cells. The enzyme treatment also increases the exposure of some antigens by reducing steric hindrance caused by surrounding molecules, thereby improving antibody uptake. Enzyme techniques are particularly good for the detection of Rh antibodies. However, antigens which are present on glycophorins, such as M, N, Fy^a, and Fy^b are destroyed by the enzyme treatment, so antibodies to these antigens cannot be detected by using enzyme techniques.

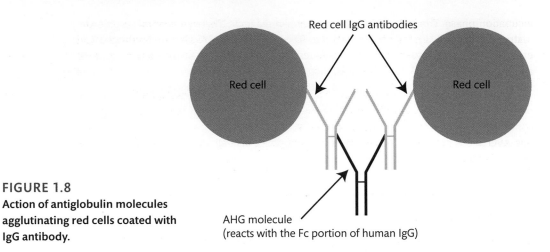

Red cell IgG antibodies

Red cell

Red cell

FIGURE 1.8
Action of antiglobulin molecules agglutinating red cells coated with IgG antibody.

AHG molecule
(reacts with the Fc portion of human IgG)

Use of anti-human globulin (AHG) reagents

By using an antibody, anti-human IgG, red cells that are coated with IgG protein can be agglutinated. The Fab portion of the anti-human globulin antibody reacts with the Fc portion of the IgG antibody present on the sensitized red cells. This therefore effectively overcomes the problem of the minimum distance between red cells, which individual IgG antibodies are incapable of spanning. See Figure 1.8.

The early AHG reagents were made by injecting a rabbit with a crude human globulin preparation so that they produced anti-human globulin antibodies. The rabbit was then bled and the serum containing the antibodies, after some manipulation, used in the *antiglobulin (Coombs) test*. These AHG reagents contained a mixture of antibodies to IgG, IgM, IgA, and to complement C3 and C4. Later work showed that C4 can be adsorbed onto red cells *in vitro* in a non-specific manner and could lead to a false positive reaction if anti-C4 were present in the AHG reagent. Modern reagents are usually made from anti-IgG raised in rabbits by using a purer IgG preparation, and a monoclonal anti-C3d; these are called *polyspecific AHG reagents*. Monospecific anti-IgG, -IgM, -IgA, C3d, and -C4 are also available and are widely used when investigating cases of immune red cell destruction.

In the *direct antiglobulin test* (DAT) red cells are taken from a patient, then washed in saline to remove all traces of plasma and immunoglobulins, except those already bound *in vivo* to the cells. The AHG reagent is then added and if bound IgG antibodies or C3 are present then the test is positive.

The *indirect antiglobulin test* (IAT) is the most widely used test in immunohaematology for the detection of antibodies in an antibody screening test and to identify the specificity of any antibodies thus found. It is also used in the serological phase of compatibility testing or crossmatching.

Plasma, or a known antibody (antiserum) is incubated with red cells, usually in a low ionic strength solution (LISS) so that any antibodies present can bind to their corresponding antigens. If a tube technique is used the cells are then washed in saline, AHG reagent added, and a positive reaction indicates the presence of antibodies. For many years antiglobulin tests were carried out in test tubes, but now column (microtube) systems are widely used. The major advantage of these systems is that there is no need to wash the red cells after the incubation phase. The cells and plasma under test are incubated in a chamber above the matrix containing the antiglobulin reagent. After incubation the cards are centrifuged and only the red cells not the plasma are forced through the matrix, and if coated with IgG they are trapped in the matrix as visible agglutinates.

These systems can be used in conjunction with columns for grouping (ABO, RhD) using IgM, directly agglutinating antibodies in the matrix either manually or in automated, computer controlled systems. Most laboratories in the UK now use some form of automation for routine ABO and D grouping, and antibody screening of patient samples for both pre-transfusion and antenatal cases.

Key points

IgM antibodies can agglutinate red cells directly in a saline medium but IgG antibodies do not and are usually detected by using the antiglobulin test or enzyme treated red cells.

1.7 Techniques

Molecular techniques are widely used for testing for human leukocyte and platelet antigens but most blood transfusion laboratories still employ serological techniques as outlined above. Although not yet widely used, DNA microarrays are available to determine the presence or absence of a wide range of blood group genes, especially single neucleotide polymorphisms (SNPs). For antibody detection the corresponding antigen, or the appropriate epitope, is required. Some recombinant blood group proteins and synthetic peptide **mimotopes** (short synthetic peptides that mimic natural epitopes of the individual blood group antigens) are being developed to be used in microarray antibody detection systems without the need for intact red cells.

Mimotopes
Short synthetic peptides that mimic natural epitopes of the individual blood group antigens that are being developed to be used in microarray antibody detection systems without the need for intact red cells.

Details of techniques have not been given in this chapter as most blood banks or transfusion departments now employ commercial test systems. Therefore the manufacturer's instructions must be followed. Each laboratory will have its own set of standard operating procedures (SOPs) that detail the techniques that have been validated for use by that laboratory. But all serological techniques follow the general principles outlined in this chapter and will be referred to in other chapters.

The basic purpose of laboratory testing pre-transfusion or transplantation is to ensure compatibility between the donor cells and the recipient. Where this cannot be achieved then any incompatibility should be as little as possible so that the advantages of the donor cells transfused or transplanted outweigh the adverse effects. Transfusion/transplantation laboratories also have to be able to investigate untoward reactions and other cases of immune cell destruction such as that found in haemolytic disease of the newborn; these are considered in the following chapters.

SELF-CHECK 1.4

What methods can be used to detect IgG antibodies?

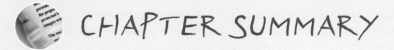

CHAPTER SUMMARY

- Although there has been a long history of attempts at transfusing blood and transplanting tissues the real advances were made in the second half of the twentieth century.

- In both transfusion and transplantation 'foreign' antigens are introduced into the body; therefore an immune response can be expected.

- The immune response can be either 'cellular' or 'humoral'.

- In the humoral response antibodies are produced in response to an external antigenic stimulus.

- The primary response is slow; IgM antibodies are produced first with the plasma cells then switching production to IgG.

- In a secondary response IgG antibodies are produced from the outset with little or no lag phase.

- Antibodies by themselves do not cause cell destruction; some can activate the complement cascade that might result in cell lysis within the circulation, intravascular lysis, or removal of cells coated with C3b by macrophages in the liver.

- Red cells coated with IgG antibody will be recognized by macrophages in the spleen and removed from the circulation; extravascular lysis.

- The main techniques used for blood grouping involve the formation and visualization of agglutination either by direct agglutination (IgM antibodies) or by using the antiglobulin test (IgG antibodies).

Answers to the questions in this chapter are provided on the book's Online Resource Centre.

 Go to www.oxfordtextbooks.co.uk/orc/knight

2

Human Erythrocyte Antigens or Blood Groups

Malcolm Needs

Learning objectives

After studying this chapter you should be able to:

- Describe what defines a blood group system.
- Describe the macromolecular structure of different blood group systems (protein or carbohydrate structure).
- Outline basic nomenclature.
- Describe antigen frequencies, particularly the differences in frequency found in different ethnicities.
- Understand basic blood group genetics.
- Understand blood group antigen functions.
- Understand basic disease association.

Introduction

The first question most people ask is, 'What is a blood group?' A blood group system can be defined as:

- **An inherited red cell *polymorphism***
- **The genes for that polymorphism are at the same location on a chromosome**
- **The resultant antigens are on the same carrier molecule**
- **The antigen can elicit an immune response**
- **An extant (existing) antiserum exists that defines the antigen**

The structures that carry the different blood group antigens all have some physiological function, not just acting as blood group antigens (see Table 2.1).

There are now 30 blood group systems recognized by the International Society of Blood Transfusion (ISBT). As a result, the terminology has become very complex. The simple names, rather than the complex numbering system, however, continue in everyday use for the different blood group systems, antigens, and antibodies. Some of the systems contain only one antigen (such as the H blood group system), while others contain many antigens (such as the Rh blood group system).

Initially, single letters were given to the blood group antigens (e.g. A, B, M, N, etc.), but as knowledge and the number of antigens expanded, a single letter could no longer be used. Two letters were then used when no **antithetical** antigen was found (e.g. Ku) but this expanded to two letters and a superscript when an antithetical antigen was found (e.g. Js^a and Js^b).

Antithetical
One of two or more alternative antigens.

Each blood group system has been given an ISBT number and the antigens within that system have also been given a number. For example, the Duffy blood group system has

TABLE 2.1 The physiological functions of the blood group systems.

Blood group system	Function	Blood group system	Function	Blood group system	Function
ABO	Unknown	Yt (Cartwright)	Possibly involved in neurotransmission	Cromer	Complement regulation
MNS	Receptor for complement, bacteria, and viruses	Xg	Adhesion	Knops	Complement regulation
P	Receptor for *Escherichia coli*	Scianna	Adhesion/receptor protein	Indian	Cellular adhesion, immune stimulation, and cell signalling
Rh	Probably structural, via ankyrin and protein 4.2	Dombrock	Possibly modification of proteins	Ok	Possibly involved in tumour metastasis
Lutheran	Probably adhesion and intracellular signalling	Colton	Water transport	RAPH	Unknown, but may be involved in kidney function
Kell	Probably a zinc endopeptidase	LW	Intracellular adhesion	JMH	Unknown
Lewis	Possibly a ligand for E-selectins	Chido/Rodgers	Inhibition of immune precipitation	I	Unknown
Duffy	Receptor for both acute and chronic inflammation pro-inflammatory chemokines	H	Possible ligand in cell adhesion	Globoside	Converts P^k to P
Kidd	Urea transporter	Kx	Possibly involved in maintenance of cell membrane integrity	GIL	Water channel and transporter of small non-ionic molecules
Diego	Anion transport and structural	Gerbich	Maintenance of cell membrane integrity *via* protein 4.1	RHAG	Neutral ion membrane transport

the symbol FY and is ISBT number 008. Within this system, the Fy^a antigen is designated FY1, or 008.001 (the system number and the zeros are redundant in this phraseology) and the Fy^b antigen is designated FY2 (008.002).

Some of the more recently described blood groups do not have a name as such, as they do not meet the *criteria* given above (e.g. the Er Blood Group Collection is known as ER or 208 and the Er^a antigen as ER1 or 208.001).

There are also seven blood group collections (Cost, Ii, Er, GLOB, Vel, and two unnamed), in which are grouped antigens that are genetically independent of all blood group systems, but which have serological, biochemical, or genetic relationships.

There is the 700 Series of Low Incidence Antigens (ten antigens) that belong to neither a blood group system, nor a blood group collection. These antigens occur in less than 1% of most populations.

Last, there is the 900 Series of High Incidence Antigens (eight antigens) that belong to neither a blood group system, nor a blood group collection. These antigens occur in more than 99% of most populations.

This situation is still evolving as more evidence comes to light, for example Duclos (of the 900 Series) and Ol^a (of the 700 Series) have, respectively, now become RHAG1 and RHAG2 of the thirtieth blood group system, RHAG.

The frequency of the different antigens can vary greatly between different ethnic groups (e.g. D negative: Basque region of Spain ~25%, China ~0.01%).

The antigens themselves tend to be formed either of an **immunodominant sugar residue** on a molecular backbone (such as the ABO antigens) or part of a protein molecule (such as the Rh antigens). If the antigen is of the sugar type, the antigen is not a direct gene product, but is the result of the *action* of the direct gene product, usually a transferase enzyme. If the antigen is of the protein type, then it is a direct gene product (although it must be remembered that there are almost always post-translational changes to any such protein).

> **Immunodominant sugar residue**
> The sugar residue that confers antigenicity on a carbohydrate antigen.

The really excellent news for the reader is that they will not be required to know about all of the antigens (of which there are now 319), the systems, the collections, or the series, but for those that are already interested, or have their curiosity aroused by this book, suggested further reading is listed at the end of the chapter.

This chapter gives an overview of what are considered to be the most important blood group systems, together with the most important antigens within those systems. Some of the blood group systems interact with each other and so will be described together, rather than separately. Indeed, the first to be considered is such an interaction of two different systems, ABO and H, the genes for which are even on different chromosomes.

2.1 The ABO, H, and Lewis blood group systems

Genes and antigens

These antigens all occur on common molecular backbones, with very slight differences in bonding. Essentially, the backbones are made up of repeating moeties of **D**-galactose, N-acetyl-**D**-glucosamine, **D**-galactose, and N-acetyl-**D**-galactosamine (for those less familiar with sugars and linkages, see Figure 2.1).

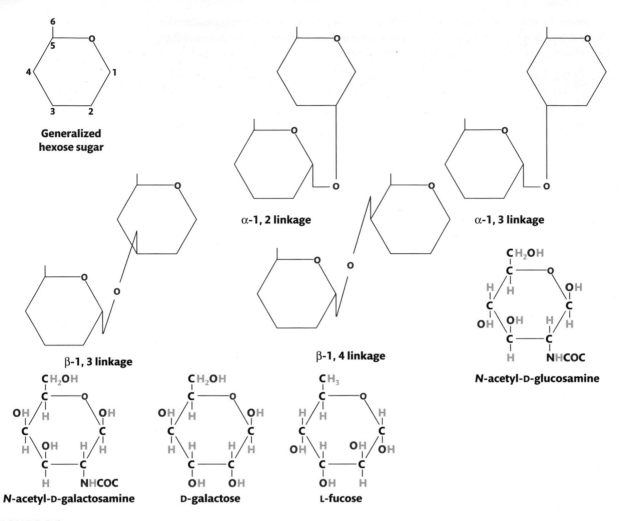

FIGURE 2.1
Various hexose sugar molecules and linkages.

At a basic level, there are two of these backbones. The first, Type 1, has a β-1, 3 linkage between the terminal **D**-galactose and the sub-terminal N-acetyl-**D**-glucosamine. This molecule is water soluble, and so is found in the plasma. The second, Type 2, has a β-1, 4 linkage between the terminal **D**-galactose and the sub-terminal N-acetyl-**D**-glucosamine. This molecule is fat soluble, and so is found as an integral part of the red cell membrane.

The ABO blood group system was the first to be described, by Karl Landsteiner in 1900, and is still regarded as the most important. This is because almost all individuals, except most newborn babies, have naturally acquired, T cell independent, IgM antibodies in their plasma, directed against any ABO and H antigens they themselves lack. Antigens within the environment, especially bacteria, such as *Escherichia coli* in the gut, stimulate these antibodies. This means that if blood of the wrong ABO group is transfused, the individual is likely to undergo a major, if not fatal, transfusion reaction.

For an individual to express ABO antigens, they must first express the H antigen. Expression of the H antigen alone means that an individual is group O. This antigen is formed by an α-1, 2 linkage of **L**-fucose to the terminal **D**-galactose on Type 1 and Type 2 backbones, by an α-1,

2-L-fucosyl transferase from a GDP-L-fucose donor. If this L-fucose, which is governed by the *H* gene (also known as *FUT1*) at 19q13.3, is not present, whatever *ABO* genes are inherited cannot be expressed and the individual is of the type O_h (sometimes, incorrectly, called the 'Bombay' phenotype). These individuals produce a, usually, potent anti-H, in addition to anti-A, anti-B and anti-A,B, whereas a group O individual (who expresses the H antigen) will only produce anti-A, anti-B, and anti-A,B.

The A antigen is formed by an α-1, 3 linkage of an *N*-acetyl-D-galactosamine to the terminal D-galactose on Type 1 and Type 2 backbones, by an α-1, 3-*N*-acetyl-D-galactosaminyl transferase from a UDP-*N*-acetyl-D-galactosamine donor.

The B antigen is formed by an α-1, 3 linkage of another D-galacose to the terminal D-galactose on Type 1 and Type 2 backbones, by an α-1, 3-D-galactosyl transferase from a UDP-D-galactose donor.

The AB blood type is formed by the presence of both the A and B antigen, formed by competitive binding of the immunodominant sugars between α-1, 3-*N*-acetyl-D-galactosaminyl transferase and α-1, 3-D-galactosyl transferase.

Humans, being what they are, this is by no means the full story. There are sub-groups of both A and B caused by numerous genetic mutations in the genes coding for the respective ABO transferase enzymes (there are also numerous genetic backgrounds to both O and O_h).

The 'wild-type' of A is A_1. This gives the strongest reaction with both anti-A and anti-A,B (from group O individuals), a strong reaction with anti-A_1, but a relatively weak reaction with anti-H.

The most common sub-type of A is A_2. This gives a slightly weaker reaction with anti-A, a strong reaction with anti-A,B, a negative reaction with anti-A_1, and a slightly stronger reaction with anti-H. Individuals of this type can produce an anti-A_1, but it is very rarely strong and it is even rarer for it to be clinically significant (i.e. reacting at $37°C$). In other words, an A_2 individual with anti-A_1 in their plasma can almost always be safely transfused with blood from an A_1 donor. Indeed, a human-derived anti-A_1 that can be used as a grouping reagent is exceptionally rare. Usually a **lectin**, produced from the seeds of *Dolichos biflorus*, which contains, essentially, a potent anti-A_1 and can be used to type red cells for the A_1 antigen.

A weaker sub-group, A_3, is rare. These red cells tend to give a mixed-field reaction with both anti-A and anti-A,B **polyclonal** reagents, but with most modern reagents this is not seen, and a negative reaction with anti-A_1 and a slightly stronger reaction still with anti-H.

The red cells from very rare A_x individuals give very weak or negative reactions with anti-A, stronger reactions with selected anti-A,B reagents, a negative reaction with anti-A_1, and a quite strong reaction with anti-H.

Numerous other sub-groups of the A antigen have been described, mostly during the years when polyclonal, rather than **monoclonal** reagents were used. There seems to be a sort of continuum of weakening of the A antigen from the strongest reactors (A_1) to the weakest that, serologically, are only distinguished from a true group O by such techniques as adsorption and elution. Although there have now been scores of different genetic mutations described that cause such sub-groups of A, it must be said that the distinction between many of these sub-groups, from the serological point of view, must be regarded as, at best, somewhat esoteric.

The sub-groups of B are, within the European population, extremely rare, although they are reported to be relatively more common within populations of Far East Asia.

ABO antigens, whilst being easily recognized serologically, are not particularly well developed at birth (e.g. an individual who may develop into an A_1B adult may appear at birth,

Lectin
A sugar-binding protein or glycoprotein of non-immune origin, which can agglutinate cells and/or precipitate glycoconjugates.

Polyclonal
Produced from more than one clone of cells.

Monoclonal
Produced from one clone of cells.

serologically, to be an A_2B). This is because the transferase enzymes that confer ABO antigenicity to the red cell are not working to their full capacity at this stage of life.

The inheritance of *ABO*, at a basic level, is quite straightforward. There are, essentially, two genes, *A* and *B*, plus a silent gene, or amorph, *O*. Assuming normal inheritance of the *H* gene, the presence of the *A* gene will result in the A antigen being expressed on the red cell surface; the presence of the *B* gene will result in the B antigen being expressed on the red cell surface; the presence of both the *A* and *B* genes will result in both the A and B antigens being expressed on the red cell surface; the absence of both the *A* and *B* genes will result in the individual being group O. Even the fact that A^1 is dominant over A^2, whilst both A^1 and A^2 are **codominant** with *B* is easily explained by the competition between the 'A' transferase and the 'B' transferase for the H substrate. The various common genotypes and phenotypes can be seen in Table 2.2.

The frequency of the ABO phenotypes differ around the world (e.g. 100% of some tribes of South American Indians are group O) and some of the various frequencies can be seen in Table 2.3.

Codominant
Allelic genes whose products are all expressed equally.

TABLE 2.2 ABO genotypes and phenotypes.

Genotypes	Phenotypes
A^1A^1	A_1
A^1A^2	
A^1O	
A^2A^2	A_2
A^2O	
BB	B
BO	
A^1B	A_1B
A^2B	A_2B
OO	O

TABLE 2.3 The approximate frequency of ABO types worldwide.

ABO group	UK	India	Taiwan	Malawi (Africa)
A	42	19	26	21
B	9	41	26	20
AB	4	9	6	4
O	45	31	42	55

Key points

The immunodominant sugar residues that confer A, B, and O antigenicity are for A: N-acetyl-**D**-galactosamine, for B: **D**-galacose and for O: **L**-fucose. In the O_h pheno-types there is no terminal **L**-fucose. Sub-groups of A and B exist, but most give good reactions with monoclonal blood grouping reagents.

Antibodies

Traditionally, because naturally acquired antibodies were thought to be IgM, it has been taught that ABO antibodies were only IgM, but many people, particularly women who have been pregnant with an ABO incompatible foetus, have a substantial concentration of IgG as well as IgM ABO antibodies. Some older types of vaccines produced in animals contained A and/or B-like antigens that led to an immune response that involved the production of IgG ABO antibodies.

ABO antibodies are very good at initiating the complement cascade and, as a result, are extremely dangerous in terms of transfusion. Indeed, most of the serious and fatal transfu-sion reactions reported to the Severe Hazards Of Transfusion (SHOT) scheme involve ABO incompatible transfusions (especially group A blood into a group O individual). The ABO groups a recipient can tolerate can be seen in Table 2.4.

Key points

ABO antibodies are mainly IgM, but IgG antibodies can also be found, and are pro-duced to the antigens that the individual lacks.

SELF-CHECK 2.1

What are the immunodominant sugar residues involved in conferring the A, B, and O blood groups? What is the genetic background of the O_h phenotype?

TABLE 2.4 The antigens found on red cells, the antibodies found in plasma, and the different ABO blood that can be given.

Antigen	Antibody(ies)	Compatible ABO group(s)
A	Anti-B	A, O and O_h
B	Anti-A	B, O and O_h
AB	None	AB, A, B, O and O_h
O	Anti-A, anti-B (anti-A,B)	O and O_h
O_h	Anti-A, anti-B, (anti-A,B) anti-H	O_h only

2.2 The Lewis blood group system and secretor

Genes and antigens

The Lewis antigens are only found on Type 1 backbone molecules and, like the H antigen, they are the result of the addition of either 1 or 2 **L**-fucose sugar residues being added to the backbone molecule. It follows, therefore, that, as they are on Type 1 molecules, those Lewis antigens detectable on red cells are there as a result of adsorption onto the red cell surface, rather than as a an integral part of the membrane.

The *Lewis* (*LE* or *FUT3*) gene has been mapped to 19p13.3. The Lewis antigens found on red cells, however, require more than just the action of this gene.

Le^a results from the action of an α-1, 4-**L**-fucosyl transferase linking an **L**-fucose to the sub-terminal *N*-acetyl-**D**-glucosamine. Le^b results from the action of an α-1, 4-**L**-fucosyl transferase linking another **L**-fucose to the sub-terminal *N*-acetyl-**D**-glucosamine (see Figure 2.2).

Keen-eyed readers will note that this is almost the H antigen on Type 1 molecules. The explanation for this lies with the interaction with yet another gene, *SE* (or *FUT2* and, like *LE* (*FUT3*) mapped to 19p13.3), although this gene does not directly encode a blood group.

ABO and H antigens may be present in saliva as soluble antigens, or ABO and H substance. If the antigens cannot be easily detected in saliva, then the individual is a non-secretor and will either be Le(a-b-) or Le(a + b-), but will not be Le(a-b+). If the antigens can easily be found in saliva, then the individual will be a secretor and either be Le(a-b-) or Le(a-b+) (but a small amount of the Le^a antigen may also be detected) (see Table 2.5).

Lewis antigens *tend* to weaken, or even disappear, because of the greater production of plasma lipoproteins during pregnancy, but return *post-partum*. Lewis antigens are not well

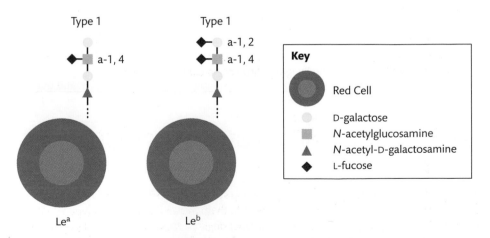

FIGURE 2.2
Le^a and Le^b (soluble) antigens.

TABLE 2.5 The inter-relationship between the *LE/FUT3* and *SE/FUT2* genes, the red cell types and the ABH secretor status.

LE / FUT3	SE / FUT2	Red cell type	ABH secretor status
lele	sese	Le(a-b-)	No
lele	SEse	Le(a-b-)	Yes
lele	SESE	Le(a-b-)	Yes
LEle	sese	Le(a+b-)	No
LELE	sese	Le(a+b-)	No
LEle	SEse	Le(a-b+)	Yes
LEle	SESE	Le(a-b+)	Yes
LELE	SEse	Le(a-b+)	Yes
LELE	SESE	Le(a-b+)	Yes

developed at birth, and an individual who will eventually become an Le(a-b+) adult may go through the following stages; Le(a-b-), Le(a+b-), Le(a+b+), and Le(a-b+).

Antibodies

Anti-Le^a is usually an IgM antibody and has only rarely been recorded as having caused a haemolytic transfusion reaction (and even then it *tends* to be self-limiting), whilst anti-Le^b, which is also usually IgM, is clinically benign. Neither antibody causes clinically significant HDNF. Both antibodies are only found in Le(a-b-) individuals, as this is the only true Le negative type, and often as a mixture of anti-Le^{a+b}.

> ### Key points
>
> The immuneodominant sugar residue that confers Le^a and Le^b antigenicity is L-fucose, one for Le^a and two for Le^b; these antigens can weaken or disappear during pregnancy. The antibodies are usually IgM of little or no clinical significance.

2.3 The MNS blood group system

Genes and antigens

There are 46 antigens within the MNS blood group system that are carried on two molecules, glycophorin A, or GYA, and glycophorin B, or GYB, both of which are described as Type 1 (COOH inside the membrane, NH_2 outside the membrane) single pass membrane sialoglycoproteins. These are encoded by two genes, *GYA* and *GYB*, both of which are located at 4q28-q31.

Most of the 46 antigens are either of very low frequency (e.g. M^v) or very high frequency (e.g. ENKT) and for the purposes of this chapter can largely be ignored. Suffice it to say that many of the antigens fall into the very low frequency category, and have usually come about by uneven crossing of the genes on GYA and GYB.

There are five antigens that will be described in more detail. These are M, N, S, s, and U. M and N are antithetical and S and s are also antithetical. The M and N antigens are located on the GYA molecule that has 131 amino acid residues. The M and N antigens are located at the extreme NH_2 terminal, residing in different amino acids in positions 1–5. The exact same five amino acid residues that make up the N antigen also appear on the GYB molecule, where the antigen is named 'N'. The S and s antigens are located on the GYB molecule that has 72 amino acid residues. The S and s antigens are differentiated by a single amino acid substitution at position 29. The amino acid residue for S is methionine, whilst that for s is threonine. Although the M and N antigens are encoded by GYA, and the S and s antigens are encoded by GYB, the genes tend to travel together. In other words, MS, Ms, NS, and Ns are inherited as a 'block', rather than as individual genes.

The frequency of the various phenotypes varies between black and white populations (see Table 2.6). From these figures it can be seen that the M and N antigens are both common and relatively equal in frequency, but that the s antigen is much more common than the S antigen (although finding S+s- blood, when it is required, is not normally a problem). What is to be noted, however, is that the phenotype S-s- is not found in the white population, but is found in the black population, albeit infrequently, and this is where the fifth antigen, U, comes into play.

All white individuals are U+, but some black individuals who are S-s- are also U-. These individuals can make anti-U. Like S and s, the U antigen is located on the GYB molecule; the amino acid residues recognizing the U antigen are between positions 33 and 39, very close to the cell membrane.

TABLE 2.6 MNS phenotype frequencies in white and black populations.

Phenotype	White population %	Black population %
M+N-S+s-	6	2
M+N-S+s+	14	7
M+N-S-s+	8	16
M+N+S+s-	4	2
M+N+S+s+	24	13
M+N+S-s+	22	33
M-N+S+s-	1	2
M-N+S+s+	6	5
M-N+S-s+	15	19
M+N-S-s-	0	0.4
M+N+S-s-	0	0.4
M-N+S-s-	0	0.7

The position of the various antigens on the GYA and GYB molecules is serologically important. The most commonly used proteolytic enzyme in routine transfusion laboratories is
papain, made from the seeds of the pawpaw fruit. This enzyme hydrolyses the C-terminal
peptide bond of argenine, lysine, and the bond next but one to phenylalanine. As a result, the
M and N, and usually the S and s antigens are destroyed by its action, but the U antigen is not.
Indeed, the reaction between the U antigen and anti-U is enhanced by the action of papain.

> ## Key points
>
> Glycophorin A is the carrier molecule of the MN antigens, and glycophorin B the SsU
> antigens. The U-phenotype appears predominately in the black population.

Antibodies

Anti-M is normally a clinically benign IgM antibody, but some examples that have an IgG
component may react *in vitro* at 37°C by the indirect antiglobulin technique. In such circumstances, type M- blood must be used for transfusion. For anti-M not reacting at 37°C, crossmatch compatible blood, but not selected as being M-, can be safely transfused.

Anti-N, again IgM, is also clinically benign. The only time that N- blood may be required is if
the patient is M+, N-, S-, s- (when the 'N' antigen will also be missing) and anti-N, reacting at
37°C is present in the plasma.

Anti-S and anti-s are both clinically significant IgG antibodies, with cases in the literature that
have caused severe transfusion reactions and severe haemolytic disease of the newborn/
foetus. Such cases are, however, extremely rare.

Anti-U, an IgG antibody, should always be regarded as potentially clinically significant. The
first example described caused fatal haemolytic disease of the newborn/foetus, and the second caused a fatal haemolytic transfusion reaction. That having been said, there are also
cases in the literature describing cases where U+ blood has been successfully transfused to
patient's with anti-U, and where healthy U+ babies have been delivered to mother's with
quite potent anti-U.

> ## Key points
>
> Anti-M can react at 37°C and be of clinical significance, but anti-N is generally benign.
> Anti-S, anti-s, and anti-U are clinically significant IgG antibodies.

2.4 The Rh, RHAG, and LW blood group systems

Genes and antigens

After the ABO blood group system, the Rh blood group system is the most important clinically. There is almost certainly more known about the Rh blood group system than any other,
but there is still much to be discovered.

The original description of the system has been the subject of a little controversy since the late 1930s, early 1940s, as two different sets of workers (Landsteiner and Wiener, and Levine and Stetson) claimed priority. Whilst in no way acting as a referee in this dispute, it would appear that Levine and Stetson described what we now know to be the D antibody in a human, whilst Landsteiner and Wiener described what we now know to be LW in an animal model (and it is this discovery of anti-LW in a guinea pig immunized with rhesus monkey red cells, that led to generations of workers in the field, and lay people, using the wrong term for the Rh blood group system, 'Rhesus' or 'rhesus').

As a result of so much being known about this extremely complex system, whole books have been written on the subject. It is beyond the remit of this chapter to go into such detail, and so only basic explanations will be given.

At one time it was thought that there were three genes encoding the Rh antigens: *D* (*d*), *Cc*, and *Ee* respectively and many textbooks still use this terminology. We now know, however, that there are just two genes that encode the Rh proteins, *RHD* and *RHCE*. Both are mapped to 1p36.13-p34.3. For the Rh proteins to be expressed on the red cell surface, another gene is needed, *RHAG*, that has been mapped to 6p11-21. Another protein encoded by the gene *LW* is also related to the Rh complex in the red cell membrane and has been mapped to 19p13.3.

There are 52 antigens within the Rh blood group system and, like the antigens within the MNS blood group system, many of these are either very high incidence antigens (such as Rh29) or very low incidence antigens (such as Rh35). Some are confined to individuals of a certain ethnic origin (for example, VS is found in 32% of the black population, but is not found in the white population). A few are **polymorphic** in all populations, but at different frequencies.

Polymorphism
The occurrence of more than one form of the antigen.

The *RHD* gene and antigen

The first Rh antigen to be described, and the most important, was D. It is also the most complex. It is the presence or absence of this antigen that determines whether an individual is Rh positive or negative. An Rh negative individual does not have either the *D* gene, or a D protein in the membrane of their red cells. In Rh negative, people of African origin do have a modified or pseudo *D* gene (*RHD*φ), but it does not result in a D protein being produced. There is no antithetical d antigen or allelic *d* gene.

The frequency of the D antigen varies between populations throughout the world. In China, for example, almost 99.99% of the population are D+, whilst in the Basque region of Spain, as many as 25% of the population are estimated to be D-. In the United Kingdom, approximately 85% of the population are D+ and 15% D-.

The mature D polypeptide is 416 amino acid residues in length that traverses the red cell membrane ten times, with both the NH_2 and COOH termini being **intracellular**. There are six extracellular loops (see Figure 2.3).

Intracellular
Within the cellular milieu.

The actual D antigen is formed of several epitopes. In basic terms, this means that there are several individual 'parts' to the antigen and an antibody can be raised against each of these individual 'parts'.

The complexity begins with the fact that certain individuals do not fall neatly within either a D+ or D- group. As can be imagined, there is huge potential for genetic mutation in a gene encoding such a large polypeptide. Some individuals have part of their *RHD* gene replaced by part of the *RHCE* gene, some have point mutations, some have multiple point mutations,

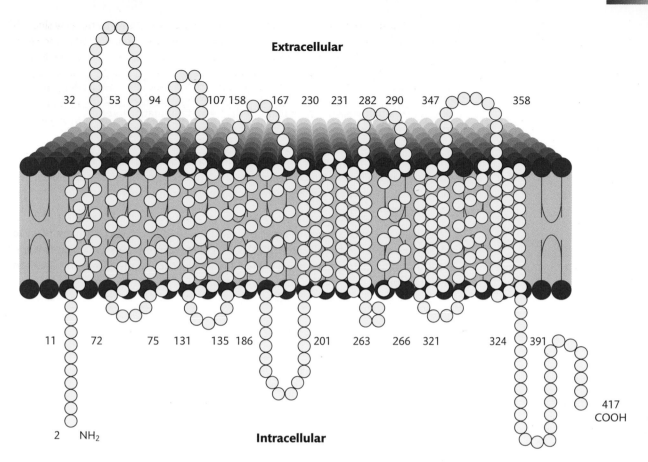

FIGURE 2.3

The mature RhD and/or RhCE polypeptide. The numbers refer to the terminal amino acid residues and those proposed to be at the inner and outer membrane surfaces.

some have pseudo-genes, some have stop **codons** in 'inappropriate' parts of the *RHD* gene. In fact, if there is a mutation that can be imagined, the mutation has probably occurred!

Another controversy is in the terminology of these mutant polypeptides. Until comparatively recently, such mutations were divided into weak D and partial D. The thought behind this was that, if a mutation was intracellular or **intra-membranous**, and so not part of the protein on the outside of the red cell, the individual expressing such a mutant D polypeptide on their red cells could not produce an alloanti-D. As the mutation often resulted in a weakening of the reaction between anti-D and the D antigens expressed, these individuals were said to express a 'weak D' antigen. It was thought to be a quantitative, rather than a qualitative difference, with fewer, but normal D antigens *per* red cell.

If, on the other hand, the mutation (or one of the mutations, in the case of more than one mutation) was extracellular, the individual expressing such a mutant D polypeptide on their red cells could (and often did) produce an alloanti-D, when stimulated so to do by transfusion with 'normal' D+ blood (or transfusion with blood from a donor with another, different, mutant D polypeptide). Very rarely indeed, such a sensitization could occur due to pregnancy. These individuals were said to express a 'partial D' antigen, but here, too, the mutation often resulted in a weakening of the antigen expression, resulting in weakened reactions between anti-D and the individual's red cells, and sometimes no visible

Codons
Three base pairs that code for a particular amino acid.

Intra-membranous
Within the cellular membrane.

serological reaction with certain anti-D reagents. This was thought to be a qualitative difference, often with an accompanying quantitative difference in terms of the number of D antigens *per* red cell.

For many years, this concept has seemed to work well. Unfortunately, individuals who express the weakened form of the D antigen have now been discovered who have produced an alloanti-D (albeit weakly). In addition, certain genetic mutations, resulting in different codons, but resulting in the same amino acid substitution, have resulted in one being categorized as a weak D and the other as a partial D. As a result of all this, there is a growing feeling that all such polypeptide mutations should be termed variant D. There is another category named D_{el}, where the D antigen is so weak (very few polypeptides on the red cell surface) that the only way to tell that there is actually an D antigen there is by adsorption and elution experiments.

To date there are over 57 well-categorized weak Ds, 66 well-categorized partial Ds, 10 incompletely categorized weak and partial Ds, 44 genetic backgrounds to D_{el} and D negative, and 5 genetic mutations resulting in the normal expression of the D antigen. No doubt more will be found.

Key points

Antigen D is the most important antigen after A and B. There are marked differences in the frequency of the D antigen in different parts of the world. Antigen D variants exist as both weak and partial D forms.

D antibodies

Immunogenic
The likelihood that an antigen will stimulate an immunological response.

The D antigen is extremely **immunogenic**. In other words, if a D- person is challenged with the D antigen, they are very likely to make anti-D. Some 20% make anti-D after just one challenge; 60% after more than one challenge, whilst 20% of such individuals seem never to make anti-D. The probable reason for this is that, in most white populations, a D negative individual will lack the complete D antigen, and the challenge of such a relatively large 'foreign' polypeptide to their immune system will easily stimulate antibody production. In addition, anti-D has been implicated in many deaths as a result of haemolytic transfusion reactions and deaths *in utero* as a result of haemolytic disease of the newborn/foetus, and despite the introduction of anti-D immunoglobulin, anti-D is still the most common cause of haemolytic disease of the newborn/foetus.

The *RHCE* gene and antigens

At a basic level, there are four more important antigens in the Rh blood group system. These are C and c (which are antithetical) and E and e (which are also antithetical). These antigens lie on the CE polypeptide that is highly *homologous* to the D polypeptide, with only some 36 amino acid differences throughout the polypeptide. There are fewer mutations to the C, c, E, and e antigens than those found within the D antigen because there are a fewer number of amino acids within the RhCE polypeptide that are directly involved in the expression of these antigens. Weak forms of all four antigens have been described, as well as variants, such as ce^S and E^w (C^w and C^x are antithetical to MAR, and are not variants of C or c).

C, c, E, and e antibodies

The c antigen and the E antigen are far more immunogenic than either the C or e antigens and antibodies to these are often found post-transfusion. Indeed, anti-E is the most commonly found alloantibody in hospital patients. Anti-c is the second most common cause of haemolytic disease of the newborn/foetus in the UK, but all four antibodies have been implicated in haemolytic disease of the newborn/foetus, albeit anti-E, anti-C, and anti-e very rarely. Anti-c has been implicated in more, and more severe, haemolytic transfusion reactions than anti-E, anti-C, or anti-e.

It is very rare for an Rh antibody of any specificity to have been naturally acquired, except for some examples of anti-E. In cases of autoimmune haemolytic anaemia, where the antibodies tend to have 'mimicking' specificities (e.g. the antibody may appear to be an anti-e, but can be totally adsorbed by e- red cells). It is even more rare for an Rh antibody to be able to initiate the complement cascade; that notwithstanding, these antibodies are usually IgG1, IgG3, or a mixture of the two sub-classes. The other common Rh antibody is anti-C^w, which is often found in mixtures with other antibodies and has, rarely, been linked with both mild transfusion reactions and haemolytic disease of the newborn/foetus. The C^w antigen (Rh8) is expressed in about 1–2% of individuals and, although most are also C+, rare examples are C-.

Key points

Anti-D, anti-C, anti-c, anti-E, and anti-e are usually IgG, clinically significant antibodies that can cause haemolytic transfusion reactions and haemolytic disease of the newborn.

SELF-CHECK 2.2

What are the main differences between the normal, weak, and partial D antigens? Which individuals can produce alloanti-D?

Inheritance of Rh

Inheritance of the *Rh* genes is relatively straightforward. However, rather in the same way that the MS, Ms, NS, and Ns antigens are passed on as a 'block', Ce, CE, ce, and cE are also passed on as a block. This is not surprising when one considers that the genes for the antigens are mapped so closely to one another, and the antigens are formed by amino acids on the same polypeptide. In addition, although the *RHD* gene is a separate entity to the *RHCE* gene, and the D antigen is on a separate polypeptide, *RHD* and *RHCE* are almost always passed on as an entity. This has resulted in there being eight 'common' **haplotypes** that, for the purposes of inheritance, can be regarded as 'single genes'. The haplotypes can be seen in Table 2.7, together with their frequency in certain populations. Note the frequency of the Dce (R_0) haplotype in the black population, compared with the other populations; the frequency of the DCe (R_1) haplotype within the Asian population, compared with the other populations; and the lack of D- in the Asian population compared with the other populations.

An individual who is DDccee (R_0/R_0) cannot be serologically distinguished from an individual who is Ddccee (R_0/r), as there is no such antibody specificity as anti-d. If the individual is

Haplotypes
Genes in a blood group system that are passed on together.

TABLE 2.7 The eight 'common' Rh haplotypes. Note that the d antigen does not exist, that the DCe (R_1) haplotype is much more common in the Asian population than the other populations, that the Dce (R_0) haplotype is much more common in the Black population than the other populations, and that D- as a whole is far less common in the Asian population than in the other populations.

Haplotype	White %	Black %	Asian %
DCe (R_1)	42	17	70
DCE (R_z)	<0.01	<0.01	1
Dce (R_0)	4	44	3
DcE (R_2)	14	11	21
dCe (r')	2	2	2
dCE (r_y)	<0.01	<0.01	<0.01
dce (r)	37	26	3
dcE (r")	1	<0.01	<0.01

white, then it is far more likely that they would be R_0r than if they were black, when R_0R_0 would be more probable.

Rh$_{null}$ phenotypes

Within the blood group systems already discussed, there are null types (O, O_h, Le(a-b-), S-s-U-, M^kM^k (not discussed, but no M, N, S, or s antigens are expressed)). Within the Rh blood group system there are two null types, one of which is directly as a result of 'missing' (mutant) *RHD* and *RHCE* genes and one of which is due to a 'missing' (mutant) *RHAG* gene. The former type of Rh$_{null}$ is termed the amorph type. This is the result of the *RHD* gene being deleted (as it is with the white form of D-), but with mutations within the *RHCE* gene that prevent the expression of any antigens on the CE polypeptide (probably as a result of the mutations preventing the insertion of this mutant polypeptide into the red cell membrane). Such individuals totally lack all Rh antigens, including Rh29, and such individuals can produce anti-Rh29, which, at a basic level, can be thought of as anti-total Rh.

The latter type of Rh$_{null}$ is termed the regulator type that is the result of a mutation at the *RHAG* gene being inherited, although normal *RHD* and *RHCE* genes may be inherited. Such a mutation within the *RHAG* gene may alter the quaternary structure of the Rh-associated glycoprotein.

It is thought that the integrity of the RhAG polypeptide is necessary for the expression of both the D and CE polypeptides on the red cell surface. Therefore, if the RhAG is not expressed, the Rh blood group system antigens cannot be expressed. Although in some cases, the Rh antigens can be detected by adsorption and elution of the respective antibodies (Rh$_{mod}$), in other cases no such antigens can be detected (Rh$_{null}$), and the individual can make anti-Rh29.

The regulator type of Rh$_{null}$ is more common than the amorph type, despite the fact that mutations within *RHAG* are not common, but both types are incredibly rare.

RHAG the Rh-associated glycoprotein

The Rh antigens are found within the Band-3-based-macrocomplex on the red cell surface, which consists of two RhAG molecules, one D and one CE polypeptide, and one LW molecule, together with a number of other proteins, for example. Band 3, Band 4.2, and ankyrin, all of which are connected to the spectrin skeleton by the ankyrin molecule. Therefore, this complex seems to play a key role in maintaining the integrity of the cell. Rh_{null} red cells that lack the Rh proteins are not the standard bi-concave discs, but mis-shapen cells called stomatocytes. There is also a mild haemolytic anaemia associated with Rh_{null}, possibly caused by an altered permeability to cations, and increased numbers of reticulocytes.

The structure of the Rh-associated glycoprotein is very similar to that of the D and CE polypeptides, but it has a complex N-glycan on the first external loop and is not palmitoylated.

LW blood group system

The LW blood group system is associated with the Rh blood group system in that D+ red cells react more strongly with anti-LW than do D- red cells. Indeed, this relationship is so strong that, on occasions, an anti-LW can be mis-typed as an anti-D. This can be very confusing when the individual producing the antibody is D positive, and the direct antiglobulin test (DAT) is negative. It is always worthwhile testing such an antibody against cord blood that is D negative, as the LW antigens are expressed strongly on cord blood, and this may help to differentiate between anti-D and anti-LW in such circumstances.

Nevertheless, D- adult red cells do carry the LW antigens, of which there are three: LW^a (LW5), LW^{ab} (LW6), and LW^b (LW7).

Very rarely, red cells are LW(a-b-), but have normal Rh antigens, but all Rh_{null} individuals are LW(a-b-). Although true LW(a-b-) red cells are rare, there are many instances recorded in the literature of individuals with a transient phenotype of LW(a-b-) producing a transient (auto-) anti-LW. This is often, but not exclusively, associated with a malignant pathology.

Neither anti-LW^a nor anti-LW^b have been implicated in clinically significant haemolytic transfusion reactions or haemolytic disease of the newborn/foetus.

> ### Key points
> The Rh antigens are expressed on two proteins, D and CE, which are associated in the red cell membrane with two RhAG and one LW protein.

2.5 The Lutheran blood group system

Genes and antigens

There are 20 antigens within the Lutheran blood group system, with another antigen (AnWj) closely associated with, but independent from the system. Within the system are four sets of antithetical antigens; Lu^a and Lu^b, Lu9 and Lu6, Lu14 and Lu8, and Au^b and Au^a. In each case the less frequent antigen is given first, although there is a frequency of >50% in all populations for Au^b, thus both antigens are polymorphic.

The frequency of the Lu^a and Lu^b antigens are, broadly speaking, similar in all populations, with the Lu^a frequency being about 8% and the Lu^b frequency being over 99%. The *LUA* and *LUB* genes are codominant. Lutheran antigens are not well expressed at birth.

The Lu(a-b-) phenotype is interesting in that there are three genetic backgrounds that can bring about this phenotype. The first to be described was the dominant type, controlled by a gene that is independent of the *LU* gene (mapped to 19q13.2-q13.3). This independent gene is termed *In(Lu)*, and is dominant over the normal *in(Lu)* gene. Inheritance of *In(Lu)* results in weakening of the Lutheran blood group system antigens to such an extent that, to all intents and purposes, the red cells are Lu(a-b-) (although this is not quite true, as the antigens can be detected serologically by adsorption and elution techniques). In addition, other antigens coded by genes independent of *LU* are also weakened. These antigens include AnWj, P$_1$, i, CD44 on which In^b is expressed, antigens of the Knops blood group system, Cs^a and MER2 of the RAPH blood group system. Such individuals do not produce anti-Lu3 (an antibody that reacts with all common Lutheran phenotypes). Although rare in itself, with a frequency of approximately 1 in 4,000 of the general population (published figures vary) this is by far and away the most common of the three types of Lu(a-b-).

The second type is the recessive Lu(a-b-). This type comes about with the homozygous inheritance of mutant *LU* genes, resulting in no Lutheran antigens being expressed. In this case, no antigens can be serologically detected by any techniques, and such individuals can produce an anti-Lu3 (indeed, detection of this antibody is the most frequent way such individuals are discovered).

The third type is the rarest of all. This is an *X*-linked form of Lu(a-b-), 'controlled' by the *XS2* gene. Like the dominant type of Lu(a-b-), extremely weak expression of Lutheran antigens can be detected by adsorption and elution techniques, but in this case the AnWj, P$_1$, i, CD44, Knops blood group antigens, Cs^a and MER2, are all expressed normally (although expression of i may be elevated). As would be expected, such individuals do not produce anti-Lu3.

The carrier molecule, which is a Type 1 single-pass membrane glycoprotein with immunoglobulin super-family domains, is found in association with a B cell adhesion molecule (B-CAM). Red cells of sickle cell patients express considerably more Lutheran glycoprotein than the red cells of the normal population. The Lutheran glycoproteins bind laminins and so, as with the LW antigens, they could be involved in the adherence of red cells to vascular endothelium and, it follows, to vascular occlusion in sickle cell disease.

Lutheran was the first system to be associated with another system, autosomal linkage, in this case secretor, the genes for both being found on chromosome 19.

Antibodies

Anti-Lu^a and anti-Lu^b have only ever been implicated in very mild, clinically insignificant haemolytic transfusion reactions and haemolytic disease of the newborn/foetus. *In vitro* reactions between Lutheran antigens and their corresponding antibodies tend to be characteristically 'stringy' and may be mistaken for rouleaux formation.

Key points

The frequency of the Lu^a and Lu^b antigens is similar in all populations; there are three different backgrounds to the Lu(a-b-) phenotype. The antibodies cause only mild haemolytic reactions.

2.6 The Kell and Kx blood group systems

Genes and antigens

The Kell blood group system is interesting in many ways—not least the fact that the first antigen/antibody to be discovered in the system was Levay (now Kp^c or KEL21) in 1945, a year before K and anti-K were described! The system probably should have been named the Levay blood group system, but as it was only discovered that it was part of the Kell blood group system in 1979, it was considered a bit late to change the name.

Thirty-two antigens are now recognized within the Kell blood group system, with the latest being KEL35 (KELP). They are encoded by genes of chromosome 7. Once again, there are several antigens that are antithetical: -K and k, Kp^a and Kp^b, Js^a and Js^b, KEL17 and KEL11, and KEL24 and KEL14. In each case the less frequent antigen is quoted first.

The K antigen/anti-K (K, *not* Kell) has the distinction of being the first antigen/antibody to be discovered by the then new indirect antiglobulin test (IAT) in 1946.

The frequencies of the various Kell antigens (see Table 2.8) vary between the white and black populations and this knowledge is, of course, important when searching for potentially compatible donors for patients with various Kell alloantibodies. One would not, for example, look for a K+k- donor amongst the black donor population as most (99%) are K-, and one would not look for a Js(a+b-) donor amongst the white population where Js^a is found in only 0.01% but in black donors where the frequency is 20%.

Until recently, it was thought that although an individual could express two of the lower incidence Kell antigens on their red cells (e.g. K+k+, Kp(a+b+)) the *K* gene and the *KPA* gene would be on different chromosomes, for example the *K* inherited from the mother and the *KPA* from the father. However, genes encoding the less frequent antigens have now been found to travel together on the same chromosome in some very rare individuals (*K* and *KPA*).

TABLE 2.8 **The various frequencies of Kell phenotypes in the white and black populations.**

Phenotype	White population %	Black population %
K-k+	91	98
K+k+	8.8	2
K+k-	0.2	<0.01
Kp(a-b+)	97.7	100
Kp(a+b+)	2.3	<0.01
Kp(a+b-)	<0.01	0
Js(a-b+)	100	80
Js(a+b+)	<0.01	19
Js(a+b-)	0	1

There are individuals who express no Kell antigens on their red cells. This null phenotype is known as K_o. Such individuals can produce anti-Ku (at a basis level, anti-total Kell) and, once this antibody is produced, can only tolerate blood from other K_o individuals.

Such individuals' red cells react more strongly with anti-Kx than do the red cells of individuals with 'common' Kell phenotypes. It was originally thought, therefore, that the Kx antigen was a precursor of the Kell antigens, rather in the same way that the H antigen is a precursor to the A and B antigens. It is now known, however, that the Kx protein is associated with the Kell glycoprotein on the red cell surface, and that it is actually a matter of steric hindrance that prevents the red cells from individuals with a 'common' Kell phenotype reacting as strongly with anti-Kx. Indeed, it has now been established that there are actually higher numbers of the Kx polypeptide expressed on the red cell surface of individuals with a 'common' Kell phenotype, than on the surface of red cells of a K_o individual.

There are individuals who do not express the Kx protein, and these have very much weakened expression of the Kell antigens. In some cases, this weakening is so profound that the red cells appear to mimic K_o red cells, until adsorption and elution techniques are carried out with Kell antibodies. This is known as the McLeod phenotype. It was shown that there is an association between the McLeod phenotype and a sex-linked condition called chronic granulomatous disease (CGD), and that far too many individuals with the McLeod phenotype also have CGD for this to be a random event. Chronic granulomatous disease manifests itself with symptoms that are like those of Duchenne's muscular dystrophy. Symptoms include muscle wasting, diminished deep tendon reflex, choreiform movements, cardiomyopathy, and increased susceptibility to infection. There is an increased level of serum creatine kinase, and the red cells are often acanthocytic.

The Kx antigen is encoded by the *XK* gene, which has been mapped to Xp21.1 (the *KEL* gene is mapped to 7q33). The gene that causes CGD is also mapped to Xp21.1 and this is why CGD is associated with the McLeod phenotype. Individuals with the McLeod phenotype and CGD can produce two alloantibodies: anti-Kx and anti-Km (originally thought to be a single antibody, anti-KL). This means that they can only be transfused with blood from another individual with the McLeod phenotype, but this has to be an individual without CGD, as those with CGD are too ill to donate.

Key points

The frequency of the Kell antigens varies in different populations. There is a complex interaction between the Kell and the Kx antigen, and an association between X-linked CGD and the McLeod phenotype.

Antibodies

The clinical significance of the Kell antibodies differs with their specificity. Both anti-K and anti-k have been implicated in very severe haemolytic transfusion reactions, whilst anti-Kp[a], anti-Kp[b], anti-Js[a], and anti-Js[b] have all been implicated in more mild episodes of haemolytic transfusion reactions. Anti-K and anti-k have been implicated in many cases of very severe haemolytic disease of the newborn/foetus (anti-k less frequently than anti-K, but this may be because anti-k is less common than anti-K). Anti-Kp[a], anti-Kp[b], anti-Js[a], and anti-Js[b] have all been implicated in serious cases of haemolytic disease of the newborn/foetus, but are much more commonly associated with a mild form of the condition.

There has been some discussion in the literature about why anti-K in particular, causes such severe haemolytic disease in some cases and not others, why titration is a poor predictor of severity and how the antibody attacks the foetal red cells. It has been suggested that an anti-K stimulated by a pregnancy more commonly causes severe haemolytic disease than that stimulated by transfusion, but this has not been substantiated.

Antibody titration is a poor predictor of severity, as much as anything, because of poor technique. It has been found that, if an individual is performing titrations on a daily basis, their precision improves immensely. Nevertheless, it does seem that anti-K is prone to cause more severe haemolytic disease at a lower titre than most other alloantibodies.

A study was undertaken with an anti-K known to have caused severe haemolytic disease and an anti-D known to have caused severe haemolytic disease and it showed that the Kell antigens appear very much earlier on the erythroid progenitors than do the Rh antigens. It seems likely that these erythroid progenitors are destroyed by anti-K before they become haemoglobinized erythroblasts (thus there is reduced hyperbilirubinaemia, erythrobastosis, and reticulocytosis in the foetus), and this mimics inhibition of foetal erythropoiesis. Anti-D, on the other hand, destroys foetal erythroblasts after haemoglobinisation, and so there is no mimicking of erythropoietic inhibition and therefore, more bilirubin is released from the destroyed cells.

> ## Key points
> All Kell antibodies are considered to be clinically significant.

SELF-CHECK 2.3

How is the McLeod phenotype associated with X-linked CGD?

2.7 The Duffy blood group system

Genes and antigens

When asked which antigens are destroyed by the action of papain, many people answer, amongst others, that the Duffy antigens are destroyed. This is not so, as only some of the Duffy antigens are destroyed by papain. There are five antigens within the Duffy blood group system, and those that are destroyed by the action of papain are Fy^a, Fy^b, and Fy6.

There was thought to be another Duffy antigen, Fy^x, but this was later found to be a very weak expression of the Fy^b antigen, although the antigen may not react with all examples of anti-Fy^b, Fy^a, and Fy^b are antithetical and *FYA* and *FYB* are co-dominant. There is also a silent gene—*FY*. The other antigens are numbered 3–6 (4 being redundant). The *FY* gene has been mapped to 1q22-q23.

The frequency of the antigens varies enormously throughout the world (see Table 2.9). There is a high frequency of the Fy(a-b-) phenotype in the black population. There is a low frequency of the Fy(a-b+) phenotype in the Chinese population and, by inference, a low frequency of the *FYB* gene in this population. Individuals who are Fy(a-b-) can make an antibody against the high frequency antigen Fy3. Very few black individuals who are transfused with Fy(a+b-), Fy(a+b+), or Fy(a-b+) blood, however, produce anti-Fy3. The reason is that

TABLE 2.9 **Frequencies of the various Duffy phenotypes in different populations. Note the high frequency of the Fy(a-b-) phenotype in the black population and the low frequency of the Fy(a-b+), and, by inference, the low frequency of the *FYB* gene, in the Chinese population.**

Phenotype	White population %	Black population %	Chinese population %
Fy(a+b-)	17	9	90.8
Fy(a+b+)	49	1	8.9
Fy(a-b+)	34	22	0.3
Fy(a-b-)	0	68	0

many of them are genetically *FYB/FYB* or *FYB/FY*, and relatively few of them are *FY/FY*. Why then, do they type as Fy(a-b-), rather than Fy(a-b+)?

Many people within the black population are homozygous for a mutation within an erythroid-specific, *GATA-1*, transcription-factor binding site, upstream of the coding region of the Duffy gene. This mutation prevents expression of the Duffy glycoprotein on red cells, but not on other cells. Duffy glycoprotein is expressed on endothelial cells lining post-capillary venules of soft tissues and splenic sinusoids. Duffy mRNA is not detected in the bone marrow of such individuals, but is present in their lung, spleen, kidneys, and colon. Therefore, the immune system of such individuals does not recognize the Fy^b antigen as 'foreign', and they will not produce anti-Fy3.

There is a selective advantage in being Fy(a-b-) in areas where certain strains of malaria are endemic as Fy(a-b-) red cells are resistant to invasion by the merozoytes of *Plasmodium knowlesi and P. vivax*. Such individuals are not, however, resistant to *P. falciparum*, which can cause more severe disease than *P. vivax*.

The Fy6 antigen is recognized only by a monoclonal antibody; no human antibody has been described. The antigen is found in 100% of the white population, but just 32% of the black population.

Antibodies

Anti-Fy^a has been implicated, on very rare occasions, in clinically significant haemolytic transfusion reactions and clinically significant haemolytic disease of the newborn/foetus, but most Duffy antibodies are only implicated in mild conditions.

Key points

There is a difference in Duffy phenotype frequencies in different ethnicities, Fy(a-b-) individuals are resistant to the *P. vivax* malarial parasite.

SELF-CHECK 2.4

Why do most black Fy(a-b-) individuals not produce anti-Fy3, even when repeatedly challenged with Fy^a and Fyb positive blood?

2.8 The Kidd blood group system

Genes and antigens

The Kidd blood group system only consists of three antigens, Jk^a, Jk^b, and the high incidence antigen JK3, and are encoded by the *JK* gene mapped to 18q11-q12. The carrier molecule is a protein of 389 amino acid residues in length, which traverses the red cell membrane ten times, giving five extracellular loops. The relative frequencies of the Kidd phenotypes are similar in European and Asian populations but Jk^a is more frequent in black populations (see Table 2.10).

There are two types of Jk(a-b-) phenotype, but both are exceptionally rare. The more common type is the amorph, *JK/JK*. Such individuals can produce anti-Jk3, as they are also negative for the high incidence antigen Jk:3. The other type is *InJk* and is, like *In(Lu)*, governed by a dominant gene preventing the expression of the Kidd antigens. Like the Lutheran antigens in the *InLu* situation, the Kidd antigens in the *InJk* situation are present, but at very low levels, requiring techniques such as adsorption and elution to be detected.

Jk(a-b-) red cells are resistant to haemolysis by 2 M urea. Like many things in science, this was a serendipitous discovery. A Samoan man with aplastic anaemia gave an unexplained high platelet count when his blood was tested on a blood counting machine. The automation relied upon the haemolysis of red cells with 2 M urea to 'visualize' the platelets. His red cells were not haemolysing within the normal one minute when exposed to 2 M urea, and this was found to be due to his Jk(a-b-) phenotype. This phenomenon was found to be common to red cells from all Jk(a-b-) individuals. Thus, a cheap screening test for the Jk(a-b-) phenotype was discovered.

The red cells from individuals heterozygous for Jk:-3 haemolyse at an intermediate rate in 2 M urea. Jk(a-b-) individuals are unable to maximally concentrate urine.

Antibodies

The antibodies, in particular anti-Jk^a, are notorious for being labile both *in vivo* and *in vitro*. Secondary immunization, however, often produces an anamnestic response, with a rapid increase in the antibody in the circulation. If the secondary stimulus is from a transfusion of Jk(a+) red cells, this might result in a severe, even fatal, delayed haemolytic transfusion reaction. Conversely, Kidd antibodies, apart from one or two isolated cases, have only been reported to cause mild haemolytic disease of the newborn and foetus. Whereas the direct antiglobulin test is positive only with a monospecific anti-IgG reagent, with the red cells of most babies sensitized with maternal antibody, in the case of Kidd antibodies it is sometimes found that an anti-C3d reagent will also produce a positive result. Kidd antibodies are usually IgG and can activate complement more readily than most other IgG red cell antibodies.

TABLE 2.10 Frequencies of the various Kidd phenotypes in certain populations.

Phenotype	White population %	Black population %	Asian population %
Jk(a+b-)	26.3	51.1	23.2
Jk(a+b+)	50.3	40.8	49.1
Jk(a-b+)	23.4	8.1	26.8

Antibodies within the Kidd blood group system often show dosage. This means that, for example, certain examples of anti-Jk^a will react more strongly with Jk(a+b-) red cells than with Jk(a+b+) red cells, and sometimes only with Jk(a+b-) red cells that have more Jk^a antigen *per* red cell than the other phenotypes.

Key points

The relative frequencies of the Kidd phenotypes are similar in most populations; there are two types of the Jk(a-b-) phenotype. Kidd antibodies often activate complement and are of clinical significance in transfusion and in HDN.

2.9 The P1PK blood group system

This system has two antigens, P1 and p^k. The main antigen is P1. Approximately 79% of the white population and 94% of the black population are P1+. When using anti-P1 derived from a human, individuals demonstrate different strengths of reaction that appears to be inherited, but this is much less obvious using mouse monoclonal anti-P1.

The antibody, anti-P1, is usually IgM, cold-reacting, causing agglutination at temperatures below 37°C and therefore, clinically benign.

Another cold reacting antibody often found reacting in room temperature tests is anti-I, or rarely anti-i. All, except a few rare individuals, have the I antigen but also anti-I as a cold reactive autoantibody. This antibody is normally benign but might increase in potency and cause cold haemagglutinin disease (see Chapter 6 for more details).

2.10 Other blood groups

This chapter has only given an overview of what are generally considered to be the more important blood group systems, but some other, selected, blood groups and miscellany will be briefly described in this section.

The Diego blood group system includes an antigen, Di^a, which is found in about 36% of South American Indians. In addition, however, it is found within the Chinese and Japanese populations, and it is interesting that the Di^a antigen can be found in European populations, in decreasing frequency, in such a way that it suggests that it was genetically spread by the Mongolian hordes of Genghis Khan.

The antibodies of the Dombrock blood group system, although sometimes clinically significant, are often too weak to be used *in vitro* as grouping reagents. As a result laboratories from NHS Blood and Transplant, together with the IBGRL have undertaken a study in which Do(a+b-) and Do(a-b+) donors were screened at a molecular level, and units of blood from these donors cryopreserved at the National Frozen Blood Bank located at the NHSBT Liverpool Centre.

The Indian blood group system is associated with CD44. It has four antigens, of which the main two are In^a and In^b, found not just on red cells but also most other cells in the body, including white blood cells. The In^a antigen has a higher incidence in not just Indians but also Arabs and Iranians. The antibodies IgG and anti-In^b have been implicated in transfusion reactions, but not haemolytic disease of the newborn.

Antigens of the Knops blood group system are found on the CR1 (complement receptor type 1) carrier molecule found on most red cells and some white cells. The antibodies, because they often only react weakly but to a high titre, are given the name HTLA—high titre, low affinity antibodies. They cause little or no *in vivo* red cell destruction but when present with other antibodies cause problems when trying to identify their specificity.

The Chido/Rodgers blood group system antigens are found on complement C4A and C4B glycoproteins that are adsorbed onto red cells. Although the IgG antibodies are not uncommon they do not cause red cell destruction and like Knops antibodies cause a good deal of frustration when attempting to determine antibody specificity.

A question often asked is do blood groups change? As antigens are an inherited characteristic then no, they cannot change, but their expression can. In some malignant diseases ABO and Rh antigens, for example, can become weakly expressed but when the patient is in remission they return to their normal expression. If someone has a bone marrow transplant then the red cells produced by the engrafted stem cells will have the blood group antigens of the donor, not the recipient, and these could be different from each other. The recipient's blood group would then have apparently changed.

There are, however, some antigens that may be *acquired*, and are recognized by antibodies present in the serum of most adults, therefore often being referred to as *polyagglutination*. These antigens, T, Tk, and acquired B, are the results of enzymes produced by bacteria *in vivo*, often associated with infections of the gut, such as necrotizing enterocolitis. Some of these organisms produce neuraminidase that cleaves sialic acid from red cells exposing the T antigen, so that the red cells can be agglutinated by the naturally acquired IgM anti-T present in most adults.

As described above, there are a number of direct associations between blood groups and disease. Over the years there have been many publications reporting other associations between blood groups and diseases, and even with personality traits. In 1927 it was suggested that 'hangovers' were more pronounced in group A people, and group B individuals 'defecate' more! Others have proposed that A_2 people have the highest IQ. However, the correlation that seems to be well substantiated is the increased incidence of cancer in group A as compared to group O individuals. And the reverse correlation is true of peptic and duodenal ulcers, more in group O than A individuals. Blood groups are also related to a number of conditions that are dealt with in Chapter 7, for example haemolytic transfusion reactions, haemolytic disease of the newborn/foetus (HDN), and autoimmune haemolytic anaemias (AIHA).

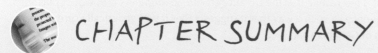

CHAPTER SUMMARY

- The 319 human erythrocyte antigens found on red cells are grouped into 30 blood group systems, five collections, and two series (high and low frequency).

- The antigens are inherited characteristics and are found on carrier molecules, usually proteins that are part of the red cell membrane and as such they have a variety of biological functions.

- Some antigens have a very varied distribution in different populations so might be of more significance in some places than in others.

- Of all the blood group systems the ABO and Rh blood group systems are the most important in blood transfusion and clinically.

- Giving a blood transfusion of the wrong ABO group could lead to the recipient suffering renal damage or even death as the result of that error.

- The D antigen is, after the A and B antigens, the most important due to its immunogenicity, its ability to induce the production of anti-D, which is still the major cause of haemolytic disease of the newborn and foetus.

- Many antibodies in the other blood group systems are clinically significant, capable of causing a haemolytic transfusion reaction or haemolytic disease of the newborn, therefore, knowledge of all the blood group systems helps when resolving problems in finding compatible blood or investigating immune red cell destruction.

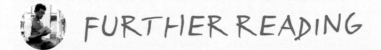

FURTHER READING

- Daniels G *Human Blood Groups*, 2nd edition. Blackwell Science, Oxford, 2002.

- Daniels G & Bromilow I *Essential Guide to Blood Groups*, 2nd edition. Blackwell Publishing Ltd, Oxford, 2010.

- Klien H & Anstee DJ *Mollison's Blood Transfusion in Clinical Medicine*, 11th edition. Blackwell Science, Oxford, 2011.

- Reid ME & Lomas-Francis CG *Blood Group Antigens Facts Book*, 2nd edition. Academic Press, New York, 2003.

Answers to the questions in this chapter are provided on the book's Online Resource Centre.

 Go to www.oxfordtextbooks.co.uk/orc/knight

Donors and Donation: Collection and Processing

Lionel Mohabir

Learning objectives

After studying this chapter you should be able to:

- Outline the criteria for the selection of blood donors in the UK.
- Describe the actions taken to reduce microbial contamination at collection.
- Understand the methods for routine blood component preparation (red cells, platelets, FFP, and cryoprecipitate).
- Understand the methods for specialist blood component preparation (e.g. for neonates, IUT).
- Understand the rationale and methods for leucodepletion and irradiation of blood components.
- Outline pathogen inactivation/reduction of blood components—theories and methodologies.
- Describe component validation and labelling criteria for blood components.
- Describe the criteria for storage of blood components.

Introduction

Many recent medical and surgical advances have relied heavily on blood component support. Thanks to the generosity of voluntary blood donors, patients with medical conditions such leukaemia, anaemia, and thalassaemia, now have an extended lifespan. Blood is rarely transfused unmodified, but is separated into red cells, platelets, and plasma components to meet specific clinical needs. Also, plasma is further processed into immunoglobulins, clotting factors, and protein fractions. The safety of blood donations is enhanced by pre-donation screening and laboratory tests for blood groups and transfusion transmitted infections (TTI).

The increasing volume and complexity of the processing and testing is accomplished with the use of automated equipment and computerization. These are all performed within a quality controlled and quality management system within blood establishments to exacting national, European, and international guidelines and regulations. In the United Kingdom, the Medicines & Healthcare products Regulatory Agency (MHRA) is the licensing authority to ensure that the guidelines/regulations are followed. Any blood establishment must comply with the Blood Safety and Quality Regulations (BSQR).

3.1 Blood donation

Blood for clinical use can be collected from:

- *Voluntary, unpaid donors*: all blood and blood components collected in the UK and most developed countries are from this group of donors. The European Directive 2002/98/EC states: 'Member States should take measures to promote Community self-sufficiency in human blood or blood components and to encourage voluntary unpaid donations of blood and blood components.'

- *Paid donors* who receive monetary payment for blood donation. This group includes commercial donors used by some of the US plasma fractionators. The financial incentive is thought to attract donors from lower socioeconomic members of the community. This population has been shown to have a higher rate of infections that can be transmitted by blood transfusions, some of which may not be detected by the mandatory screening assays that all donations are subjected to and could, therefore, infect recipients.

- *Replacement donors* provide blood for the patient being transfused, usually a relative. These are essentially voluntary donors but they may feel coerced to donate so that the relative can receive the necessary medical intervention. Sometimes the family use professional, paid donors as replacement. A higher incidence of transfusion transmitted infections has been reported in replacement donors.

- *Donors who receive non-financial incentives* such as cholesterol testing, time off from work, etc. are used by some blood services to increase blood collections. There is conflicting evidence on the effectiveness of this method of attracting blood donors.

Pre-donation screening

In the UK, the rules for the collection, testing, and production of blood components are to be found in *The Guidelines for the Blood Transfusion Services in the United Kingdom*, commonly referred to, because of the colour of its cover, as the Red Book .

The acceptable age for blood donation in the UK is 17–65, but regular donors can donate beyond this with the approval of the medical staff at the blood establishment. The minimum weight for donation is 50 kg. Body weight is related to blood volume so that smaller donors are more likely to suffer adverse reactions such as dizziness and fainting after donation. Before a donation of blood or blood component is collected, a series of pre-donation screening checks must be completed to:

- Protect the donor by reducing any adverse effects as a result of donating blood.
- Protect the recipient by reducing the possibility of contaminated blood entering the blood supply.

Pre-donation screening allows potential donors to self-exclude if they think that their blood will present a risk to the blood supply. This is accomplished by:

- Reading a leaflet which states the reasons why you should never give blood, such as:
  - you are HIV positive
  - you are HTLV positive
  - you are a hepatitis B positive and/or carrier
  - you are a hepatitis C carrier
  - you have been paid for sex, either financially or with drugs
  - you have injected or have been injected with non-medically prescribed drugs.

- Reading a leaflet which states the reasons why you must not give blood for at least 12 months after protected or unprotected sex:
  - you are a man who has oral or anal sex with men in the last 12 months even if you used a condom
  - if your partner is, or you think they are HIV or HTLV positive or a hepatitis B or C carrier
  - for women whose male partner has ever had sex with another man
  - if your partner has ever received money or drugs for sex
  - if your partner has ever injected or been injected with non-medically prescribed drugs
  - if your partner has or you think may have been sexually active in parts of the world where HIV/AIDS is very common, such as, most African countries

- Completing a 'yes/no' donor health check questionnaire, which will enable the prospective donor and the blood collection team to determine suitability of the donation and any adverse effect on the donor by donating.

- Having an oral interview with a member of the blood collection team to confirm some of the answers and to get further information on questions to which the answer is 'yes'.

- Having a haemoglobin (Hb) screen to ensure you have met the minimum requirement to donate. The reason for this is that by donating blood or blood components your blood volume should not be reduced by more than 13%. The haemoglobin is assessed in most blood collection sites in the UK using a copper sulphate test with a specific gravity of 1.053 for females and 1.055 for males. A drop of blood from a finger prick should fall through the copper sulphate solution within 15 seconds if the minimum Hb is 12.5 g/l for female or 13.5 g/l for male is met. Blood samples are taken from donors who have not passed the copper sulphate test for an accurate haemoglobin assessment at the blood transfusion centre. Automated equipment for measuring haemoglobin at blood collection sites is being introduced.

The donor health check questionnaire must be signed by the donor, together with a qualified healthcare professional who obtained the health history before a blood donation was taken. This is to affirm that:

- The donor has read and understood the educational materials provided.
- The donor has been given the opportunity to ask questions and was satisfied with the responses.
- To the best of their knowledge the information provided was true.

It confirms that consent has been given for a donation to be taken and tested.

Donors in some countries are asked confidentially if their donation should not be transfused to others, a procedure known as **confidential unit exclusion**. This is to allow donors, who

Confidential unit exclusion
This allows donors whose behaviour puts them at increased risk of acquiring HIV (or other TTI) who cannot avoid donating to confidentially indicate that their blood should not be transfused.

because of peer pressure, felt obligated to donate and are given the option to opt out at the donor session. This intervention was shown to have minimal impact on blood safety especially with the introduction of nucleic acid testing.

The pre-donation or donor screening is an inexpensive and effective method of deferring donors who may pose a risk to the blood supply either because their blood may transmit an infection or the medication taken may have an adverse effect on the recipient. It is also the only means of increasing transfusion safety from diseases for which there are currently no laboratory tests, such as Creutzfeldt–Jakob disease (vCJD).

Donors who are deferred through questioning will contain a population who are infectious and a proportion who are non-infectious and are inappropriately deferred (false positive deferrals). Similarly, acceptable donors will also contain a small proportion who are infectious (false negative), but the majority will be non-infectious (true negative screening). The majority of those who are potentially infectious will be detected when their donation is tested in the laboratory, but an extremely small number of donations from donors in the window period phase of infection will pass both the donor and donation screening and will be made available for transfusion (see Chapter 4).

Donors who have recently visited areas where malaria and Chagas disease are endemic are offered an antibody test at least six months after their return or if they are displaying symptoms of infection. In the absence of a test, the donor is deferred for 12 months for malaria risk and indefinitely for Chagas. This is based on evidence that within six months the overwhelming majority of people exposed to one of these infections would have made antibodies that will be detectable in screening tests.

Donors who have had tattoos, body piercing, and acupuncture are deferred for 12 months but those who have had endoscopy are suspended for six months. However, a donation may be taken from these donors at least four months after the procedure if a validated anti-HBc test (and HBV NAT) is negative. The blood group must be confirmed on the donation and all other microbiology and red cell antibody screen must also be negative. Donors who are positive for anti-HBc may be accepted if they have been shown to have an anti-HBs titre of 100 iu or greater.

As an additional safety precaution, donors are asked to telephone the blood transfusion centre to report any additional medical information that might come to mind after the donation or if they fell ill within a few days following donation. Most of these telephone calls are to report an acute illness which would not affect the donation but they occasionally report risk factors which were not disclosed at the donor session. Sometimes, information is received from third parties, which has to be carefully evaluated before a decision on the fate of the donation is taken.

Key points

Pre-donation screening is an inexpensive way of deferring donors who may pose a risk to themselves and reduces the risk of contaminated blood entering the blood supply.

SELF-CHECK 3.1

What pre-donation screening is performed?

SELF-CHECK 3.2

What is the purpose of pre-donation screening?

Donation process

A donation of blood is taken from those who have passed the donor screening and copper sulphate/haemoglobin tests. The donation record form (session form), blood collection and satellite bags and sample tubes are labelled with the same unique ISBT 128 barcoded number (see below). The donor is asked to confirm his/her identity and the arm is cleansed with 2% chlorhexidine gluconate and 70% isopropyl alcohol, which has been shown to be superior to alcohol or iodine based swab in destroying microorganism skin contamination. The needle from the blood bag is inserted into the donor's vein and a minimum of 20 ml of blood is diverted to a sample pouch to remove any remnant skin contamination (through the skin plug). This sample pouch is then sealed and the blood flows into the main pack which contains the **anticoagulant**. The main bag is either kept on an automatic mixer or periodically manually mixed to prevent the blood from clotting. The blood donation is usually completed in about ten minutes, when approximately 450 ± 45 ml of blood is collected. If it takes longer than this, the blood is not used for platelet production but the red cells and plasma are suitable for use. Three (or more) samples are taken from the sample pouch for testing.

After donating, the donor is required to rest for about ten minutes and advised not to undertake any strenuous or hazardous activity for the remainder of the day. They are offered biscuits, tea, coffee, or a cold drink before they leave the session.

Anticoagulant
A substance which when it is added to the blood inhibits clotting

---

Key points

Decontamination of the donor's arm and diverting the first 30 ml of donated blood into a sample pouch for testing further reduces the risk of microorganisms contaminating the bag of blood.

BOX 3.1 ISBT 128 format

ISBT 128 is an international standard used to securely identify human blood, tissue, and organs for transfusion or transplantation. The blood donation number has a barcode and a 14 digit eye readable number. The format of the number is:

AAAAAYYNNNNNNC, where

AAAAA is the country code,

YY is the year,

NNNNNN is a six-digit number, and

C is a check character, which is the output of a mathematical calculation on the preceding digits to eliminate transcription and transposition errors. When the barcode is scanned or read by a barcode reader, it is displayed as a 15-digit number because the eye readable check character is two digits.

The use of the ISBT 128 number format makes the donation number unique and supports the safe transfer and transfusion across national and international borders. This format can also be used for other information printed on the blood component label.

Anticoagulants and additives

If blood was collected into a container without any anticoagulant it would clot and be unsuitable for transfusion. Sodium citrate was discovered as an anticoagulant in 1914–15 and was a major advance in transfusion during the First World War.

During the Second World War a mixture of sodium citrate and glucose or dextrose was used as both the anticoagulant and the storage medium for whole blood. To prevent bacterial growth, the solution was sterilized by autoclaving, but the pH was adjusted with the addition of citric acid to below 5.8 to prevent caramelization of the dextrose when heated. This solution is known as acid citrate dextrose (ACD).

The citrate chelates calcium ions in the plasma and prevents coagulation, whilst glucose/dextrose serves as nutrient for red cell metabolism. Blood can be stored in ACD for three weeks at 4°C with a 75% 24-hour post-transfusion recovery.

Phosphate is gradually lost from the red cells of ACD suspended blood and this affects ATP production, especially during the third week of storage. Addition of phosphate to the storage solution maintains ATP production and the post-transfusion red cell recovery at the end of the shelf-life . Therefore phosphate was added to the solution—citrate phosphate dextrose (CPD)—which does not affect the anticoagulant activity but increases the shelf-life of whole blood and red cells to four weeks.

The loss of ATP has been shown to be related to loss of red cell viability. Addition of adenine or inosine to stored red cells restored their shape, and improved red cell recovery and osmotic fragility. Collection of whole blood in citrate phosphate dextrose that contains adenine (CPDA-1) extended the shelf-life to five weeks. The post-transfusion red cell recovery at five weeks averaged 81% for whole blood and 72% for red cells from which most of the plasma has been removed.

During the manufacturing process of packed red cells, dextrose and adenine are removed with the plasma, but these can be added to the red cells by using an additive solution containing saline, adenine, and glucose (SAG). This restores the nutrients and enables longer storage, lower viscosity, and better flow of red cells as they are less packed.

Red cells in blood stored in SAG have a 24-hour *in vivo* recovery of $83 \pm 7\%$ and an average haemolysis of $0.58 \pm 0.15\%$. Addition of mannitol reduces the haemolysis and increases the shelf-life by a week. Mannitol has been shown to be a free radical scavenger and stabilizes cell membranes. Red cells can be stored in a solution of saline adenine glucose mannitol (SAGM) after the removal of plasma and have a six-week shelf-life. Donations from which SAGM suspended red cells are produced are collected into a standard CPD anticoagulant as the additives are not required to be present in the plasma or in platelet preparations.

There is a concern of renal toxicity associated with transfusion of high concentrations of adenine and mannitol to low birth weight infants and during exchange transfusions. Mannitol is also a potent diuretic and can cause fluctuation in cerebral blood flow in neonates. Because of this, blood for exchange or large volume transfusions to neonates is collected in CPD but the red cells are not processed by adding SAGM. Blood stored in SAGM is suitable for smaller 'top up' transfusions for these patients.

Key points

Anticoagulants are used to prevent the donated blood from clotting. Additives are used to improve the shelf-life of blood components and the post-transfusion viability by providing some essential nutrients.

BOX 3.2 2,3 diphosphoglycerate (2,3 DPG)

2,3 diphosphoglycerate is an intermediate product of glycolysis and plays a role in the release of oxygen from the red cells to the tissues. In the red cells there is an interaction between haemoglobin, 2,3 DPG, and oxygen. With low levels of 2,3 DPG, the affinity of haemoglobin for oxygen increases. This dynamic is reversed with normal levels of 2,3 DPG leading to the release of oxygen from the haemoglobin. During red cell storage, 2,3 DPG becomes depleted in about two weeks but the levels return to normal within 24 hours of transfusion.

BOX 3.3 Changes which occur during storage of blood

Storage lesions are changes occurring in stored blood which affect their functions *in vivo*:

- There is a progressive loss in red cell viability which affects their survival in recipients when transfused. The depletion of red cell ATP was shown to be related to the loss of membrane lipid, change in shape from discoid to spheres, and increase in red cell rigidity. The rate of loss of red cell viability and hence the 24-hour survival varies with the storage solution used.

- Depletion of 2,3 DPG which leads to increased affinity of haemoglobin for oxygen and decreased oxygen release.

- Release of potassium from red cells.

- Release of leucocyte enzymes as a result of leucocyte deterioration.

- Release of cytokines, histamines, and lipids, which are associated with febrile transfusion reactions and transfusion-related acute lung injury (TRALI).

- Release of microaggregates and procoagulants, which can cause TRALI.

- Platelet viability is quickly lost during storage as whole blood.

SELF-CHECK 3.3

Why are anticoagulants and additives used in blood collection?

SELF-CHECK 3.4

Why is 2,3 DPG important?

3.2 Donor/donation linking

Each donor is given a unique donor number. With every donation, the bag of blood, all samples collected, and the session form is given the same unique donation number. In the UK, the ISBT 128 barcode format is used for donation numbers. The donation number is linked to the corresponding donor number usually through the use of computers to allow traceability.

Use of computers

Computers play an essential part of blood transfusion centre activities. They are used for storing donor and donation information, generating statistics, and running queries, amongst other uses. Some of the specific uses of computers in a blood transfusion environment are:

- Recording donor demographics such as name, date of birth, address, and other contact details
- Scheduling collection sites and donors
- Donation numbers, including date of collection and collection location linked to the corresponding donor
- Preparing schedules for blood collection
- Producing letters for donor recruitment
- Components prepared, by whom, and the equipment used
- Test performed and results
- Component validation and labelling
- Quality assurance
- Inventory management
- Fate of donation/component, that is, where the component was issued to
- Searching for specific components
- Invoicing, if required
- Provide an audit trail
- Used for sample tracking
- Providing statistics on blood and blood components

Login donation for processing

Before a donation is processed, the donation number and pack type is logged into the host computer. This is to ensure that all satellite packs are accounted for at the end of the production process. This also ensures that should the manufacturer find a problem with a particular lot of blood bags they have prepared then all donations for this lot can be recalled.

3.3 Component preparation

Donations of whole blood can be separated into:

- Red cell concentrate
- Platelets
- Fresh frozen plasma
- Occasionally leucocytes are prepared from **buffy coats** when requested for named patients
- Cryoprecipitate can be prepared from fresh frozen plasma

Buffy coat
The layer of WBC sitting on top of the red cell layer after centrifugation.

Whole blood for red cells, platelets, and plasma is normally collected in bottom and top (BAT) packs that can be processed on automated blood component extractors such as Fenwall Optipress II, NPBI Compomat, and Pall Bagpress. In blood transfusion services where this sort of automation is not available, blood packs with satellite bags connected at the top are used.

Separation of whole blood into selected components is by **differential centrifugation**. Red blood cells are the densest component of blood, followed by white blood cells or leucocytes, platelets, and plasma. During centrifugation red blood cells move to the bottom of the bag, with plasma at the top. A 'buffy coat' containing leucocytes and platelets separates between the red cells and plasma.

Large temperature-controlled computerized centrifuges are used to separate blood components. Before each centrifuge is put into routine use, it must be validated for, among other things, temperature, rotor speed, and time, to determine the optimum conditions for producing the highest yield of viable components being prepared.

Whole blood packs, together with all the attached satellite packs and **leucodepletion** filters (if used), must be carefully packaged into the centrifuge buckets, ensuring that they are balanced.

The centrifuge will spin on a validated programme setting (the correct speed and time) and when it has stopped, the donations are placed on automated or manual blood component extractors to separate the donation into the component parts.

Differential centrifugation
Subjecting a sample or donation of blood to accelerating force based on relative centrifugal force (or g force) and time to separate components according to size and density.

Leucodepletion
A process for removals of white blood cells from blood components to less that 5×10^6 per unit through an in-line filter.

SELF-CHECK 3.5

Name four components that can be prepared from whole blood.

Separation of components

METHOD *Buffy coat preparation*

- Whole blood for buffy coat preparation is bled into the donation pack which has a tube at the top leading to a transfer pack for plasma, and a transfer pack for red cells, filter, and SAG-M at the bottom (see Figure 3.1).

- The whole blood is centrifuged at ~5,000 g for ~7 minute (a hard spin) at 22 ± 2°C to sediment the red cells, platelets, and leucocytes. Platelets and leucocytes settle at the interface of the red cells and plasma.

- The Optipress II (shown in Figure 3.2) is used to separate plasma, red cells, and buffy coat from the BAT packs. After switching the power on, selecting the correct programme, and inserting the appropriate back plate to the system, the centrifuged whole blood pack is placed onto the extractor as shown in Figure 3.2.

- The satellite pack for plasma (pack B in Figure 3.1) is placed on top of the Optipress with the connecting tubing passed through a sealing clamp.

- The red cell transfer pack (C), SAGM pack (D), and leucodepletion filter is placed on a weighing scale next to the Optipress with the connecting tubing located through the sealing clamp at the bottom of the expressor.

- After pressing the start button, the system prompts for the entry of the donation number barcode and the operator code.

- The internal cannulae at the bottom and top of the main BAT pack are broken to allow red cells and plasma to flow into their respective transfer packs.

- Buffy coat containing platelets, leucocytes, and some red cells, remain in the main pack.

- The transfer tubes are sealed and the components separated.

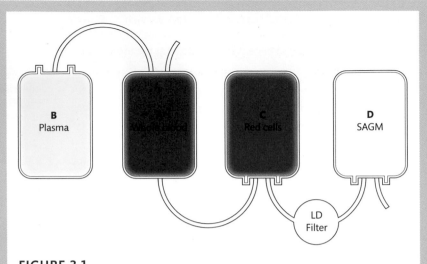
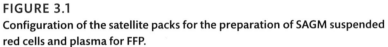

FIGURE 3.1
Configuration of the satellite packs for the preparation of SAGM suspended red cells and plasma for FFP.

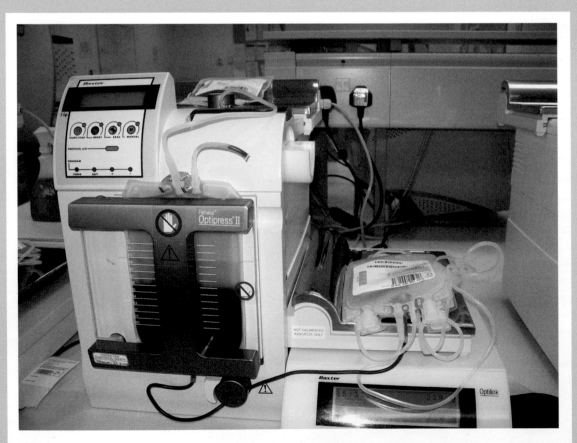

FIGURE 3.2
Use the Optipress to separate plasma and red cells and leaving the buffy coat in the main pack.

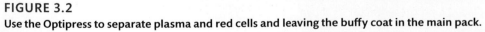

METHOD *Platelet preparation*

In the UK, platelets are either obtained through apheresis or pooled buffy coats. Single donation platelet concentrate is used in other countries as well as apheresis and buffy coat-derived pooled platelets.

Buffy coat derived platelets

- A sterile connecting device (see Figure 3.3) is used to serially connect four buffy coats of the same ABO and RhD groups to a platelet pack with a leucodepletion filter (see Figure 3.4). For CMV negative platelets, all the donations in the pool must be CMV negative.

- The most remote buffy coat (pack B in Figure 3.4) must still be connected to its plasma pack (A) which is usually from a male donor, an intervention to reduce transfusion-related acute lung injury (TRALI).

- The donation numbers of the buffy coats and plasma are entered to the host computer. A platelet pool number is computer generated which must be attached to the platelet pack.

- Flush the first three buffy coats and the plasma into the last buffy coat container (pack E in Figure 3.4) next to the platelet pack.

- Seal and separate the three empty buffy coat packs and discard.

- Centrifuge the pooled buffy coat using a slow spin to sediment the red cells and leucocytes with the platelets remaining in the plasma.

- Separate the pooled platelet-rich plasma into the platelet storage pack (F) through the leucodepletion filter using the automated component extractor.

- The pooled platelet pack is sealed, separated, and labelled and the contents are then constantly mixed until required.

- Prior to bacterial testing, the pooled platelet pack is thoroughly mixed and a sample of platelet-rich plasma is transferred to the small satellite pack (G). This sample is used to test for bacterial contamination of the pooled platelets.

Single donation platelet concentrate

- Blood donation intended for the preparation of single donation platelet concentrate is collected in a multiple bag system consisting of the main donation pack, with a satellite pack containing red cell additive and two packs for the platelet preparation.

- The donation is subjected to a slow spin (~2,000 g for ~3 minutes) at $22 \pm 2°C$ to sediment the red cells while retaining the platelets in the plasma.

- The platelet-rich plasma is expressed into a satellite pack which is connected to an empty pack. The platelet rich plasma and the empty bag are separated from the main red cell pack.

- The red cell additive solution is transferred to the red cell pack and the tube connecting the two is sealed and separated. The red cell pack is mixed with the additive solution and stored at $4 \pm 2°C$. The empty red cell additive pack is discarded.

- The platelet-rich plasma (and satellite pack) is subjected to a hard spin in a centrifuge set at $22 \pm 2°C$ to sediment the platelets.

- All the plasma, except for about 50 ml, is expressed into the satellite pack, leaving the platelet concentrate behind.

- The platelet concentrate is allowed to rest for three hours at $22 \pm 2°C$ and then constantly mixed.

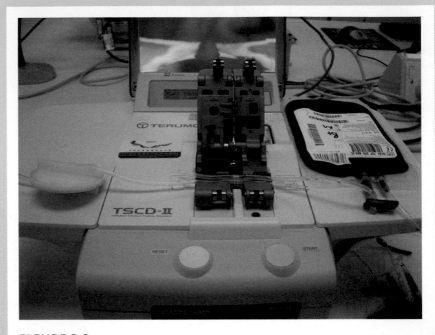

FIGURE 3.3
The Terumo TSCD-II showing the sterile connection of a leucodepletion filter tube to a buffy coat pack.

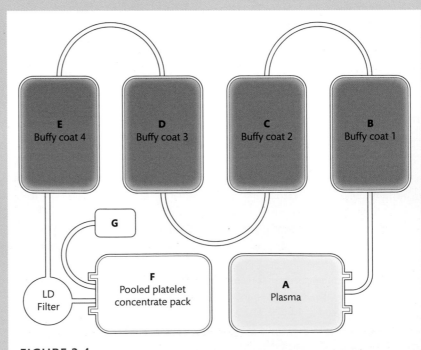

FIGURE 3.4
Serial sterile connection of the four buffy coat and plasma pack to the platelet pack with leucodepletion filter and satellite pack.

METHOD Red cells and FFP

Red cells are produced:

- **As part of the buffy coat process.** After the buffy coat separation, the red cell pack is detached. The red cells pack is attached via a leucodepletion filter to a satellite pack containing SAG-M. The SAG-M pack is hung on a rack and the cannula broken to allow the SAG-M to flow through the filter into the red cells. This is to prime the filter and aids the leucodepletion of the red cells by reducing the viscosity. The red cells are thoroughly mixed with the SAG-M. The pack is then hung on the rack to allow the SAG-M suspended red cells to flow though the filter into the original SAG-M pack and is leucodepleted in the process. The tubing connected to the filter is sealed and the red cell pack is detached. It is labelled with the component code, blood group, date bled, expiry date, and any additional information, such as red cell phenotypes, and stored at 2–6°C.

- **In the preparation of FFP.** Whole blood collected in CPD is used for the preparation of red cells and FFP. The main pack is attached through integral tubing to three satellite packs, one of which contains SAG-M and there is also an in-line filter (see Figure 3.5). During the first part of the process, the whole blood (pack A) is filtered (leucodepleted) into one of the satellite packs (B). The tubing to the filter is sealed and the filter and the empty pack is detached and discarded. The leucodepleted whole blood with the remaining two satellite packs are centrifuged, then placed on the Optipress. Using the appropriate programme and back plate, the plasma is expressed into a satellite pack (C) which is then sealed and detached. It is then rapidly frozen to achieve a core temperature of −30°C or below. It is then labelled and vacuum packed and stored below −25°C. The SAG-M in the other satellite pack (D) is allowed to flow into the red cells and thoroughly mixed. The empty pack is sealed and detached and the red cell pack is labelled and stored at 2–6°C.

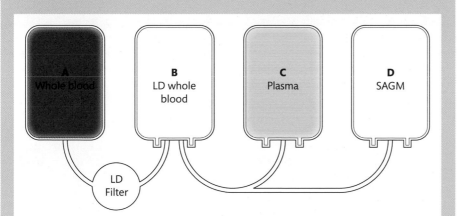

FIGURE 3.5
Configuration of the satellite packs for the preparation of SAGM suspended red cells and plasma for FFP.

- **For neonatal use.** Whole blood collected in CPD is used for the preparation of red cells for neonatal use. The main pack is attached through integral tubing to three satellite packs and an in-line filter. During the first part of the process, the whole blood is filtered (leucodepleted) into one of the satellite packs. The tubing to the filter is sealed and the filter and the empty pack is detached and discarded. The leucodepleted whole blood with the remaining two satellite packs are centrifuged then placed on the Optipress. Using the appropriate programme and back plate, some of the plasma is expressed into a satellite pack which is then sealed. The plasma pack and the remaining satellite pack are detached and discarded. The red cells suspended in plasma, with a haematocrit of 60–70%, are labelled and stored at 2–6°C.

Key points

Blood components are prepared from donated whole blood by differential centrifugation. The densest component, red cells, separate out first, followed by leucocytes and platelets, with plasma on top.

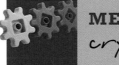

METHOD Preparation of cryoprecipitate

Cryoprecipitate contains concentrated factor VIII: C, von Willebrand factor, fibrinogen, factor XIII, and fibronectin. It is prepared from the plasma from the red cells and FFP component production. However, instead of the plasma pack being detached from the red cells and SAG-M packs, the SAG-M is emptied into the red cells. The red cell pack is sealed and detached, leaving the plasma pack connected to the empty SAG-M pack. This is rapidly frozen to achieve a core temperature of –25°C or below. The FFP is placed in a 4 ± 2°C refrigerator for 12–18 hours to thaw, then centrifuged to sediment the cryoprecipitate. The cryosupernatant plasma (CSP) is expressed into the attached SAG-M pack leaving the cryoprecipitate and 20–40 ml of CSP. The cryoprecipitate is resuspended and is either:

- Rapid frozen to –25°C or below within two hours of preparation, then labelled and stored at –25°C, or below
- Pooled in batches of five donations using a sterile connecting device to join the cryoprecipitate bags. The pooled cryoprecipitate is rapidly frozen to –30°C or below within two hours, then labelled and stored –25°C or below.

SELF-CHECK 3.6

What is the principle for separating the components in whole blood?

SELF-CHECK 3.7

Why are sterile connecting devices used?

Components for neonatal use

Blood for neonatal transfusion must be negative for anti-CMV and must be tested for atypical red cell antibodies by an antiglobulin test. The donation should also be tested negative for high titre anti-A/B. The Red Book recommends that high titre anti-A/B should be tested for using a 1 in 128 dilution of the donation plasma/serum by a saline agglutination test or an equivalent dilution by other techniques. Because of the smaller blood volume of neonates, low titre antibodies, which may be tolerated by adult patients, can cause transfusion reactions with potentially harmful consequences.

Red cells for exchange transfusion should not be processed as SAGM units or be more than five days old at transfusion as the increasing concentration of potassium in the supernatant plasma in older donations can be harmful to neonates.

Blood transfusion services provide red cells of nominal volume of 35 ml for top up transfusion for neonatal patients. These smaller red cell packs are prepared by splitting adult red cell components into up to eight paediatric packs. Similarly, adult apheresis platelet donations are split into four paediatric packs. Smaller volumes of methylene blue treated FFP are also available for these patients.

SELF-CHECK 3.8

What are the additional test requirements for blood components intended for neonatal use?

Leucodepletion

Universal leucocyte reduction (leucodepletion) was introduced in the UK in November 1999 as a measure to reduce the risk of transmission of vCJD after it was shown that leucocytes are a reservoir of prions. Other reported benefits of leucodepletion are:

- Reduction in febrile non-haemolytic transfusion reactions (FNHTR) to platelet and red cell transfusion
- Lower bacterial rate of contamination of red cell concentrates
- Decrease in the risk of CMV transmission
- Reduction in HLA alloimmunization and refractoriness to random platelet transfusion

The benefits of universal leucodepletion are contested. Some experts agree that transfusion of leucodepleted blood components to some patient groups such as those with haematological malignancies has prevented FNHTR, HLA immunization, and CMV disease but do not agree that it should be extended to all transfused patients.

The Red Book recommends that at least 99% of cellular leucodepleted components (except granulocytes) should contain less than 5×10^6 leucocytes with a 95% confidence limit, and more than 90% should contain less than 1×10^6 leucocytes. The Red Book recommends testing at least 1% of all components produced. If ten or less of these components are produced monthly then all the components need to be checked.

Key points

Leucodepletion is a filtration method to reduce the number of viable white cells as a risk reduction for vCJD transmission.

Apheresis

Apheresis is increasingly being used to extract individual blood components from donors' boold for transfusion. Automated instruments use centrifugation to separate the blood components based on the differences in their density. Sterile containers and harnesses are used in these instruments to collect blood from the donor arm to which anticoagulant is added. The container is centrifuged and the components separated out in layers based on their density. The desired component layer is then removed into a collection pack and the remaining components returned to the donor.

Automated apheresis instruments operate either using continuous or intermittent flow. With continuous flow instruments, blood is removed from one arm into the centrifugation container. After the removal of the desired component, the unwanted components are returned to the same or the other arm of the donor. The process is continued until the desired volume or concentration of component is obtained.

With intermittent flow apheresis instruments, blood is collected from the vein of one arm of the donor into the centrifugation container. When the container is full and the components are separated, the desired fraction is removed and the remainder is returned to the same access site of the donor. This process is repeated until the desired volume of component is achieved.

This process is used to produce platelets, granulocytes, red cells, plasma, and stem cells. One to three adult doses of platelets can be obtained during one procedure, which is beneficial to patients who require repeat transfusions as they are exposed to blood components from fewer donors. Plateletpheresis donors should not donate more than twice per month and no more than 24 times per year.

Two units of red cells can be collected during a single procedure, but the donors must be at least 70 kg in weight with haemoglobin of 14.0 g/l. Double donations of red cells should not be collected more than a six-monthly unless iron supplement is taken by the donor.

Donors must be between 18 and 60 years of age for the first apheresis session but can continue until 65. These donors have to meet other criteria, depending on the blood component, which can be found in the Red Book.

SELF-CHECK 3.9

Why was universal leucodepletion introduced in the UK?

SELF-CHECK 3.10

What are the other benefits of leucodepletion?

Irradiation of blood components

Irradiated cellular blood components are recommended for neonates and other immunocompetent or immunocompromised patients such as transplant recipients. These components often contain viable lymphocytes which, if partially HLA identical to the recipient, can cause transfusion-associated graft versus host disease (TA-GVHD). The recipient may be unable to reject the lymphocyte graft because of their suppressed or immature immune status. Thus the transfused viable lymphocytes can engraft and multiply and attack the recipient cells which they regard as foreign. Patients with TA-GVHD can display symptoms such as fever, skin rash, bone marrow suppression, diarrhoea, and abnormal liver function test. The condition is uncommon and can be fatal.

Gamma **irradiation** of the cellular blood components with a dose 25 Gy damages DNA and renders the lymphocyte DNA incapable of replication with little or no effect on the function of the red cells, platelets, or granulocytes. Thus, irradiated cellular components will reduce the risk of TA-GVHD. However, irradiation has been shown to cause red cell membrane leakage, resulting in an increase in haemoglobin and potassium in the suspending medium and a decrease in ATP and 2,3 DPG. As a result, the shelf-life of irradiated red cells has been reduced to a maximum of 14 days after irradiation and only RBCs up to 14 days old should be subjected to irradiation.

An alternative to gamma irradiation is X-ray radiation, which is generated by X-ray tubes by bombarding targets with electrons accelerated in vacuum through a high voltage electric field. An X-ray dose of 25 Gy has been shown to be as effective as gamma radiation. There are indicator tags for both gamma and X-ray radiators to show that the components have been successfully irradiated.

> **Irradiation**
> A process for inactivating donor lymphocytes using gamma (or X-ray) irradiation to prevent transfusion-associated graft versus host disease (TA-GVHD), a rare but potentially fatal consequence of blood transfusion.

Key points

Irradiation damages the DNA of lymphocytes and prevents them from replicating and causing graft versus host disease.

SELF-CHECK 3.11

Why are blood components irradiated?

3.4 **Pathogen reduction**

In accordance with the Red Book guidelines, all blood donations are tested for hepatitis B and C, HIV-1 and 2, HTLV, and antibodies to syphilis. There are, however, other pathogens that can be transmitted by blood transfusion requiring other strategies to further reduce the risk of disease transmission.

Current strategy on blood safety relies on:

- Education, questioning, and exclusion of donors
- Donor arm cleansing
- Testing and elimination of infected or potentially infected blood donations and components
- Preventing deferred donors known to have transfusion transmissible infections from donating or ensuring that their donations are discarded through the use of computers, and
- Irradiation of blood components to reduce transfusion-associated graft versus host disease (TA-GVHD)

The post-donation testing strategy is designed to reduce the possibility of blood with transfusion transmissible infection from entering the blood supply. The tests performed in industrialized countries have reduced the risk of transfusing an infected blood component to miniscule levels. But there are also viruses, bacteria, and protozoan infections which can be transmitted

Pathogen inactivation
A process for removal of infectious agents in blood components/products through chemical or heat treatment and filtration.

Pathogen reduction
Process for reducing or eliminating most infectious agents in blood components/products.

by blood that are not currently screened for and **pathogen inactivation/reduction** technologies offer the promise of an even safer blood supply. For emerging infections, pathogen reduction (PR) will considerably reduce the chance of patients being infected as a result of blood transfusion before a test is introduced. In addition, this technology can be effective in preventing TA-GVHD by preventing the replication of any remaining leucocytes in the blood component and can inactivate most bacteria.

Whilst PR offers the hope of an even safer blood supply, it has several disadvantages:

- The chemicals used to inactivate the pathogens may be toxic.
- They may not completely inactivate all the pathogens (pathogen reduction), thus the component may still be infectious.
- There may be a reduction in clinical efficacy of the treated blood component, for example reduction in coagulation anticoagulant factors in PR FFP.
- Reduction in component viability and survival.
- Development of antibodies to neo-antigens.

Chemical pathogen inactivation

Psoralens

Psoralens, such as metoxypsoralen (MOP) and trimethypsoralen (TMP) that occur naturally in plant products such as limes, celery, and parsnips, and UV light are used to treat psoriasis and are approved for the treatment of cutaneous T cell lymphomas.

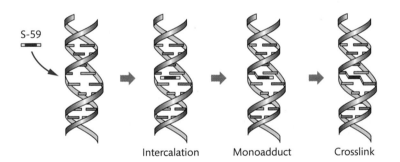

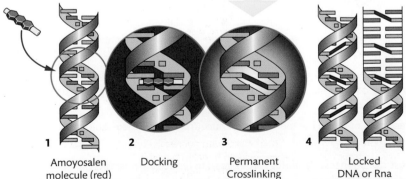

FIGURE 3.6
The Intercept Helinx™ photochemical technology. (© Cerus Corporation, used with permission.)

An example of such a system is that produced by the Cerus Corporation (California, USA) that uses a psoralen derivative, amotosalen hydrochloride (S-59) in their patented Helinx™ photochemical technology (PCT) for pathogen reduction (PR). S-59 works first by intercalating into the helix of the nucleic acid. When this is activated by UV-A, S-59 is covalently linked to one strand of the nucleic acid (see Figure 3.6). Further exposure to UV-A, results in S-59 covalently binding to the second strand of the nucleic acid to form a diaduct or interstrand cross-link. S-59 forms an irreversible cross-link with approximately 1 in 83 base pairs and this is sufficient to completely prevent replication.

METHOD *The Intercept photochemical technology system*

The PCT with S-59 is used for the pathogen inactivation of platelets and plasma components. Platelets and plasma in transparent plastic containers are mixed with S-59 solution, then illuminated with UV-A (with excitation of 320–400 nm). Because of possible side effects, the Intercept blood system which uses the Helinx™ has a compound adsorption device (CAD) to remove any excess S-59. The plasma or platelets are then transferred to another container for storage and use.

Any materials or components that absorb UV light will reduce the effectiveness of the PCT process and these techniques are unsuitable for PI of red cell components. A frangible anchor linker effector (FRALE) was developed for pathogen inactivation of red cells without the requirement for light inactivation.

Riboflavin

Riboflavin or vitamin B2 has been widely investigated and shown to be safe. Riboflavin requires UV light and oxygen to inactivate pathogens (see Figure 3.7). Nucleic acid can be damaged by direct action of UV light. The reaction of light with riboflavin generates

Direct effect of UV light

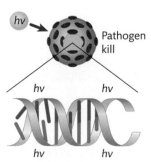

In blood products, viral, bacterial, parasitic and leukocytic nucleic acids absorb low wavelength photons resulting in nucleic damage

RB–guanine electron-transfer

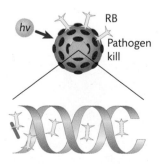

RB interacts with nucleic acids, causing additional irreversible nucleic acid damage through electron transfer chemistry, primarily between RB and guanine

FIGURE 3.7
The Mirasol PRT system.
(Copyright CaridianBCT, 2012.
Used with permission.)

superoxide anion radicals O_2^- and HO_2 which damage nucleic acid. Singlet oxygen is also produced which can lead to photo-oxidation of guanine and hence damage to nucleic acids.

Limited studies have shown that any reduction in the haematological parameters of platelets or plasma as a result of riboflavin treatment is within clinically acceptable limits. The pathogen reduction of blood components spiked with infectious agents is marked. However, further studies are required to establish the safety of the by-products of riboflavin and the clinical efficacy of the treated blood components.

Solvent detergent

The solvent detergent process was introduced in 1985 for the viral inactivation of plasma components. It was shown to be effective in achieving 5–6 $\log_{10}$ reduction in viral load of spiked samples with minimal loss of component activity. The most common combination of solvent detergent in use is tri-(n-butyl)-phosphate (TNBP) an organic solvent and Triton X-100 a non-ionic detergent. The treatment works by disrupting the membranes of enveloped virus, bacteria, and eukaryotes resulting in a loss of infectivity. It is not effective against non-enveloped viruses such as hepatitis A. Triton X-100 disrupts the lipid bilayers of the pathogens and stabilizes TNBP. TNBP extracts and sequesters the lipids into a separate colloidal phase. The technology is used for treatment of FFP and commercial fractionated plasma components such as coagulation factors VII, VIII, IX, XI, prothrombin complex, fibrinogen, protein C, fibrin glue, and immunoglobulins.

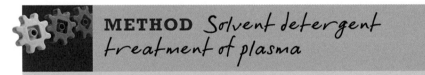

METHOD *Solvent detergent treatment of plasma*

SD-FFP is prepared in pools of frozen/thawed plasma from 380 to 5,000 donors (up to 1,250 litres).

- The rapid thawed plasma is passed through a 1μm filter to remove cells, cell fragments and membrane-associated viruses.
- One per cent TNBP and 1% Triton X-10 is added and incubated for four hours at 30°C.
- TNBP is removed using castor oil extraction and phase separation, followed by a clear filtration.
- Triton X-100 is removed by hydrophobic interaction chromatography.
- The components are sterile filtered by passing through a 0.2 μm filter.
- This is then aliquoted into 200 ml volumes, fast frozen at −60°C, and then stored at −30°C.

There is a 15–20% reduction of the activity of clotting factors in SD-FFP. This may lead to an increased number of transfusions of SD-FFP to achieve the same clinical benefit as untreated FFP. However, studies have concluded that as 30% activity is required to maintain haemostasis, the loss of coagulation factors seen as a result of SD treatment is not clinically significant. There is also 35–76% reduction in anticoagulation factors in SD-FFP. This can cause increased clotting risks in patients who are deficient in these factors.

No adverse effects were reported in Europe but the occurrence of thrombosis and/or haemorrhage with the use of solvent detergent treated FFP (SD-FFP) was reported in the USA. A decreased incidence of transfusion-related acute lung injury (TRALI) has been reported with the use of SD-FFP.

Methylene blue

Methylene blue (phenothiazine dyes) (MB) has been used as oral antiseptic, disinfectant, treatment for methaemoglobinemia, and as an antidote for nitrate poisoning amongst other conditions. It has also been reported as a cure for malaria. Its use for pathogen inactivation was reported in 1991.

Methylene blue binds preferentially to nucleic acids and negatively charged lipids and can also bind to viral core proteins. It binds either to the outside of DNA or intercalate between the rungs of the double helix. On exposure to light, guanine specific cleavage occurs, resulting in the inactivation of the nucleic acid. This process is enhanced in the presence of oxygen.

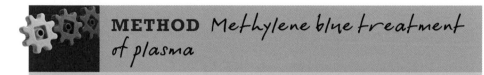

METHOD *Methylene blue treatment of plasma*

Methylene blue treatment involves thawing a unit of plasma and filtering through a 0.65 μm membrane filtration system to remove residual leukocytes and intracellular organisms. Methylene blue to 1 μmol/l concentration is introduced and the bag is exposed to UV light at 590 nm. The treated plasma is then filtered to reduce the MB to less than 0.1 μmol/l prior to storage at or below −30°C.

Methylene blue has been shown to inactivate enveloped viruses. Some non-enveloped viruses, bacteria (especially Gram negative), and protozoa survive this inactivation process. Intracellular pathogens and white blood cells are not inactivated as MB has difficulty in penetrating plasma membranes. When MB is used to treat red blood cell component, there is an increase in lysis and ion leakage.

The toxicological properties of MB have not been fully investigated. However, toxicity appears to be minimal at the concentration used for pathogen inactivation of FFP. No adverse events were reported with over two million units of MB treated FFP transfused.

Key points

Pathogen reduction technologies reduce the numbers of viable pathogens and hence the risk of transfusion transmissible infections. They work either by damaging the membranes or genomes, or by removal by filtration.

SELF-CHECK 3.12

What is the benefit of pathogen reduction?

3.5 Component validation and labelling

All components must be labelled with the following information as a minimum:

- Donation number in eye readable and barcoded format
- Component type

TABLE 3.1 Storage and transportation temperature and shelf-life on blood components.

Component	Storage temperature	Shelf-life	Transportation temperature
Red cells in SAGM	4 ± 2°C	42 days	2–10°C
Red cells in CPD	4 ± 2°C	28 days	2–10°C
Apheresis platelets	22 ± 2°C with continuous gentle agitation	5 days*	22 ± 2°C
Pooled platelets	22 ± 2°C with continuous gentle agitation	5 days*	22 ± 2°C
Granulocytes	22 ± 2°C	24 hours	22 ± 2°C
FFP	−25°C or below	24 months	−25°C or below
Cryoprecipitate	−25°C or below	24 months	−25°C or below

* Seven days permitted if bacterial detection or PR is employed.

- ABO and RhD blood groups (although the RhD type is not required for FFP in the UK)
- Date bled
- Expiry date

Other information such as CMV and irradiated status, suitability for neonatal use, and red cell phenotypes may also be printed on the label.

The use of computer generated component pack labels considerably enhances the safety and security of the component validation/labelling process and blood stock management. After labelling, the components should be stored at the correct temperature (see Table 3.1) until they are issued from stock.

Component issue and transportation

A computerized system increases the security of issuing blood components, enables printing of an issue sheet, stores the destination, and removes the units from stock. Appropriate insulated boxes should be used to maintain the components at the correct temperature (see Table 3.1) during transportation to the receiving hospital. These boxes should be validated for use at the required temperature and periodically verified to ensure that the conditions are maintained for the appropriate time. The validation should be performed at extreme transport temperatures such as in summer and winter.

In order to complete the audit trail, a record must be kept of the date, time, and person transporting the container and the person who received it at the destination.

Key points

Blood components must be transported in validated containers to avoid deterioration during transit.

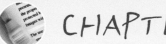

CHAPTER SUMMARY

■ Blood is collected primarily from voluntary unpaid donors either as whole blood or selected components using automated systems.

■ Blood collected from paid donors is associated with an increased risk of transfusion transmissible infections.

■ Pre-donation screening is an essential risk reduction measure aimed at protecting the donors and reduces the risk of collecting blood from individuals with transfusion transmissible infections.

■ Blood is collected into a pack containing an anticoagulant to prevent it from clotting. The main blood pack may have several satellite packs for component production.

■ The main blood pack and all satellite packs have the same unique ISBT 128 number to allow traceability and are associated with the donor.

■ Whole blood can be separated into red cells, platelets (in the buffy coat layer), and plasma, using differential centrifugation. Use of specialized centrifuges, automated component separators, and sterile connecting devices to maintain closed systems are essential.

■ Pooled platelets are prepared from four or five single donation buffy coats and suspended in plasma from one of the male donations to reduce the risk of TRALI.

■ Two or three adult doses of platelets can be collected from a donor at one time using automated blood separating machines.

■ The additive/storage solution used for red cells can affect the shelf-life of the product, for example 28 days for CPD and 42 days for SAGM.

■ Changes occur during the storage of blood which affects the viability of the components. For example, red cell ATP and 2,3 DPG levels decline during storage, with formation of microaggregates and procoagulants, release of cytokines, lipids, histamine, and haemolysis.

■ Gamma or X-ray irradiation is used to render DNA of leucocyte in platelets and red cell components incapable of replication so as to reduce the risk of transfusion-associated graft versus host disease.

■ Pathogen reduction methods such as methylene blue, solvent detergent treatment, and Intercept Helix™ Photochemical Technology are used to destroy the replicating ability of DNA and RNA of infectious agents and reduce the risk of their transmission by blood transfusion. This process also removes the need for irradiation of the treated components.

■ The use of a computerized system ensures that an audit trail is kept of the complete process and increases the security of component labelling and issue.

■ Boxes used to transport blood components should be capable of maintaining the correct temperature for the duration the component is out of controlled temperature storage refrigerators or freezers.

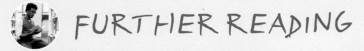

FURTHER READING

- **Barbara JAJ & Regan FAM, Contreras MC (eds)** *Transfusion Microbiology*. **Cambridge University Press, Cambridge, 2008.**

- **British Blood Transfusion Society** *An Introduction to Blood Transfusion Science and Blood Bank Practice*, **5th edition. British Blood Transfusion Society, Manchester, 2009. www.bbts.org.uk.**

- **Medicines Control Agency** *Rules and Guidance for Pharmaceutical Manufacturers and Distributors 2002*, **6th edition. The Stationery Office, Norwich, 2002.**

- **UK Blood Transfusion and Tissue Transplantation Services** *Guidelines for the Blood Transfusion Services in the United Kingdom*, **7th edition. The Stationery Office, Norwich, 2005. www.tsoshop.co.uk or at http://www.transfusionguidelines.org.uk.**

Answers to the questions in this chapter are provided on the book's Online Resource Centre.

 Go to www.oxfordtextbooks.co.uk/orc/knight

Blood Donation Testing

Lionel Mohabir

Learning objectives

After studying this chapter you should be able to:

- Understand validation of equipment and processes.
- Describe the mandatory testing requirements.
- Describe methods for blood grouping of donations.
- Describe methods for antibody screening of donations.
- Understand the aetiology of transfusion transmitted infections—HBV, HCV, HIV, and HTLV.
- Understand the aetiology of other transfusion transmitted infections—syphilis, malaria, and Chagas disease.
- Understand how prions and vCJD are relevant to transfusion/transplant.
- Outline how to reduce bacterial contamination of blood and components.
- Understand the algorithms for microbiology testing and donor re-instatement.
- Understand the principles and use of automated/semi-automated test systems for microbiology tests.
- Understand the principles of ELISA, chemiluminescence, and NAT testing.

Introduction

Pre-donation screening prior to blood donation is an essential step in reducing the number of potentially infective donations collected. Post donation, in addition to ABO and RhD typing, an increasing number of serological, nucleic acid test (NAT), and bacterial screening tests have been introduced to ensure the microbiological safety of the donated blood and blood components.

Testing is usually performed on automated equipment with on-line data/result transfer to the host computer. As with blood collection and processing (Chapter 3), testing is performed within a quality controlled and quality management system in blood establishments. The laboratories are also subjected to two-yearly audits by the Medicines and Healthcare products Regulatory Agency (MHRA). Also blood establishments must comply with the Blood Safety and Quality Regulations (BSQR).

4.1 Mandatory testing

The *Guidelines for the Blood Transfusion Services in the United Kingdom* (the Red Book) states that all blood components must be tested for the following disease markers and satisfactory results obtained before blood and blood components can be released from quarantine for use:

- ABO and RhD blood groups
- Red cell antibody screening
- HBsAg
- Anti-HIV
- Anti-HCV
- Anti-syphilis
- Nucleic acid testing for HCV RNA*
- Anti-HTLV*

Blood grouping

Validated
Having documentary evidence to show that a system/equipment or process meets pre-defined requirements for its intended use.

The ABO and RhD blood groups are required for all blood components except for fresh frozen plasma (FFP) when only the ABO is necessary. The tests must be performed on a **validated** automated test system using reagents that are CE marked in accordance with the EU In Vitro Diagnostics Device Directive (IVDD) and have been subjected to batch pre-acceptance testing. Manual tests can be used to resolve any persistent automated failures. The Red Book requires that:

- Samples taken with the current donation of *known* donors should be tested once for the ABO and Rh blood groups. The blood grouping results should be the same as the existing computerized record. The minimum requirements for ABO and Rh are tests with anti-A, anti-B, and an anti-D or a blended anti-D that are able to detect weak D, and the partial D types—D^{IV}, D^V, and D^{VI}.

- Samples taken with the current donation of *new* donors should have two separate blood group tests performed and the results sent on-line to the host computer. The minimum requirements for ABO and Rh are tests with anti-A, anti-B, and two anti-D, which between them can detect partial D types—D^{IV}, D^V, and D^{VI}. The blood group results should only be accepted if both results are in agreement. Any discrepancies must be identified and investigated and a decision taken on the fate of the donation.

Key points

Before a blood component can be labelled, two identical blood group results are required, one of which can be from a previous donation (computer record). New donors must be tested twice for ABO and Rh blood groups.

* These tests can be performed using a pool of plasma from several donations, whereas all the other tests are performed on individual donations.

Additional phenotyping

Some blood services test all donations for the other major Rh types, C, c, E, e, and K. All will test a selection of units for other red cell phenotypes such as S, s, Fy^a, Fy^b; and Jk^a, Jk^b.

Red cell antibody screening

The Red Book requires that as a minimum all blood donations must be tested for antibodies to Rh and K antigens using a test with a minimum sensitivity of 0.5 iu/ml anti-D. In the majority of blood establishments, this is achieved by using an enzyme technique on the Beckman Coulter blood testing analyser, at the same time as the blood group is performed. Blood components targeted for neonatal use must be screened for red cell antibodies using at least a two-cell panel by an antiglobulin test which can detect 0.1 iu/ml anti-D; this test is also used to test patient samples prior to blood transfusion.

Donations with a positive antibody screen should be further investigated to identify the specificity of the antibody. Dilutions of the plasma should then be tested by anti-human globulin test (AHG) to determine the fate of the components prepared from the donation. The Red Book recommends the following:

- Components for neonatal transfusion must have a negative antibody screen by AHG using undiluted plasma.

- Fresh frozen plasma can be used if there is a negative antibody screen by AHG in a 1 in 10 dilution of plasma.

- Red cells in SAG-M can be used if there is a negative antibody screen by AHG in a 1 in 50 dilution of plasma.

METHOD Beckman Coulter method

Tests on the Beckman Coulter fully automated blood pre-transfusion testing system are performed in a patented microplate consisting of 10 x 12 wells. Ten samples can be tested in one microplate, with up to 12 tests per sample. A unique feature of the microplate is the V-shaped wells with terraces/grooves to trap agglutinates (see Figure 4.1). A positive reaction is indicated by an even carpet of cells across the well and a negative reaction by a button of cells at the bottom of the well.

- The system dilutes the samples and dispenses them, together with reagents, into pre-defined positions in the microplate.

- The microplate is transferred to an incubation elevator at a temperature of approximately 30°C for 60 minutes, both of which are configured by the operator.

- After incubation, the microplate moves into the reading position where the differences in light transmission are captured by a CCD camera.

- The CCD image is converted into data points or pixels which are used to generate the following image analysis measurements:

  - the pixels in the peripheral region of the well (P)

  - the darkest 256 pixels in the centre of the well (C)

  - the ratio of light transmitted between the periphery and centre of the well (P/C)

  - the sharpness at the edge of the cell button between the periphery and centre regions of the well (SPC)

  - the low intensity area (LIA) obtained by counting the dark pixels at the centre of the well

- The above information is compared to pre-set values to determine if the reaction is positive, negative, or indeterminate.

- In addition, a calculation is performed to determine if the well is empty.

- The software compares the reactions in each of the wells for a sample against a pre-set configuration to determine the final result(s).

- The results are printed but there is an option to upload the results to the host computer.

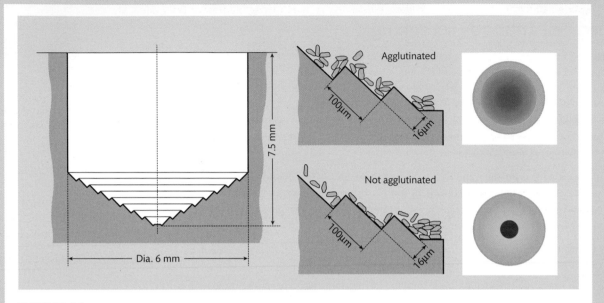

FIGURE 4.1
Diagrammatic representation of the Olympus terraced microplate well with positive (agglutinated) and negative reactions (reproduced with permission of Beckman Coulter).

High titre anti-A/B

Passive transfer of anti-A/B to recipients through ABO mis-match through transfusion of plasma rich components such as pooled or apheresis platelets can result in acute haemolysis. This can be worse for neonates because of their small blood volume. Most of such **transfusion reactions** occur when group O blood components are transfused to group A or B recipients. The Red Book recommends that each blood service should have a policy for testing and issuing high titre anti-A/B blood components. Where the test is necessary, a negative result must be obtained on a 1/128 dilution of the plasma by a saline agglutination test or an equivalent dilution by another technique. Some blood transfusion centres perform this test on Beckman Coulter blood testing analysers. A national high titre anti-A/B control is available which must give a positive reaction for the batch of test results to be valid.

> **SELF-CHECK 4.1**
>
> What tests must be performed before a blood component can be labelled for issue?

Generic principles of transfusion microbiology testing

Following an infection, the virus replicates within the host and can reach a high titre or viral load before there is an **immune response**. The speed of replication, or doubling time, and the

---

Transfusion reactions
This is a systemic response produced by the body to the infusion of blood or blood components/products. The adverse reaction may be to proteins in the blood or incompatible cellular components such as leucocytes, platelets, or erythrocytes.

Immune response
The body's ability to recognize and defend itself against substances that appear foreign and harmful such as bacteria and viruses.

viral load reached varies with the different infectious agents. The formation of IgM antibodies followed by IgG results in a decline in the viral load, often to below the level of detection. The antibodies persist in the patients for varying times depending on the virus and the host immune competence.

The period between inoculation and detection of the infection using laboratory tests is termed the '**window period**' (WP) (Table 4.1 and Figure 4.2). This is normally measured in days or weeks and would depend on the test used and the **sensitivity**:

- Nucleic acid test (NAT) detects the DNA or RNA of the virus whilst it is replicating and has the shortest window phase.
- Antigen assay will become positive later in the infection.
- Antibody assay becomes positive after there is an immune response. If this is the only test used, then the window period will be longer and some infected donations will not be detected.

During the NAT window period there is an eclipse phase when the donation is not infective. After the eclipse phase but before the NAT test becomes positive, the donation may be infectious but the risk is extremely low.

SELF-CHECK 4.2

What is the window period?

Window period
This is the period between the onset of the infection and the appearance of the detectable infectious agent or antibodies to it. For a virus, the window period is shorter for the detection of the viral RNA/DNA than antibodies which are produced later in the infection.

Sensitivity
This is the proportion of people who have a disease/infection (or products such as antibodies to it) which is correctly identified by a screening test.

Hepatitis B (HBV)

Australia antigen was discovered by Blumberg in 1965 in the serum of an Australian aborigine, which formed precipitin lines in an immunodiffusion assay with serum from a multi-transfused haemophiliac patient. It was subsequently called hepatitis B surface antigen (HBsAg). In 1970, Dane and co-workers identified the infectious agent of HBV (Dane particle) using electron microscopy. More than 400 million people in the world are infected with HBV, with the highest prevalence of between 8–20% in South-East Asia, China, and Africa.

HBV belongs to the hepadnavirus family. The Dane particle is the complete virion and contains the DNA which is enclosed in the nucleocapsid. A large excess of envelope material in

TABLE 4.1 Window period reduction for microbiology serology and NAT.

Disease marker	WP for serology test	WP for NAT
HBV	36 days	15 days for ID NAT 28 days for mini-pools of 8 samples
HCV	65 days	5 days for ID NAT 5 days for mini-pools of 8 samples
HIV	15 days for anti-HIV 11 days for combined antibody/antigen test	5 days for ID NAT 7 days for mini-pools of 8 samples
HTLV	45 days	Not available

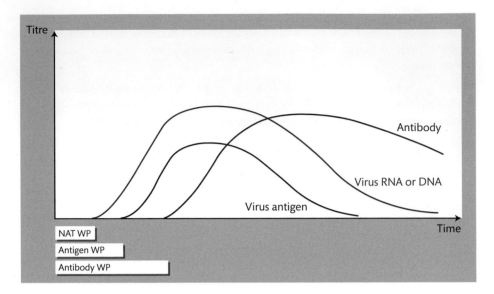

FIGURE 4.2
Response to viral infections.

the form of small spheres and rods of average width of 22 nm is produced as a result of HBV infection. These small particles lack DNA and are not infectious. The Dane particle is 42 nm in diameter and consists of:

- An outer lipid layer—HBsAg, which contains embedded proteins responsible for binding and entry into liver cells.
- An inner nucleocapsid core—hepatitis B core antigen (HBcAg). The nucleocapsid is composed of protein and encloses the partially double-stranded circular viral DNA and DNA polymerase.
- The partially double stranded circular viral DNA of approximately 3,200 base pairs codes for four genes called C, P, S, and X.

The modes of transmission of HBV include:

- Blood transfusion (or transplants) but this is extremely rare in countries where screening for HBsAg (and HBV NAT) and viral inactivation of plasma products is the normal practice.
- Sexual contact with a chronically infected person.
- Infants born to infected mothers.
- Intravenous drug abusers.
- Acupuncture, tattooing, and body piercing using infected needles.
- Occupational contact in healthcare professionals.
- Haemodialysis patients if the equipment is not properly sterilized.
- Household contacts of HBV infected individuals.
- Institutionalized individuals such as prisoners and mental patients.

Hepatitis B virus infects the hepatocytes of liver but does not usually cause direct damage to these cells. The host cellular immune response to HBV is the cause of liver damage—the more vigorous the immune response, the greater the resulting damage. This can lead to complete viral clearance and the development of anti-HBs to prevent re-infection.

However, due to inadequate immune response and host factors, the infection may persist in some individuals.

Clinical course of infection

The onset of HBV infection is usually insidious:

- There is an incubation period of 60–90 days but this can be as long as 180 days. This is dependent on the viral dose, route of infection, and host factors.

- There is a period of acute infection during which HBsAg and HBeAg (derived from the core gene, modified and exported from the liver) are detectable. Patients may present with symptoms such as mild fever, fatigue, nausea, anorexia, vomiting, dark urine, skin rashes, and abdominal, muscle, and joint pains. Jaundice is found in 30–50% of individuals who are infected when over five years of age, but in less than 10% of those infected under the age of five.

- Most HBV infected adults will recover and develop immunity. Anti-HBs, anti-HBc, and anti-HBe can be detected. Some individuals with HBV will develop chronic infection which is age related. The risk of progression to chronic infection is approximately 90% for neonates and children under one year, 30% for children aged 1–5 years and 2% for those over five years old.

Genotypes and mutants

Eight genotypes have been identified (genotypes A–H). In addition, there are several subtypes of HBV.

HBV replicates by the use of reverse transcriptase (RT) to form an RNA intermediate. Reverse transcriptase lacks proof-reading capability and therefore error in transcription is not detected and corrected. This can lead to mutant strains of HBV which, if the conditions are right, can result in its survival along the wild-type or replace it. Mutant strains can also spontaneously evolve. HBV escape mutants are increasingly being seen in individuals who have been vaccinated and have high levels of anti-HBs.

Tests

Sensitive ELISA and chemiluminescence assays for the detection of hepatitis B surface antigens (HBsAg) are available for blood donation screening. A multiplex NAT for HBV, HCV, and HIV has been introduced in the UK blood services for blood donation screening in pools of 24 samples.

Tests on serial samples for anti-HBs, HBeAg, and anti-HBe from HBsAg positive patients are useful as an indication of the chronicity or infectivity.

- The presence of HBsAg for more than six months would indicate a chronic infection.

- Seroconversion from HBsAg to anti-HBs suggests a resolution of the disease and establishment of immunity.

- HBeAg positive indicates infectivity.

- Seroconversion from HBeAg to anti-HBe indicates progression to the resolution of the disease.

Discretionary testing for anti-HBc is performed on samples from donors who have body piercing/tattoos, acupunctures, and endoscopy at least four months after the procedure or the donors are suspended for 12 months (six months for endoscopy).

> *Key points*
>
> **HBV is a partially double-stranded DNA virus which infects the hepatocytes of the liver. The damage to the infected cells is due to the host cellular immune response. Many genotypes, sub-types, and mutants have been described.**

Hepatitis C (HCV)

Hepatitis C (HCV) was the first virus to be identified by molecular cloning methods by Choo and co-workers in 1989. It was previously referred to as non-A non-B hepatitis virus. HCV infects only humans and chimpanzees, and is a member of the *Flaviviridae* family. It is a small, lipid enveloped virus with a single positive stranded RNA.

According to the World Health Organization (WHO), up to 3% of the world population, that is, more than 170 million people are infected with HCV. The prevalence rate of HCV infection in the developed world ranges from 0.5–2%, with 6.5% in parts of Equatorial Africa and up to 20% in Egypt. There are six main HCV genotypes (genotypes 1–6) with geographical associations.

The modes of HCV transmission are:

- Intravenous drug abuse
- Blood transfusion and transplant, although this is rare in developed countries where a blood test is used
- Sexual intercourse
- Needlestick injury (in healthcare workers)
- Perinatal infection—from infected mother to baby
- Acupuncture, tattooing, and body piercing using infected needles.
- Haemodialysis
- Sharing household objects such as toothbrush or razor, if contaminated with blood

Clinical course of infection

The onset of infection with HCV usually goes unnoticed: 60–70% of infected people are asymptomatic, with only 10–20% developing non-specific symptoms such as malaise, fatigue, and abdominal pain. The average incubation period is 6–7 weeks, but can vary from 2–26 weeks or more. In 10–30% of infected individuals, the infection is self-limiting, leading to recovery. The remainder will develop chronic hepatitis, with 10–20% developing cirrhosis. Between 1–5% of the chronically infected patients will develop hepatocellular carcinoma over a period of 20–30 years.

The liver is the major site for HCV infection, where it multiplies rapidly, with up to 10^{12} viruses produced daily. There is evidence of HCV reservoirs outside the liver in the peripheral blood lymphocytes, epithelial cells in the gut, and the central nervous system.

> *Key points*
>
> **HCV is a small single stranded RNA virus which mainly infects the liver cells. Approximately 3% of the world population is infected with this virus.**

Tests

An antibody test for HCV was first introduced in the UK for blood donation screening in 1991. This has resulted in a significant reduction in transmission of this virus by blood transfusion. The assay (ELISA and chemiluminescence) has since been enhanced to marginally increase the sensitivity and **specificity**. Any samples which are repeatedly reactive are confirmed by testing with an alternative ELISA and recombinant immunoblot assays (RIBA). Nucleic acid testing (NAT) for HCV (and HBV and HIV-1) is performed on all donor samples in the UK.

Specificity
This is the proportion of people who are correctly identified by a screening test as negative for the disease/infection.

Human immunodeficiency virus (HIV)

In 1981, the Center for Disease Control in Atlanta, USA, reported cases of homosexual patients suffering from previously rare conditions such as pneumocystis pneumonia and Kaposi's sarcoma. This condition, called acquired immunodeficiency syndrome (AIDS), was shown in 1983 to be caused by a newly recognized human immunodeficiency virus (HIV-1). HIV-2 was later reported in West African patients as another cause of AIDS.

There are more that 40 million HIV-infected individuals worldwide, with nearly equal number of infected men and women. The majority of these are in resource poor countries such as Sub-Saharan Africa, Asia, and South America.

Three HIV-1 groups have been known for some time: M (for main), O (outlier), and N. A rare fourth HIV-1 group, P, has been identified in Cameroonians living in Paris. Groups O and N are rare and are found predominantly in Cameroon in Central Africa. Nine sub-types have been recognized in group M. They are A, B, C, D, F, G, H, J, and K. In addition, there are the recombinant forms which are the results of recombinations of two or more group M sub-types. Genotype B is the main one found in the developed countries but genotype C is prevalent in most of the world.

HIV has two copies of positive single-stranded RNA which codes for the virus's nine genes. It is amongst the most variable of all human pathogen. The variability arises because:

- The RNA has to be transcribed into DNA using an enzyme reverse transcriptase (RT) which lacks proof reading. As a result, errors are introduced at an average rate of one substitution per genome per replication round.
- The virus replicates rapidly *in vivo*, generating approximately 10^{10} virions per day.
- During recombination, RT copies the two viral RNA molecules which are packaged together in a viron. As a result of 7–30 cross over per replication round, mosaic genomes are produced.

The main routes of HIV transmission are:

- Unprotected sex with an infected individual; the risk increases with repetitive sexual contacts. The risk of infection also increases in the presence of other sexually transmitted disease.
- Intravenous drug use by sharing of unsterilized injection syringes and needles with infected individuals.
- Transmission from mother to baby (maternofoetal transfer). An estimated 15–30% of HIV-infected mothers will transmit the infection to their babies during pregnancy and delivery in the absence of any intervention. Latent HIV transmission is rare in patients on anti-retroviral prophylaxis and elective Caesarian delivery.
- Transfusion of contaminated blood products. This is now a rare event in countries where the screening of donated blood for HIV is mandated.
- Needlestick injury in healthcare workers.

Clinical course of infection

HIV-1 is an RNA retrovirus belonging to the lentivirus family. These viruses typically have a long period of clinical latency during which there is virus replication and central nervous system involvement. Following HIV infection, the virus targets the CD4+ T cells where it enters the cells and multiplies. This is the acute phase of infection and can last up to eight weeks, during which:

- The infected individuals may be asymptomatic or display flu-like symptoms. Symptoms resembling infectious mononucleosis have also been described. The symptoms last for 7–10 days but rarely more than 14 days.
- As a result of intense replication, viral loads of 100 million copies of HIV-1 RNA/ml can be reached.
- There is seeding of virus into a range of tissue reservoirs, particularly in the lymphoid tissues of the gut.
- There is destruction of CD4+ T cells leading to a decline in counts, sometimes to levels that allow development of opportunistic infections.

Following the host immune response and antibody production (seroconversion), there is a rapid decline in the viral load and the CD4+ T cell count starts to rise but never reaches the pre-infection levels.

Equilibrium between viral replication and the host immune response or viral setpoint is reached, which is a strong predictor of long-term disease progression. This chronic phase or period of clinical latency can last for 8–10 years or longer. During this period, there is a high turnover of virus, with the resultant destruction and decline of CD4+ T cells.

Host factors mainly determine how rapidly the decline into AIDS occurs. A CD4+ T cell count of less than 200 increases the risks of AIDS defining illnesses such as opportunistic infections.

Tests

Early detection of HIV infection will enable the patient to benefit from appropriate therapeutic treatment and prevent transmission of infection. Fourth generation ELISA and chemiluminescent immunoassay (CLIA) screening tests will detect antibodies to HIV-1, including most sub-types, and HIV-2 and will also detect p24 antigen of the virus particle, thus reducing the window period. Donated blood in the UK is also tested in pools of 24 samples by multiplex HBV, HCV, and HIV NAT.

Key points

HIV has two positive single strands RNA and it infects CD4+ T cells. Destruction of the infected CD4+ T cells can lead to opportunistic infections. The progression from infection to AIDS is dependent on host factors as well as response to treatment.

Syphilis

Syphilis is caused by a spirochete bacterium, *Treponema pallidum*. It is estimated that worldwide, there are 10–12 million new infections each year. Penicillin is very effective at treating this infection, although other treatments are available. If untreated, the course of infection is classified into the following stages:

- Primary syphilis—usually a painless lesion (chancre) develops at the site of infection after around 9–90 days (usually 2–3 weeks) with local, tender lymphadenopathy. Occasionally multiple painful lesions develop. The lesion(s) spontaneously heal after 4–5 weeks.

- Secondary syphilis—this usually occurs 4–8 weeks after primary syphilis. The symptoms include fever, malaise, generalized lymphadenopathy, and a diffuse rash, typically on the palms, soles, and scalp. There may be other clinical presentations and complications in a small percentage of patients. These patients spontaneously improve, but a quarter may relapse into secondary syphilis. These relapses are rare after one year.

- Early latent syphilis—this is less than two years' duration and the patients are asymptomatic but still infectious.

- Late latent syphilis—this is an asymptomatic, non-infectious stage of more than two years' duration.

- Tertiary syphilis—this occurs 3–20 years after exposure. About 35% of patients will develop tertiary syphilis. Three main manifestations are neurosyphilis, cardiovascular syphilis, and gummatous syphilis.

Syphilis can also be transmitted transplacentally from infected mother to baby. This happens mostly during the first two years of infection, although there have been cases of transmission during late latent syphilis. A third of the pregnancies will result in miscarriage or stillbirth, and a third with congenital syphilis. The remaining third of babies will be born without infection. There is a two to five-fold increase in risk of acquiring HIV infection in individuals who are infected with syphilis. This is because the genital sores provide an entry point for the HIV virus during sexual contact.

The immune response to syphilis involves a 'non-specific' antibody response to a broad range of antigens such as cardiolipin, and specific anti-treponemal antibodies. Specific anti-treponemal IgM antibodies are developed towards the end of the second week of infection and become undetectable 3–9 months after treatment of early syphilis. Anti-treponemal IgG antibodies appear at about four weeks.

Tests

Serological tests for syphilis are classified into:

- Non-treponemal (non-specific)—for example Venereal Diseases Research Laboratory (VDRL) and Rapid Plasma Reagin (RPR) tests. Sensitivity of these tests is estimated to be 78–86% for primary infections and 95–100% for secondary and latent infections with specificity of 85–99%.

- Treponemal (specific)—for example *Treponema pallidum* haemagglutination assay (TPHA) and *Treponema pallidum* particle agglutination assay (TPPA). Fluorescent treponemal antibody-absorbed (FTA-abs) has a specificity of 96% and a sensitivity of 84% for detecting primary syphilis and 100% for the other stages of infection. Enzyme immunoassay (EIA)—this is rapidly becoming the screening test of choice because of the high sensitivity (98.5–100%) and specificity (97–100%) and can be automated.

Key points

Syphilis is caused by the *Treponema pallidum* spirochetes. If left untreated, patients can develop tertiary syphilis which manifests as neurosyphilis, cardiovascular syphilis, and/or gummatous syphilis. The risk of being infected with HIV is increased in individuals with syphilis.

Human T cell lymphotropic virus

Human T cell lymphotropic virus type I (HTLV-I) is a retrovirus which infects T cells. The virus was first isolated in a patient with cutaneous T cell leukemia in 1980. The infection is asymptomatic in the majority of individuals, but they are infectious for life.

Human T cell lymphotropic virus type I is endemic in Japan, the Caribbean, Africa, and South America. It is also found in southern India, northern Iran and aboriginal populations of northern Australia. There are an estimated 10–20 million people worldwide who are infected with this virus. In Europe and North America HTLV-I is found predominantly in migrants from endemic areas and intravenous drug users.

Human T cell lymphotropic virus type I is the causative agent of adult T cell leukemia/lymphoma, which is a very aggressive T cell malignancy. The mean age at diagnosis is 60 years in Japan but 40 years in the Caribbean and Brazil. For ATL, men are more commonly affected, with an M:F ratio of 1.5:1.

Human T cell lymphotropic virus type I also causes a variety of chronic inflammatory syndromes such as HTLV-I associated myelopathy (HAM) or tropical spastic paraparesis (TSP). This is an inflammation of the nerves in the spinal cord and causes stiffness, weakness in the legs, low back pain, incontinence, and constipation, though all the symptoms may not be present in the same patient. The mean age at onset for HAM/TSP is 40 years and women are two to three times more likely to be affected than men.

Human T cell lymphotropic virus type II was identified in the 1980s. It is not linked with any disease but has been associated with several cases of HAM/TSP.

The routes of transmission are:

- From infected mother to baby mostly through breastfeeding. One in four babies born to infected mother acquires the infection this way.
- Unprotected sex, with the risk of acquiring the infection from a man greater than from a woman.
- Through blood transfusion of whole blood and cellular components. Transmission is rare by plasma transfusion and leucodepletion has decreased the transmission of this virus. The use of an antibody test has significantly reduced transmission through this route.
- Through sharing needles and syringes.

Tests

Enzyme immunoassay is used to screen for HTLV-I and HTLV-II infections on all donations and immunoblot for confirmation. The EIA tests are performed on pools of 24 samples in the UK blood services.

> ## Key points
> HTLV-I is a retrovirus which is endemic in Japan, Africa, the Caribbean, and South America. It can cause T cell leukaemia/lymphoma, HTLV-I associated myelopathy and tropical spastic paraparesis.

Cytomegalovirus

Cytomegalovirus (CMV) is a member of the herpes group of viruses. The virus has a double stranded DNA, 160–180 nm in diameter and replicates in leucocytes and other haemopoietic cells. In healthy individuals CMV infection may not be apparent or they may exhibit mild flu-like symptoms. However, in immunologically compromised or immunosuppressed patients (low birth weight infants, transplant recipients, and AIDS patients) it can be a life-threatening condition.

After primary infection, there is an incubation period of 22–40 days during which IgM and then IgG antibodies are formed. Among blood donors, between 50–70% have antibodies to CMV. Following infection, the CMV DNA becomes integrated into the human host genome, where it remains latent. During the latency period, the individual is normally free of infectious virus. The virus can be activated when the immune system is compromised, for example as a result of pregnancy and immunosuppressive therapy.

The routes of CMV transmission are:

- Pre-natal (congenital) where the sources of infections are semen, maternal cell bound viraema, and ascending genital infection. This is determined by the presence of CMV in urine by cell culture during the first week of life.
- Perinatal infection during delivery, possibly from cervical secretions or during breast-feeding. Cytomegalovirus is not isolated from the urine during the first week of life but can be detected in the urine and/or saliva from two weeks to six months after delivery.
- Sexual contact.
- Blood transfusion.

Testing

In the UK, all blood components are leucodepleted. Because CMV resides in the white cells, there is reduction in the risk of transmission by blood transfusion. However, the risk reduction is not sufficient to remove the need for CMV testing. Thus, blood components for intra-uterine transfusions, neonates up to 28 days post expected date of delivery, pregnant women, and for granulocyte transfusions are screened for antibodies to CMV usually using an ELISA test and those tested as CMV antibody negative are considered 'safe' from latent CMV. In practice, blood services will flag CMV antibody reactive donors on their computerized records and will not retest further donations.

Key points

Cytomegalovirus is a double-stranded DNA virus which can cause severe disease or fatality in immunosuppressed or immunocompromised patients.

4.2 Additional (discretionary) testing

Malaria

Malaria is a blood-borne infection which is transmitted from one person to another by female Anopheles mosquitoes. The infection is caused by a protozoan *Plasmodium* parasite of which the four common species are:

- *P. falciparum*
- *P. vivax*
- *P. malariae*
- *P. ovale*

A fifth species *Plasmodium knowlesi* which has been known for a long time in primates has been identified in humans.

Human malaria is found predominantly in the tropical and subtropical regions of the world. There are 300–500 million cases of malaria resulting in between 1.5 to 2.7 million deaths annually. *P. falciparum* and *P. vivax* are the dominant species worldwide and are responsible for the more severe and lethal infections. The existence of the *Plasmodium* species in different parts of the world depends on the vector (mosquito) and biological and environmental factors such as humidity and temperature. For example, *P. vivax* stops developing below 60°F, whereas the temperature for *P. falciparum* is higher.

The parasite spends part of its life cycle in mosquitoes which transmit the infection to a human host while feeding on blood. The second part of the life cycle is in humans, where the parasite first invades the liver cells and multiplies. It may remain dormant in the liver for months. It is then released into the blood stream and infects the red blood cells, which cause the cells to burst. The symptoms of malarial infection, which occur 10–16 days after the mosquito bite, are chills, fever, and sweating. Sufferers may also experience headaches, nausea, and vomiting. Patients may suffer recurrent attacks, that is, every two days for *P. vivax* and *P. ovale* and every three days for *P. malariae*, which coincides with the infection and bursting of many red blood cells at the same time.

Apart from mosquitoes, malaria can also be transmitted through:

- Blood transfusion
- Sharing of needles to inject intravenous drugs, and
- From an infected mother to baby

Tests for malaria include:

- Stained thick and thin smears of blood on a microscope slide to screen and identify the Plasmodium specie. This is regarded as the 'gold standard' and is useful for current infection and to aid appropriate treatment.
- 'Dipstick' tests which detect products of plasmodial metabolism (such as LDH) and plasmodial antigens (such as histidine rich protein 2). These tests are easy and quick to perform and require little technical skill.
- ELISA and immunofluorescence tests are used to detect immunity to Plasmodium species. ELISA tests are used in the UK blood transfusion services to screen donors for malaria antibodies between 6 and 12 months after return from a malarial endemic area.
- PCR techniques which can detect less than ten parasites in 10μl of blood. This requires specialized equipment, trained staff, and takes longer to perform.

Key points

Malaria is caused by four species of the *Plasmodium* parasite—*P. falciparum*, *P. vivax*, *P. malariae*, and *P. ovale*. The disease is spread through the bite of the female Anopheles mosquitoes and is transmissible through blood transfusion.

Trypanosoma cruzi (Chagas disease)

Chagas disease was discovered by Carlos Chagas in 1909 and is caused by the protozoan parasite *Trypanosoma cruzi (T. cruzi)*. The disease is endemic in southern Mexico and South and Central America, where about 8–11 million people are infected. The parasite is transmitted to people and animals by insects of the Triatoma genus and the family *Reduviidae*, often referred to as reduviid or 'kissing bugs'. The reduviid bugs live in the cracks in walls and roofs of houses made of mud, straw, adobe, and palm thatch in the rural areas of the endemic countries. They emerge at night to feed on the faces of people while they are asleep. After biting the victim, they ingest their blood then defecate. *T. cruzi* is excreted in the faeces of the reduviid bug and is unknowingly rubbed into the bite wound, eyes, and mouth of the unsuspecting host.

The acute phase of infection is usually asymptomatic, or the patient may exhibit mild symptoms such as fever, body ache, fatigue, headache, rash, loss of appetite, diarrhoea, and vomiting. If untreated, the infection is likely to resolve within a few weeks or months. However, the infection can cause death in children and immunocompromised people as a result of inflammation of the heart muscle and brain. There is a chronic phase during which the infection remains dormant for decades or life. About 10–30% of patients develop cardiac and/or intestinal complications which can be fatal.

T. cruzi can be transmitted through:

- Insect bites with the vector in the faeces
- Congenital transmission—from mother to baby
- Organ transplant
- Blood transfusion in southern Mexico and South and Central America
- Accidental laboratory exposure, and
- Consumption of uncooked food which is contaminated with faeces from infected reduviid bugs

Testing

In the acute phase of infection when there are circulating parasites, diagnosis of Chagas disease can be made by examination of Giemsa-stained blood films. Diagnosis in the chronic phase is made by testing with two serological assays to detect antibodies to the *T. cruzi* parasite. Antibody tests used are indirect fluorescent antibody (IFA) and enzyme immunoassay (EIA).

In the UK, blood from donors who have lived or work in rural areas of Chagas endemic countries (for four weeks or more) must be negative for antibodies to *T. cruzi* at least six months after their return using an EIA. This includes donors whose mothers were born in southern Mexico, South and Central America. In the absence of a test, the donor is deferred indefinitely.

Key points

T. cruzi is transmitted through the faeces of the reduviid bug which live in mud huts in South and Central America. The infection can cause the death of children and immunocompromised people.

SELF-CHECK 4.3

Why are tests for antibodies to malaria and Chagas performed on selected donors?

4.3 Microbiology serology testing

Two test systems are used within the UK blood services:

- Abbott PRISM for HIV (antibody or combination antigen antibody test), anti-HCV, and HBsAg detection. The tests are performed in dedicated channels for HIV, HCV, HBsAg, anti-HBc, and anti-HTLV. There is a sixth channel which is used as a backup in case of failure of any of the dedicated channels. A chemiluminescent immunoassay (CLIA) is used for the detection of the test markers or analytes.

- Ortho Summit is also used for HIV (antibody or combination antigen antibody test), anti-HCV, and HBsAg detection. The tests are performed in microplates using enzyme linked immunosorbent assay (ELISA).

Antibodies to syphilis are mostly tested for using a Treponema pallidum haemagglutination assay (TPHA) or Treponema pallidum particle assay (TPPA) on the Beckman Coulter blood testing analyser. ELISA test for anti-syphilis is sometimes used in routine blood donation screening. Anti-HTLV ELISA test is performed in pools of 24 samples.

METHOD Chemiluminescent immunoassay (CLIA) methods

Three methods used on the Abbott PRISM are three-step sandwich assays, two-step sandwich, and two-step competitive assay. The tests are performed on microparticles in specially designed black reaction trays which each have two sets of eight wells. The microparticles are coated with antigens and/or antibodies, depending on the analyte being detected. The tests are incubated at 37°C in heated channels of the PRISM.

Three-step sandwich assays

- The first step of the assay is the incubation of the sample and microparticles in the incubation well of the reaction tray. Analyte(s) in the sample will bind to the corresponding antigen and/or antibody on the microparticles.

- The incubation mixture is washed into a reaction well where the microparticles with or without bound analytes are trapped on a glass fibre matrix. Any unbound material is washed through to an absorbent material contained in the reaction tray.

- Further reactions take place on the microparticles on the glass fibre matrix.

- A biotinylated probe is added to the reaction well and incubated. The probe will bind to the free arm of antibody (from sample or control) attached to the microparticles. Unbound probe is washed away.

- Acridinium labelled conjugate is added to the reaction well and after incubation unbound conjugate is washed away.

- A background reading is taken, then activator is added to the reaction well. The activator will cause acridinium to emit light (photons) which is measured. This reading is corrected for the background and compared with the cut-off to determine if the reaction is positive or negative.

Three-step sandwich assay

This is the same as the three-step sandwich assay but the step involving the incubation with a biotinylated probe is omitted.

Two-step competitive/blocking assay

This is same as the two-step sandwich assay but the conjugate attaches to any binding site on the microparticles that are not occupied by antigens or antibody from the sample.

 METHOD *ELISA methods*

Sandwich assay

ELISA is usually performed in 96 well microplates. Antigens and/or antibodies are coated to the bottom of the microplate well. Incubation temperatures vary with assay types.

- Sample is added to the microplate well and incubated, allowing the analyte to bind to the coated microplate well. Unbound sample is washed away, usually using an automated plate washer.
- Conjugate (usually an antibody to the analyte conjugated to an enzyme such as horseradish peroxidase or alkaline phosphatase) is added to the well and incubated. The conjugate will bind to any bound analyte from the sample. Unbound conjugate is washed away.
- A substrate is added which will be cleaved by the enzyme on the conjugate (if present) to coloured substance. The reaction is stopped with an acid after a fixed time, usually resulting in a change in colour, the optical density of which can be measured in a microplate reader. The colour change indicates a positive reaction.

Competitive ELISA method

- Sample and conjugate are added to the microplate well and incubated. The conjugate is the analyte conjugated to an enzyme such as horseradish peroxidase or alkaline phosphatase and will compete with the analyte being tested for to bind to the coated microplate well. Unbound sample and conjugate is washed away.
- The substrate is added and after a period of incubation, the reaction is stopped with an acid and the microplate read.
- A negative reaction is indicated by a high optical density as in the absence of the analyte from the sample, the conjugate will bind to the coated wells.

Because there are only two incubation steps, the assay is quicker to perform than the sandwich assay.

What serological tests are performed for detection of HBV, HCV, and HIV contamination of blood donation?

Nucleic acid testing (NAT)

Following the transmission of HCV through a commercial intravenous immunoglobulin (IvIg) preparation, the European Committee for Proprietary Medicinal Products recommended that from 1999 HCV RNA negative plasma is used for intravenous immunoglobulin (IvIg) preparation if there is not a viral inactivation step. HCV RNA (HCV NAT) test using polymerase chain reaction (PCR) was introduced in the UK. The test was initially performed on pools of 96 plasma samples and then subsequently on pools of 48 samples. Cross-pools were prepared and tested on positive pools to identify the infected donation(s).

Hepatitis C NAT has been extended to include all blood components with a shelf-life of greater than 24 hours. Fully automated NAT for HBV, HCV, and HIV has been implemented in the UK in pools of 24 samples, increasing further the safety of the blood supply. For a positive mini-pool, cross-pools are prepared to identify the infected donation. The use of mini-pools can be justified in countries where the prevalence of the tested virus is low. However, in countries where there is a high prevalence of the tested virus (such as HIV) it would be prudent to perform individual donation NAT (ID NAT). The reduction of the window period for microbiology serology and NAT is shown in Table 4.1.

The principle of NAT is:

- Concentration, extraction, and purification of the nucleic acid (DNA and RNA). In some cases the sample is centrifuged at high speed to concentrate the nucleic acid containing cells and increase the sensitivity of the test. The cells are mixed with a lysis buffer to disrupt the cell wall and release the nucleic acid. The nucleic acid is then captured on a solid phase such as silica or using sequence specific probes. After washing away the impurities, the nucleic acid is re-suspended.

- Amplification of the nucleic acid to increase the number of copies and hence, the sensitivity of the test.

- Detection of the specific component of the DNA or RNA.

An internal control is included in each pool of samples (or each sample for ID NAT) to ensure that the extraction, amplification, and detection have taken place. The internal control must be positive for the test to be valid.

A fully automated commercial NAT system, Roche cobas s201 is in use in the UK Blood Services for the detection of HBV, HCV, and HIV. This system uses real-time PCR, where the products of amplification are measured during the reaction. The sample with added internal control is pre-treated in the sample preparation unit (SPU) to lyse the viral envelope and the released RNA or DNA bind to the positively charged silica surface of magnetic glass particles. The magnetic glass particles (with or without captured nucleic acid) are transferred to an S tube for genome amplification and detection and the end result is the emission of light for a positive reaction which is measurable.

An alternative commercial NAT system is the fully automated Chiron Tigris which uses a patented transcription mediated amplification technology (TMA) for multiplex HBV, HCV, and HIV-1 detection. The viral genome capture, amplification, and detection take place in a single tube at the same temperature as described below:

- Samples (or pools) with internal control are lysed to release the RNA/DNA in a multi-tube unit (MTU). Capture probes hybridize to targeted nucleic acid which then attach to magnetic particles by their tail sequence. Any unbound material is washed away.

- Amplification reagent containing a reverse transcriptase, RNA polymerase, and primers is added to the MTU. The primers bind to targeted RNA/DNA and are used by the reverse transcriptase to create DNA copies of viral RNA. A second complementary copy of DNA is produced to form a double stranded DNA duplex. The RNA polymerase makes multiple copies of RNA amplicons from the DNA template. The reaction continues until all the reagents are used up, resulting in billions of copies in one hour.

- A single-stranded nucleic acid probe labelled with acridinium ester is added to the mixture and hybridizes to complementary amplicon. Unhybridized probes are inactivated to reduce background noise. Hybridized probes produce a chemiluminescent signal which is measured in a luminometer.

METHOD Basic PCR method (Figure 4.3)

1. PCR can amplify and detect DNA sequences directly. However, for RNA viruses such as HCV, a reverse transcription step using the enzyme reverse transcriptase is necessary to produce complementary DNA (cDNA) which can be used as a template for PCR.

2. The purified DNA (or cDNA) is mixed with a thermostable DNA polymerase (taq polymerase), two oligonucleotide primers, deoxynucleotide triphosphate (dNTPs), reaction buffer, and magnesium. Other additives may be included. The following reactions take place in a thermocycler which automatically changes the temperature for preset times.

3. The reaction mixture is heated to 95°C to denature the DNA, causing each double strand to separate into two single strands (sense and antisense).

4. The temperature is lowered to 50–65°C to allow the oligonucleotide primers to bind to the complementary sequence of the DNA.

5. The temperature is then raised to 72°C for the taq polymerase to cause the primers to 'grow' along the single stranded DNA to produce two amplicons (and two double stranded DNA).

6. The cycle is repeated many times by alternating the temperature to 95°C, then 50–65°C, and then 72°C to produce millions or billions of copies of DNA.

7. The end product can be visualized using the fluorescent dye, ethidium bromide after gel electrophoresis.

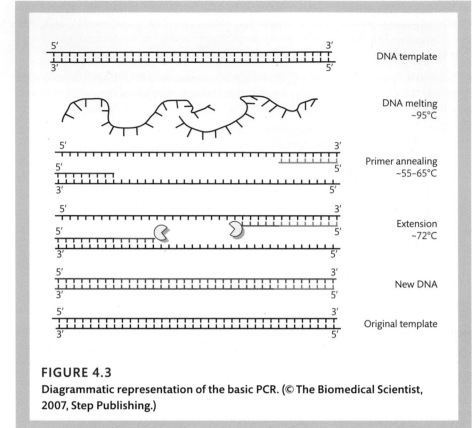

FIGURE 4.3
Diagrammatic representation of the basic PCR. (© The Biomedical Scientist, 2007, Step Publishing.)

Key points

Serological tests were first introduced to detect antibodies and antigens from infectious agents. Introduction of NAT further reduced the risk of transmission of infectious agents through blood transfusions.

4.4 **Microbiology positive screen and confirmatory testing**

Donations which are negative for the mandatory tests and the required additional markers can be released to stock if all the required blood group serology tests are satisfactory. The Red Book requires that any donor sample which is positive for any microbiology marker (initial reactive samples) is retested in duplicate. All blood and components derived from that donation must be quarantined to prevent inadvertent issue. The duplicate test must be performed using the same assay which was used in the original test. Thus:

- If the duplicate repeat results are non-reactive (negative), all components prepared from the donation can be released to stock if the blood group serology tests are satisfactory.

- If one or both of the repeat tests are repeat reactive (positive):

  · All components prepared from the donation must be labelled 'Not for transfusion' and discarded.

  · The donor record must be flagged for confirmatory testing. Sample(s) from the donation must be referred to a reference centre for confirmatory testing. The reference centre should be independent of the microbiology screening laboratory. The assays used for confirmatory testing should (where possible) be at least as sensitive as the screening assay. The confirmatory testing is necessary because all microbiology test kits have a small percentage of false positive reactions. By testing with different test kits/assays or additional tests for that marker, the true infectivity of the sample can be determined.

  · If the reference centre confirms the result as positive, the donor must be permanently excluded from further donation. The donor should be offered counselling and an additional sample taken to confirm the infection.

  · If the reference centre result is negative or indeterminate, the donor record should be flagged for repeat testing after 12 weeks (see re-instatement algorithm).

Re-instatement algorithm for reference centre negative or indeterminate results

Samples should be taken from the donor at least 12 weeks after the previous donation was found to be repeatedly reactive. This is to allow any infection in the 'window period' or early seroconversion to reach a detectable level. The 12-week follow-up sample is tested at the BTS and the reference centre and if the results are:

  · Non-reactive for that microbiology marker at both the BTS and reference centre, the donor can be returned to the active donor panel. The next donation can be used if all mandatory and additional tests are satisfactory.

  · Non-reactive at the BTS for that microbiology marker but reactive or indeterminate at the reference centre and considered to be a false positive reaction, the donor can be returned to the active donor panel. The next donation can be used if all mandatory and additional tests are satisfactory.

  · Still reactive for that microbiology marker by the current assay but non-reactive by an alternative assay of equivalent sensitivity at the BTS but non-reactive or indeterminate at the reference centre and considered to be a false positive reaction, it can be re-tested using an alternative screening assay. The next donation can be used if all mandatory and additional tests are satisfactory. Procedures must be in place at the BTS to ensure that the donor sample is tested using the alternative screening assay for the offending infectious disease marker.

  · If the use of an alternative is not feasible, the donor must be deferred from further donations and a letter sent to explain the false reactivity.

- For a repeat reactive donation, any components from the previous donation(s) which are still in stock (e.g. fresh frozen plasma or cryoprecipitate) should be quarantined until the infectious nature of the current donation is determined. This is a precautionary measure as it is possible, but unlikely, for the previous donation to be in the 'window phase' and could transmit the infection even though the screening tests for the mandatory microbiology markers were negative at the time.

SELF-CHECK 4.6

Why was nucleic acid test (NAT) introduced?

4.5 **Bacterial contamination**

Mandatory transfusion microbiology screening of donated blood has reduced the risk of transmission by transfusion of these viral contaminants to miniscule proportions (see Table 4.2). Bacterial contamination of blood and blood components remains the main infectious cause of transfusion reactions resulting in sepsis and death.

Fatalities due to bacterial contaminated blood components are extremely rare. The majority of these are due to Gram negative bacteria such as *Serratia liquifaciens* and *Yersinia enterocolitica* and also Gram positive coagulase-negative *staphylococci*. These organisms can proliferate at 2–6°C, the storage temperature of red cell components. The patients usually develop high temperature and chills during or shortly after transfusion, and death can occur within 24 hours.

Surveillance studies have shown that 1 in 1,000–2,000 units of platelets are contaminated with bacteria. However, the risk of death from bacterially contaminated platelet transfusion is between 1 in 7,500 and 1 in 100,000. Fatality due to whole blood derived platelets is higher than that of single donor apheresis platelets. Passive surveillance studies in the UK, USA, and France show that Gram positive bacteria account for 71% of transfusion transmission but Gram negative organisms were implicated in 82% of the fatalities.

Fresh frozen plasma and cryoprecipitate are rarely associated with transfusion-transmitted bacterial infections. There are reports of both of these components acquiring bacterial infections when they were thawed in a contaminated water bath.

BOX 4.1 *Bacteria implicated in transfusion transmission by red cell and platelets*

Red cells	Platelets
Gram-positive bacteria	**Gram-positive bacteria**
Bacillus cereus	*Bacillus cereus*
Coagulase-negative staphylococcus	Coagulase-negative staphylococcus
Enterococcus faecalis	*Enterococcus faecalis*
Group B streptococcus	Group B streptococcus
Staphylococcus epidermidis	*Proprionibacterium acnes*
Proprionibacterium acnes	*Staphylococcus epidermidis*
Streptococcus species	*Staphylococcus aureus*
	Streptococcus species
Gram-negative bacteria	**Gram-negative bacteria**
Acinetobacter species	Acinetobacter species
Enterobacter species	Enterobacter species
Escherichia species	Escherichia species
Klebsiella species	Klebsiella species
Morganella morganii	Pseudomonas species
Proteus species	Proteus species
Serratia species	Serratia species
Yersinia enterocolitica	*Yersinia enterocolitica*

TABLE 4.2 Estimates of the risks of infectious donations issued for transfusion in the UK for 2007–2009 (Safe supplies: Testing the Nation Annual review 2009 (www.hpa.org. uk/webc/HPAwebFile/HPAweb_C/128146241976)).

Risk (1 per x million) due to:	HBV	HCV	HIV	HTLV-I
All donations	0.67	82.78	5.13	17.74
New donors	0.19	16.58	3.73	3.41

The sources of blood component bacterial contamination are:

- Skin contamination—this is due to inadequate decontamination of the skin prior to phlebotomy. On occasions, there may be subcutaneous bacterial infection which is unaffected by the skin cleansing. During blood collection, the skin core or plug may become detached by the collection needle and contaminate the blood pack. Diversion of the first 20–30 ml of the donation into a sample pouch (used for blood grouping and microbiology screening) will reduce the contamination of the main pack.

- Asymptomatic donors—the donors are transiently infected as shown by elevated IgM or IgG antibody titres to bacteria, notably *Y. enterocolitica*.

- Contaminated blood bag—*S. marcescens* found in the dust of the manufacturing plant is thought to contaminate the outside of the blood collection bag. These multiply in the presence of moisture and nutrient, and possibly gain entry into the inside of the bag.

- Contaminated water bath—*Pseudomonas cepacia* and *P. aeruginosa* in water baths used for thawing FFP and cryoprecipitate have been cultured from these components.

- Contamination during processing—this is extremely rare with the use of sterile connecting devices and integrated blood and satellite packs.

Screening for bacterial contamination

The detection of the bacteria in blood components depends on:

- Timing of sampling—low level contamination may not be detectable on the day of collection. These bacteria may proliferate over the succeeding days to sufficiently high numbers to cause severe adverse reactions in recipients. A decision has to be made on the day of sampling post collection, where the majority of bacterial contamination will be detected but still retain a reasonable shelf-life. This is usually a day or two after collection.

- Storage temperature of the blood component—most bacteria proliferate more rapidly at 20–24°C (for platelets) than at 2–6°C (for red cells).

- Sensitivity of the test system.

- Volume of the test sample—a larger volume is required to detect low level bacterial contamination.

Test systems

1. BacT/ALERT (BioMérieux, France)—this is an automated liquid culture system. It uses a broth bottle into which the sample is injected. The bottle has a colourimetric sensor which changes from blue to yellow with increasing CO_2 concentration as a result of bacterial proliferation. There are separate bottles for aerobic and anaerobic bacterial detection. Because the majority of fatalities are due to aerobic bacterial contamination and cost, there is a preference for testing for aerobic bacteria only in some services.

2. Pall enhanced Bacterial Detection System (eBDS)—this is a closed culture system which relies on the consumption of oxygen as a result of bacteria proliferation.

Key points

Transfusions of blood components, predominantly platelets, contaminated with bacteria have been responsible for several fatalities. Some blood establishments have introduced automated blood culture systems to detect bacterial contamination of platelet components.

SELF-CHECK 4.7

Which blood component is more likely to transmit bacterial infections and why?

4.6 West Nile virus (WNV)

Since its isolation in 1937, WNV is responsible for epidemics in Southern Europe, Africa, the Middle East, Russia, western and south Asia and more recently in America. It is transmitted by a wide range of female mosquito species of which the *Culex* is the most predominant vector. It is a member of the *Flaviviridae* family and genus *Flavivirus*. West Nile virus is a small, spherical, lipid-enveloped virus which contains a single-stranded, positive-sense RNA virus.

An estimated 20–30% of infected individuals display symptoms such as fever, headache, rash, nausea, vomiting, eye pain, myalgia, flaccid paralysis, and lymphadenopathy. A small proportion of these progress to a more severe disease, culminating in encephalitis and meningoencephalitis.

The virus was transmitted by transfusion of red cells, platelets, and fresh frozen plasma. It is unlikely to be transmitted by fractionated plasma products because of the heat and solvent detergent treatment used. West Nile virus was also transmitted by solid organ transplant and breastfeeding. The transfusion transmission of WNV has prompted blood centres in the USA to defer donors for 28 days if they display symptoms of WNV infection. On 1 July 2003, mini-pool NAT for WNV was introduced in the USA and Canada. Low titre viraemic donations may not be detected by the mini-pool NAT.

The only known risk of WNV entering the UK blood supply is from returning travellers from affected areas who may be incubating the virus and FFP imported from the USA. The following are in place to reduce the risk:

- Asymptomatic donors are deferred for 28 days after leaving an endemic area with ongoing WNV transmission in humans. Alternatively, a validated WNV NAT on the donation must be negative. The NHSBT has introduced mini-pool (pools of 6 samples) NAT for WNV from May 2012 for donors who are returning from affected areas.

- Donors with a history of WNV and/or a positive WNV NAT test should be temporarily deferred for clinical microbiology investigations. These donors may donate after six months without the requirement for a WNV NAT test.

- A negative WNV NAT test is required for all FFP imported from the USA. They are also subjected to methylene blue treatment which has been shown to reduce the WNV viral load by at least 6.5 $\log_{10}$.

Key points

Transfusion transmitted West Nile virus has been implicated in the deaths of patients in North America. This virus is not currently a risk to the UK blood supply.

4.7 Other threats to the blood supply

Transmissible spongiform encephalitis, prions and variant Creutzfeldt–Jakob disease

The first case of a variant CJD (vCJD) was described in 1996. Accumulated clinical, neurological, epidemiological, and scientific evidence points to an abnormal prion protein being the causative agent and is of the same strain as bovine spongiform encephalitis (BSE).

Prion protein normally exists as PrP^c (cellular form) predominantly in nerve cells where it may help to maintain neuronal function. It can also be found in varying concentrations in plasma, platelets, white cells, and erythrocytes. Abnormal prions (or PrP^{sc} after scrapie) are the infectious protein particles lacking in nucleic acid which can invariably cause fatal neuro-degenerative diseases. Prion diseases have been found in sheep, cats, cattle, mink, mule deer, elk, greater kudu, nyala, onyx, and also in humans, and are associated with an accumulation of abnormal prion protein in the brain.

Human prion disease can be classified into the following categories:

1. *Sporadic CJD*: this is the most common form of CJD, with an annual incidence of one in a million worldwide. The cause of sporadic CJD is unknown, but a popular theory is that it may arise from spontaneous conversion of normal prion protein in the brain to the abnormal form. The average age of onset of the disease is 65, with progressive dementia and death within about six months.

2. *Acquired CJD*: this includes accidental exposure to abnormal prion through medical and surgical procedure (iatrogenic CJD) such as human growth hormones and gonadotropin, inadequately sterilized electrodes, corneal transplants, and dura mater grafts. It is also transmitted through cannibalistic funereal rites of the Fore tribe of Papua New Guinea, resulting in a disease called kuru. This practice has since stopped, which resulted in a reduction in the number of kuru cases.

3. *Inherited CJD*: this accounts for about 15% of human prion disease and is caused by an inherited abnormal gene. At least 20 different mutations in the human prion protein gene (PRNP) have been found.

4. *Variant CJD (vCJD)*: as of 11 June 2012, there have been 176 deaths due to definite or probable cases of vCJD in the UK. Forty-nine fatal cases have been identified in other parts of the world, including 25 in France.

The possibility of transmission of vCJD by blood transfusion was raised following the first reported case of the disease. The UK Spongiform Encephalopathy Advisory Committee (SEAC) advised the use of universal leucoreduction as a precautionary measure to reduce the theoretical risk of transfusion transmitted vCJD infection. Experiments have previously shown prion infectivity in buffy coat. Also, donors who have two or more members in the family with familial CJD or were transfused since 1 January 1980 cannot donate. The UK also started importing plasma for fractionation predominantly from the USA and from other countries from October 1999.

To date there have been three cases of transmissions of vCJD by blood transfusions. Two cases have been associated with two donations from the same donor. A screening test for abnormal prion is under development, and there is a CE marked RBC prion reduction filter under evaluation.

Key points

Variant CJD is caused by an abnormal prion protein which was transmitted through contaminated meat products and has resulted in over 200 deaths worldwide, mostly in the UK. The abnormal prion is also transmitted through blood transfusion and procedures to reduce the risk are being developed or undergoing clinical trial.

SELF-CHECK 4.8

What is the causative agent of vCJD and how is it transmitted from one individual to another?

Chikungunya virus

Chikungunya virus (also known as CHIKV) was first isolated in Tanzania in 1952 and has since been found in several African countries, India, South-East Asia, Saudi Arabia, and Mediterranean countries. Since 2004 there have been outbreaks in Indian Ocean islands and north-eastern Italy.

Chikungunya virus is an alphavirus which is transmitted to humans by several species of mosquitoes, usually *Aedes aegypti* and *A. albopictus*. Infections may be asymptomatic or patients may present with symptoms such as fever, headache, vomiting, rash, thrombocytopenia, muscle and joint pain, and weakness. In rare cases other complications such as encephalitis, fulminant liver failure, and death have been reported.

It is possible for CHIKV to be transmitted by blood transfusion or tissue or organ transplantation. Visitors to most Chikungunya endemic areas will be excluded from donating for six months under the current malaria guidelines. In most Chikungunya endemic areas where malaria is not a problem, visitors must not donate:

- For six months after their return to the UK if they have been or may have been infected with the virus, or
- For four weeks if they have not presented with symptoms of infection.

4.8 Quality control/British working standards

The overwhelming majority of donor samples will be non-reactive for the mandatory microbiology markers. To increase confidence that rare weakly reactive samples are detected, microbiology test kits should meet nationally agreed minimum criteria for specificity and sensitivity. The National Blood Service Microbiology Kit Evaluation Group with representatives from the UK BTS and the Health Protection Agency (HPA) evaluate microbiology kits and integrated test systems for their suitability for donation testing.

Each batch of tests must include the manufacturer's positive and negative controls for which the correct results must be obtained for the sample test results to be valid. In addition, a British Working Standard (BWS) is included in each batch of tests to demonstrate that an acceptable level of sensitivity is achieved. The BWS is produced by the National Institute of Biological Standards and Controls (NIBSC) but controls available from the HPA or an in-house control can be used. The BWS, HPA, or in-house controls if used, should be reactive for the test results to be valid.

Statistical process control is used to monitor the performance of the microbiology assays by plotting the sample optical density to cut-off ratio (S/CO) of the working standard on a Shewhart chart. Commercial software is available to automate this process and display the points on a chart with 'warning' and 'out of control' limits set at 2 and 3 standard deviations. Plotting the S/CO of the working standards daily will give an early warning when the assay performance is deviating from normal. Thus, the operator can investigate the cause of the deviation and correct it before the assay fails.

The S/CO of the BWS and reagent batch number are reported to NIBSC and are used to compare the performance of each test equipment/assay of the transfusion centre with each other. A report of the analysis is sent to the transfusion centre so that they are aware of how the equipment/assay performance compares with others and take appropriate actions, if necessary.

SELF-CHECK 4.9

Why are internal and external controls used?

Batch pre-acceptance testing (BPAT)

Before each batch of microbiology or other assay kits are used, routinely **batch pre-acceptance testing** (BPAT) is performed to ensure that:

- It meets the minimum standard of sensitivity and specificity,
- It has not deteriorated during transportation, and
- It provide information on batch to batch variation.

Batch pre-acceptance testing
Tests performed to show batch of test kits/reagents received meets pre-defined criteria such as sensitivity and specificity and has not deteriorated during transportation.

In the NHSBT, lot release testing is centrally performed at the National Transfusion Microbiology Reference Laboratory (NTMRL) before delivery of the kits to the transfusion centres. If the kits have passed the lot release test, the BTS will perform a delivery acceptance test before the kits are used for donation (or patient) testing. The delivery acceptance test is required to show that the kits have not deteriorated during transportation and that the specificity is within the contracted level.

Assay kits which fail lot release or delivery acceptance test should not be used for routine testing but returned to the supplier.

SELF-CHECK 4.10

Why is pre-acceptance testing performed?

Infection surveillance

All blood transfusion centres in the UK report the number of initial and repeat reactive, new and known donors, and confirmed positives each month to the NHSBT/HPA Infection

Surveillance Unit. The manufacturers of the kits and batch numbers are also collected. This information is used to prepare a monthly report which allows the users to compare equipment performance for each batch of kits, batch to batch variation, and is also used to estimate the risk of an infected donation being transfused (see Table 4.2).

Sample archive

Blood transfusion centres in the UK maintain sample archives either in the form of deep well microplate (for 96 samples with up to 1 ml of plasma/serum per sample) format or in the original PPT tubes. The sample archives are kept below –20°C either at in-house or commercial storage for a minimum of three years. The main reason for retaining an archive sample is to allow retesting if a recipient develops a transfusion transmissible infection following transfusion.

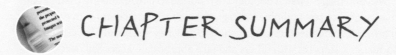

CHAPTER SUMMARY

- The mandatory tests for the release of blood and blood components in the UK are ABO and RhD blood group, red cell antibody screen, HBsAg, anti-HIV, anti-HCV, anti-syphilis, anti-HTLV, and NAT for HCV RNA.

- Discretionary tests are performed for anti-CMV, anti-malaria, anti-Chagas (*T. cruzi*), and anti-HBc.

- All tests are performed on individual donations except for NAT and anti-HTLV which are tested on pools of 24 samples (or less).

- The tests are performed on automated systems using ISBT 128 barcoded samples and the results are uploaded to the host computer on-line to reduce transcription errors.

- Some blood transfusion centres perform high titre anti-A/B on all donations while others restrict this to donations intended for neonatal transfusions or components with high plasma content. Components from high titre anti-A/B negative donations are labelled as such. This is to reduce the chance of transfusion reactions with ABO mis-match transfusions, such as group O platelets given to group A or B recipients.

- Tests for syphilis are either performed on an Beckman Coulter blood testing analyser by TPHA or TPPA, or by ELISA.

- All other serology tests are performed on automated systems using ELISA or chemiluminescent methods.

- In the UK, NAT is performed on the Roche cobas s201 using a multiplex assay for HBV DNA and HCV, and HIV RNA.

- All reagents used are subjected to batch pre-acceptance testing to ensure that they meet minimum standards of quality.

- External or in-house controls should be included in each batch of tests.

- Any donation which is serologically reactive (initial reactive) is retested in duplicate on the same system and manufacturer assay. If both duplicate tests are negative, the donation and all components can be released for transfusion. Otherwise, all components from that donation must be discarded and a sample referred to a reference centre for confirmatory tests.

■ Donors who are confirmed by the reference centre as microbiology positive for any marker must be removed from the donor panel.

■ The commonest microbiological risk to the blood supply is bacterial contamination. Some blood transfusion centres test platelet components for these using automated culture systems.

■ Test for West Nile virus is not a requirement for blood collected in the UK, but plasma products imported from the USA must be negative WNV NAT.

■ Variant CJD is a threat to the UK blood supply and leucodepletion has been introduced as a precaution to reduce transfusion transmission. Also, donors who have two or more members in the family with familial CJD or were transfused since 1 January 1980 cannot donate. A test is not currently available but is in development and CE marked prion reduction filters for RBCs are under evaluation.

 # FURTHER READING

● **Barbara JAJ, Regan FAM, & Contreras MC (eds)** *Transfusion Microbiology*. **Cambridge University Press, Cambridge, 2008.**

● **British Blood Transfusion Society** *An Introduction to Blood Transfusion Science and Blood Bank Practice*, **5th edition. British Blood Transfusion Society, Manchester, 2009. www.bbts.org.uk.**

● **Medicines Control Agency** *Rules and Guidance for Pharmaceutical Manufacturers and Distributors 2002*, **6th edition. The Stationery Office, Norwich, 2002.**

● *Safe Supplies: Testing the Nation*. **Annual review from the NHS Blood and Transplant/ Health Protection Agency Centre for Infections Epidemiology unit, 2009. London, August 2010. www.hpa.org.uk/Topics/InfectiousDiseases/ReferenceLibrary/BIBD/ References/.**

● **UK Blood Transfusion and Tissue Transplantation Services** *Guidelines for the Blood Transfusion Services in the United Kingdom*, **7th edition. The Stationery Office, Norwich, 2005. www.tsoshop.co.uk or at www.transfusionguidelines.org.uk.**

Answers to the questions in this chapter are provided on the book's Online Resource Centre.

 Go to www.oxfordtextbooks.co.uk/orc/knight

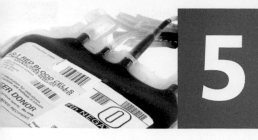

5

Clinical Use of Blood Components

Karen Madgwick and Bill Chaffe

Learning objectives

After studying this chapter you should be able to:

- Understand basic circulatory physiology and the structure and function of the components of blood.

- Understand the normal physiological response to anaemia and/or bleeding and how different patient groups may respond.

- Describe the different blood components available and their appropriate and inappropriate use based on best practice national guidelines.

- Understand the benefits of transfusion therapy and the alternatives available to using allogeneic blood.

- Outline how best to manage the use of the precious resource—blood.

- Understand how good communication, standards, audit, and review of product use will aid appropriate use of blood components.

- Outline national initiatives designed to facilitate the appropriate use of blood.

Introduction

This chapter covers the function of blood *in vivo* and the body's response to anaemia and bleeding. Having gained an understanding of what blood is needed for within the body the reader can then consider how to best support patients by choosing the most appropriate replacement therapies. This chapter does not contain detailed information about blood components themselves, their manufacture, preparation for use, or the appropriate groups to be issued; for this the reader should refer to Chapter 3 on blood components and Chapter 6 on compatibility testing. This chapter also considers the alternatives available to traditional transfusion therapies based on donor (allogeneic) blood.

5.1 Structure and function of blood

It is important to understand the function of the individual components *in vivo* before considering the therapeutic use of the blood components currently available. Blood is a complex fluid which is essential for life, carrying oxygen, nutrients, chemical messages, and waste products to and from the tissues and organs of the body, and playing a significant role in regulating the body's temperature and preventing disease and blood loss. The arteries transport blood away from the heart towards tissues and organs, the thin walled capillaries allow exchange between the tissues and the blood circulating. The veins return the blood back to the heart. The different organs of the body have different circulatory requirements, with cardiac output being adjusted depending on individual needs, for example when exercising the usually high requirement of the digestive systems and the kidneys is diverted to skeletal muscle.

When blood is removed from the body and not allowed to clot it will slowly separate into three distinct layers:

- Erythrocytes (red cells) are at the bottom; these cells transport gases. An adult will have over 20 trillion red cells, each with a lifespan of about 120 days. Red cell production is triggered by a reduction in oxygen delivery to the kidneys, which secrete the hormone erythropoietin. Erythropoietin stimulates the bone marrow into producing more red cells whose primary function is the transport of oxygen.

- The buffy coat, containing leucocyctes (white cells) and thrombocytes (platelets) forms the middle layer. The leucocytes defend the body against invasion by microorganisms and foreign antigens. The thrombocytes are fragments of larger cells, megakarocytes, and play a major role in the formation of blood clots following injury.

- The plasma is the top layer. The plasma contains salts and proteins (albumin, globulins, and clotting factors) dissolved in water, and carries nutrients, wastes, and hormones. Albumin is a large, 'sticky' protein which cannot easily cross the capillary walls. Albumin molecules bind salts, bilirubin, and some drugs for transportation around the circulation but also play a significant role in maintaining the osmotic pressure of the vessels, by pulling in or repelling water. The globulins are proteins that are involved with transporting ions and vitamins and (gamma globulins) the body's defences.

The volume of blood present depends on the size and weight of the individual, but in an adult is usually around four to six litres, of which approximately 55% will be plasma and 45% red cells.

5.2 Normal physiological response to anaemia and/or bleeding

Oxygen is delivered to the tissues by the haemoglobin (Hb) inside the red cells. The oxygen transport system normally operates to maintain constant oxygen consumption (although this will vary depending on the individual needs of each tissue/organ). Oxygen delivery is the product of cardiac output and the oxygen content of the arterial blood. When oxygen delivery to the tissues decreases, oxygen extraction from the lungs increases. The oxygen dissociation curve is a graphical plot that shows the proportion of saturated haemoglobin against the oxygen tension. This determines how readily the haemgloblin will release the oxygen molecules to the tissues. When this compensation cannot occur hypoxia (low oxygen) results and this can cause tissue damage and even, in extreme conditions, organ death. Whilst a patient's haemoglobin level is helpful when deciding whether a patient needs transfusion, the individual's vascular system, cardiac, lung, and bone marrow function will greatly affect the decision whether or not to transfuse.

Other factors that affect oxygen delivery include body temperature, acid base status, 2,3-diphosphoglycerate (2,3 DPG) levels, and the structure of the haemoglobin molecule itself (i.e. anything other than 'normal' Hb AA can affect oxygen carrying and delivery).

In a patient, transfusion of red cells may be considered because a fall in the number of red cells (drop in haemoglobin) has been observed. The drop in haemoglobin may be caused by loss (bleeding), decreased survival time (increased destruction), or decrease in production (bone marrow failure). Acute blood loss is not always visible as blood can accumulate in body cavities and can be very difficult to identify clinically, particularly in children.

In summary, it is important to consider each patient individually, taking into account all of the above factors, when deciding whether to transfuse.

Key points

Maintaining the supply of oxygen to the tissues by red cells is vital as hypoxia can lead to tissue damage.

5.3 Blood components available and their appropriate use

Blood products should only be given when it will benefit the patient and the decision to transfuse should be based on clinical guidelines, although it is sometimes necessary to modify the guidance according to individual patient needs. It is important that the reason for giving the blood product is recorded on the request form and clearly documented in the patient's clinical notes. At the time of writing, all blood products in the UK (with the exception of granu-locyte preparations) are leucodepleted (the majority of white cells are removed by filtration).

Red cells

The majority of red cell products produced in the UK meet the following criteria:

- Red cells (leucocyte depleted) in additive solution
- Volume of 270 ± 50 ml
- Greater than 40 g Hb per unit
- Haematocrit 0.55–0.75
- Thirty-five-day shelf-life
- Storage temperature 2–6°C
- Transfusion over a maximum of four hours from removal from controlled storage

See Figure 5.1.

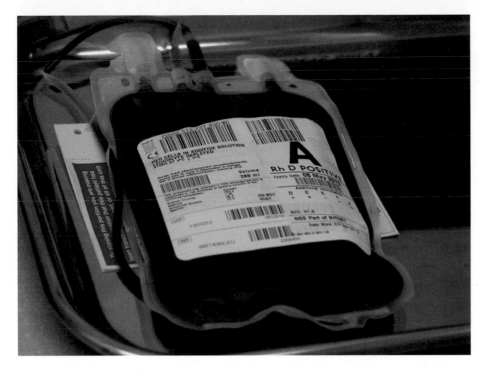

FIGURE 5.1

A unit of red blood cells (in additive, leucocyte depleted) provided by National Health Service Blood and Transplant (NHSBT). The unit number is displayed on the top left of the label, below which is the product and storage conditions. The ABO and Rh D group of the product is displayed on the top right of the label, below which is the expiry date and below that is additional information on red cell phenotypes and CMV (Cytomeglavirus) status.

The usual reason for transfusing red blood cells is to increase the patient's oxygen carrying capacity, which may have decreased either due to loss or lack of production of the patient's own red cells. The clinical reason for transfusion may be due to the primary diagnosis such as haemoglobinopathy, cancer, anaemia of chronic disease (i.e. ineffective production of red cells), or bleeding (i.e. increased loss of red cells). Prior to the decision to transfuse, the level of bone marrow function and the need for the patient to maintain an appropriate activity level must be considered. In accordance with the British Committee for Standards in Haematology (BCSH) guidelines, an adult patient should not be transfused if the Hb is above 100 g/l, but there is a strong indication for transfusion if the Hb is below 70 g/l, and transfusion will usually become essential when the Hb falls to below 50 g/l. It is thought that an Hb between 80 and 100 g/l is a safe level even for those patients with significant cardiorespiratory disease, although transfusion may need to be considered when a patient is symptomatic (is short of breath, suffers from angina, is weak, or very tired). However, these triggers can vary greatly, depending on the primary reason for the anaemia, for example a thalassaemia patient may require a maintenance Hb of >100 g/l in order to suppress the bone marrow and a patient with sickle cell disease (Hb SS) may be symptom free with an Hb of 70 g/l. It is difficult to state a formula for the volume of red cells to be transfused in a non-bleeding patient. The BCSH guidelines recommend that depending on the starting haemoglobin (Hb) one or two units should be transfused and then the patient's Hb and symptoms should be reassessed to see if more red cells are required. The age of the product, the weight of the patient and the volume of red cells transfused will all affect the incremental rise in haemoglobin. However, as a rough guide, one unit will give an incremental rise of approximately 10 g/l in an adult. In patients who are bleeding, prompt action and good communication are key, with the maintenance of tissue perfusion being vital to prevent shock. As above, it is rarely necessary to use red cell products where the patient's haemoglobin is above 100 g/l, but where possible the aim should be to maintain the haemoglobin above 80 g/l.

Whilst most of the concepts of red cell transfusion considered above apply equally to the treatment of both adults and children, the product chosen for administration can be different as there are a number of small volume paediatric and neonatal red cell products available.

Key points

The main reason for transfusing red cells is to maintain or increase the oxygen carrying capacity of the blood. However, not all individuals need to have the same Hb level to prevent hypoxia; an Hb of >80 g/l is usually sufficient.

SELF-CHECK 5.1

Name three factors that may affect the expected haemoglobin rise (10 g/l) post transfusion of one unit of blood to a patient who is not bleeding.

Fresh frozen plasma (FFP) and cryoprecipitate (cryo)

Fresh frozen plasma (FFP) is comprised of 90% water, and 8% proteins and carbohydrates. It is prepared from anticoagulated whole blood within six hours of collection, and it contains high levels of all coagulation proteins, including the labile factors V and VIII. FFP is made, where possible, from male donors as female donors with a history of pregnancy may have HLA antibodies in their plasma which has been shown to increases the incidence of transfusion-related acute lung injury (TRALI). See Figures 5.2 and 5.3.

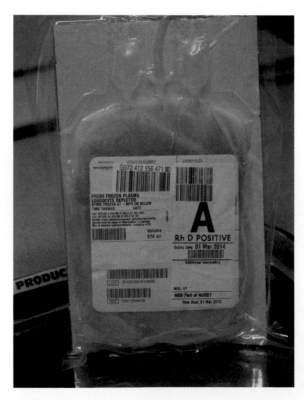

FIGURE 5.2

A unit of FFP for neonatal use that has been methylene blue treated provided by National Health Service Blood and Transplant (NHSBT). This unit of fresh frozen plasma has been treated with methylene blue in order to reduce the risk of transmission of pathogens. Currently the product is recommended for use in children born after 1996. The volume of the unit indicated in the middle of the label is 65 ml.

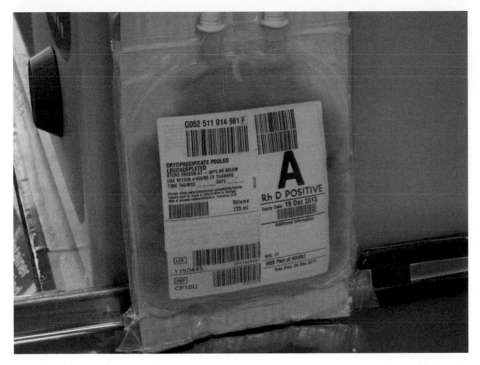

FIGURE 5.3
Example of a unit of plasma, cryo depleted leucocyte depleted, provided by National Health Service Blood and Transplant (NHSBT). A unit of cryoprecipitate depleted frozen plasma (the supernatant left when producing cryoprecipitate) is a product that is used for to plasma exchange during the treatment for thrombotic thrombocytopenic purpura (TTP).

Each 150–300 ml pack of FFP contains 2–5 mg/ml fibrinogen, >0.7 iu/ml Factor VIII, and other clotting factors. Cryoprecipitate (cryo) is made by thawing FFP slowly at 4°C and re-suspending the precipitate in 10–20 ml of plasma and contains 150–300 mg fibrinogen and 80–120 iu Factor VIII per pack. The possible adverse effects of using FFP include allergic reactions, fluid overload, TRALI, and immune suppression. When it is decided to use FFP, giving the patient an adequate dose is really important. Usually 12–15 ml/kg is the accepted starting dose, depending on the clinical situation. Therefore, a therapeutic dose in a 60 kg women will be approximately 900 ml and in an 80 kg male 1,200 ml. Where requests for FFP are made for an adult below 900 ml the weight of the patient should be queried with the requesting clinician. Packs with a smaller volume of FFP are available for infants and children.

Clinical situations where FFP has been shown not to be of benefit are in formula replacement (for example giving one unit of FFP for every two units of red cells). However, in a patient suffering from massive haemorrhage it is accepted that additional clotting factors will be required when the patient has had the equivalent of one body volume replaced by donor blood. In this instance clotting tests, to determine the extent of the coagulopathy, may take too long and FFP should be given as soon as possible. Also, in the treatment of hypovolaemia (low fluid volume) crystalloids or colloids are more suitable, and where bleeding is significant red cells should be given. In accordance with the BCSH guidelines FFP should not be used for the reversal of warfarin overdose in the presence of bleeding where an alternative prothrombin complex is available. A patient with a moderately prolonged INR in the absence of bleeding should be corrected by giving intravenous vitamin K at a dose between 0.5 and 2 mg. In patients with disseminated intravascular coagulation (DIC) treatment should be directed at the cause. However, FFP is recommended where there is haemorrhage and an abnormality of coagulation.

In massive transfusion there is no evidence that prophylactic replacement prevents the onset of abnormal bleeding but where the PT >19.5 and/or APTT >48 seconds, FFP is recommended, starting at a dose of 15 ml/kg. In patients where the fibrinogen level is less than 1.0 g/l cryoprecipitate is indicated.

In adults, cryoprecipitate is usually given as one therapeutic dose (two pooled packs) and then the fibrinogen level repeated to ensure that the patient's fibrinogen is >1.0 g/l. When the patient is having a massive transfusion it is important to repeat haematological and biochemical tests regularly in order to monitor the patient's progress and assess the need for products. In liver disease the risk of bleeding may be increased due to *thrombocytopenia* and increased levels of tissue plasminogen activation. Fresh frozen plasma may be indicated if the patient is bleeding or where surgery is proposed. However, complete correction is virtually impossible. In summary, therefore, FFP and cryoprecipitate should only be used having considered both the clinical and laboratory findings.

SELF-CHECK 5.2

According to the BCSH guidelines, what is the recommended dose for an adult requiring fresh frozen plasma (FFP)?

Platelets

A platelet concentrate may be produced either from several whole blood donations or by apheresis of a single donor. Apart from exposing the patient to fewer donors, the apheresis donation has the same specification as a platelet pool. After production, platelets are stored for up to five days, at 20–24°C in plastic packs designed for gaseous exchange, and on equipment designed to continuously agitate the product. One adult 'pack/dose' is provided in <300 ml plasma containing >240 × 10^9 platelets. See Figure 5.4.

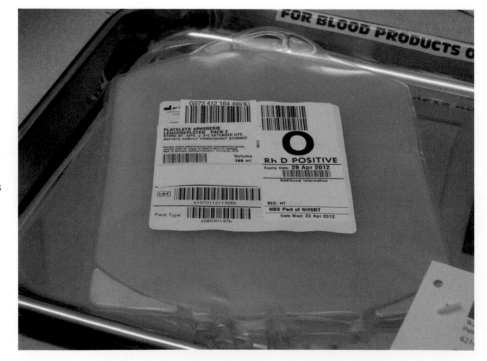

FIGURE 5.4

Example of a unit pooled leucocyte depleted platelets provided by National Health Service Blood and Transplant (NHSBT). This unit of platelets has been produced by pooling the platelets from several whole blood donations. As part of the storage information (below the unit number on the left hand side of the label) it is stated that the product requires gentle agitation on storage.

Adverse effects of transfusing platelets include a slightly higher risk of bacterial contamination than red cells, due to their being stored at 22°C, and the possible risk of alloimmunization due to the presence of a small number of red cell fragments.

In patients with a low platelet count, the cause of thrombocytopenia should be established prior to transfusion. In accordance with the BCSH guidelines, the transfusion of platelets is indicated to prevent and treat haemorrhage in patients with thrombocytopenia or platelet function defects. This product is not usually indicated in ITP (idiopathic thrombocytopenia) and is contraindicated in TTP (thrombotic thrombocytopenic purpura). In patients with bone marrow failure, prophylactic platelet transfusions have been shown to decrease morbidity and in such patients the platelet count should be maintained above $10 \times 10^9/l$ to reduce the risk of haemorrhage. Where the patient is haemorrhaging and receiving a massive blood transfusion, the platelet count should be maintained above $75 \times 10^9/l$. In patients with disseminated intravascular coagulation (DIC), platelets are indicated where bleeding is associated with thrombocytopenia. The more controversial area of platelet transfusion is where thrombocytopenic patients require a surgical procedure. The guidelines state that biopsy may be performed, provided adequate surface pressure is applied, in patients with severe thrombocytopenia without platelet support. For more invasive surgical procedures the platelet count should be raised to $100 \times 10^9/l$ for operations in critical sites such as the brain or eyes, and to at least $50 \times 10^9/l$ for other procedures. Dosage will depend on the required incremental rise, with one adult dose of platelets expected to raise the platelet count by $20 \times 10^9/l$.

Granulocyte preparations

While there is no good data to show that transfusing white cells is clinically effective, some clinicians will use granulocyte preparations for patients with very low neutrophil counts who have an overwhelming infection that is not responding to drug therapy.

Key points

All blood components should only be transfused if there is a clinical indication. Fresh frozen plasma is not to be used as a plasma expander. Platelets should be used to correct a low platelet count in cases of bone marrow suppression or failure, but not for cases of ITP or TTP.

5.4 Blood products

Human albumin solutions

Human albumin solutions (HAS) were first produced in the Second World War as a resuscitation fluid. There is a lot of debate as to their clinical effectiveness. Human albumin solutions were produced from large quantities of pooled plasma which was then fractionated and heat treated. These products have an excellent safety record. Human albumin solutions are usually available as 20, 4.5, or 5% solutions in various volumes. Whilst there is debate regarding the use of these products, with the recommendation that alternatives (crystalloid or artificial colloid) should be used whenever possible. HASs are still used in resuscitation, management of renal disease, replacement fluid in severe hypovolemia, draining of significant ascites, and in burns (although not in the first 24 hours). Whether HAS or artificial colloids should be used will depend on the patient's renal function, sodium/potassium levels, and the risk of oedema.

Factor concentrates

These include Factor VIII, IX; Factor II, VII, IX, and X; prothrombin complex concentrate (PCC) and recombinant Factor VIIa. These products are usually recombinant licensed pharmaceutical products used in the treatment of patients with inherited coagulation deficiencies. Prothrombin complex concentrate and recombinant VIIa may also be used in life-threatening bleeds.

Human immunoglobulins

Immunoglobulins are produced from normal pooled plasma, either to produce a specific immunoglobulin such as anti-D (see below) or non-specific, which can be used to replace immunoglobulins in patients with antibody disorders. Pooled immunoglobulins are provided in intravenous (IVIg) and subcuteanous (SCIg) formats, with the dose being monitored to achieve the required levels of immunoglobulin (IgG) in the patient's serum.

Anti-D immunoglobulin

Anti-D immunoglobulin is prepared from human donors with high levels of alloimmune anti-D antibodies. Preparations are available from a number of companies in a number of different doses. As the use of this product is very specific the manufacturer's instructions must be followed within the guidance given in the British Committee for Standards in Haematology (BCSH) guidelines on the use of anti-D immunoglobulin.

5.5 Special requirements

Irradiated blood components

Cellular blood components potentially contain T lymphocytes and require irradiation prior to administration to patients who may be immunocompromised, in order to prevent transfusion-associated graft versus host disease. Patients with inherited or acquired immune disorders (Hodgkin's disease), patients who have received treatment with purine analogues, individuals who have had a bone marrow/stem cell transplant, unborn babies, and babies requiring exchange transfusion should all receive irradiated cellular products. For more detailed guidance the reader may refer to the relevant British Committee for Standards in Haematology (BCSH) guidelines.

Cytomegalovirus (CMV) negative products

The transfusion of cellular blood components containing lymphocytes has been shown to transmit cytomegalovirus (CMV). Whilst CMV infection tends to be asymptomatic in most individuals it can lead to problems in immunocompromised individuals. Although the risk of CMV transmission is now very low due to the majority of cellular products being leucocyte depleted, it is recommended that components indicated as being CMV negative are issued to vulnerable patients such as pregnant women, neonates, and transplant patients whose CMV status is unknown or who are CMV negative.

5.6 Decision making, who needs a transfusion, risks and benefits

Whilst transfusion can be essential for some patients, blood components are sometimes transfused without understanding the exact clinical benefit. It is important that the normal physiological response to anaemia and/or bleeding, along with the body's ability to produce the cells quickly if necessary are considered in the decision to transfuse. Although transfusion is very safe, particularly in comparison to other risks during a hospital stay, it is not risk free. Therefore, it is very important that a critical approach is taken to prescribing blood products. Where possible, patients must be informed about the benefits, risks, and alternative choices available to them. There is also the issue of managing a valuable, precious, and potentially scarce resource. Blood components and products must be used wisely to ensure sufficient availability for those patients that have life-threatening problems. There are risks to being transfused as highlighted in the annual Serious Hazards Of Transfusion (SHOT) adverse incident reporting scheme reports. Transfusion transmitted infections, acute or delayed reactions due to serological incompatibilities, or receiving blood intended for someone else, as a result of human error, are amongst the risks discussed in these reports. Allogeneic blood components should only be used when there are good reasons to believe that the benefits will outweigh the risks. It is important that there is some clinical benefit to the patient, improving their condition and/or quality of life. Decisions also need to be made about whether suitable alternatives (autologous or pharmacological) are available that may have the same beneficial outcome without exposing the patient to the risks of autologous transfusion, as even when blood is considered safe by current standards it may contain unknown pathogens.

When the patient is bleeding it is very difficult to quantify how much blood is being lost. Blood may be spilt onto bed sheets, drapes, the floor, doctors, nurses, as well as into drains and suction devices often along with other bodily fluids. It is essential that there are good policies and procedures (both clinical and within the laboratory) to manage such patients appropriately and quickly. When significant blood loss occurs, the fall in oxygen carrying capacity, together with the reduction in blood volume, cause a fall in oxygen delivery. If intravenous therapy (crystalloid or colloid) maintains a normal blood volume, an increase in cardiac output may occur, enabling adequate oxygenation of the tissues. The resultant haemodilution reduces the viscosity of the blood, improving capillary flow and enhancing the supply of oxygen to the tissues. Although when the haemoglobin falls below 7 g/dl it is unlikely that increased cardiac output alone will maintain adequate oxygenation of all tissues. In bleeding patients, the decision to transfuse should be based on the clinical condition of the patient (in particular their heart and lung function) and their ability to compensate for a reduction in oxygen supply. However, in surgical patients the duration of the bleeding/anaemia is generally short, with the haemoglobin (number of red cells) expected to rise rapidly in the post-operative period. In medical patients, the anaemia may be expected to remain for months or even permanently. It should be clear that product selection, and transfusion triggers and transfusion regimes will be very different in different patient groups as well as within individual patients within the same patient group.

An example of poor decision making is shown in Table 5.1.

Table 5.1 shows the results of two patients under the care of the gynaecology department. They were both for elective surgery, one for a myomectomy and one for a hysterectomy. Blood taken at a pre-admission clinic four weeks before the operation showed that both patients had a haemoglobin level below ten and both were iron deficient. The patients were

TABLE 5.1 Poor decision making

Pre-op Hb	MCV	Fe deficient?	Operation	Red cells txed	Post-op Hb
9.2 g/dl	66.4	Yes	Myomectomy	1 unit	10.4 g/dl
9.3 g/dl	65.6	Yes	Total abdominal hysterectomy	2 units	11.1 g/dl

transfused intra-operatively and both were discharged with a haemoglobin level higher than it was pre-operatively. These two patients should have received iron therapy prior to their admission for such an elective procedure. It could also be argued that they should not have had a higher haemoglobin post-operatively than they started with, and that the transfusion intra-operatively was unnecessary.

Reducing the need for transfusion

It is important to understand how good communication, adherence to standards, audit, and review of product use will aid the appropriate use of blood components and thus manage this precious resource. Improving practice requires a planned, consistent approach. Unless there is local dissemination and implementation with supportive education a change in practice will not be achieved. So how can inappropriate transfusions be prevented? There are a number of national and local initiatives:

- Adherence to national guidelines when introducing local policies and procedures to ensure appropriate use of the blood products.

- The use of hospital transfusion teams (which include the blood bank manager, a transfusion practitioner, and a medical consultant lead) to give guidance, implement policy, provide an educational and training resource, and audit/review performance.

- The investigation and reporting of errors and near misses both locally and nationally provides data and information which can be used to improve practice. It is a requirement of the Blood Safety and Quality Regulations that all errors and incidents are appropriately reported, with all incidents involving laboratory errors or errors resulting in patient potential or actual harm being reported externally to the Medicines and Health products Regulatory Authority (MHRA).

- Audit is a valuable tool to ensure that the predefined standard of care is being met and that blood component use is appropriate. Audits may be local, regional, or national. Local audits may be used to ensure compliance to local guidelines, whereas participation in national audits allows comparison to other similar establishments. Audits of practice compared to a 'standard' provide clinical staff with relevant information and can aid in education, understanding, and subsequently modifying behaviour.

- It is important that, where possible, patients are well informed of both the risks and the benefits of the treatment they are to receive. It is equally important that they are advised of any alternative treatment options that may be available so that an informed choice may be made about whether they wish to receive a blood transfusion.

- The use of performance indicators, such as those provided by the Blood Stocks Management Scheme (BSMS) allow transfusion teams to monitor product use and product wastage. Whilst this, in itself, may not reduce the number of patients receiving blood, it does provide valuable information on hospital stock levels and wastage, which can be compared to 'national averages', ensuring that individual sites control stocks effectively.

Key points

There are many risks associated with transfusions and these have to be taken into account when deciding whether to transfuse, or use a suitable alternatives.

SELF-CHECK 5.3

Suggest four local/national initiatives which help to ensure the appropriate use of blood and blood products.

5.7 **Alternatives to donor blood**

Appropriately used donor blood is essential for many medical treatments and can save lives. However, donated blood is a limited resource and the potential impact of variant Creutzfeldt–Jakob disease (vCJD) and a decreasing donor population is affecting the blood supply. The health service circulars *Better Blood Transfusion* encourage hospitals to ensure blood transfusion is an integral part of patients' care and that the use of effective alternatives to donor blood and where appropriate, the use of autologous blood is offered to patients. Autologous blood is an individual's own blood, whereas allogenic blood is blood or components from another individual.

The emergence of HIV/AIDS in the 1980s highlighted the need for better screening and made the public more aware of the risks of receiving an allogenic transfusion. However, the development of 'auto transfusion' came from the USA in the early 1970s mainly in response to the growth of coronary artery and other surgeries, leading to an ever-increasing demand for blood. It is possible that oxygen carrying resuscitation fluids may become available within the next few years; however, 'artificial blood' is probably many years away. With a decreasing blood supply (due to the elderly population, 'bird' and other flu viruses, and vCJD) there is an urgent need for successful blood conservation strategies in order to maintain a healthy blood supply for those patients where autologous transfusion is not an option.

Conservation strategies

Some of the strategies for blood conservation in surgical and/or bleeding patients are considered below. Conservation in medical patients is not considered, as strategies are limited and vary greatly depending on the clinical diagnosis and the type of transfusion required.

Early assessment (pre admissions)

An early full blood count assessment and advice on good diet or supplements in the months prior to planned surgery can ensure that when the patient attends for surgery their haemoglobin is at a good level. In patients where iron or B12/folate deficiency is identified, the patient should be sent for assessment and treatment prior to admittance for surgery. Oral haematinics (oral iron or B12/folate supplements) take time to have an effect but are cheap, safe, and effective. The higher the haemoglobin prior to surgery the lower the chance of requiring transfusion of donor red cells. Also required is a planned approach to surgery, for example not taking aspirin or non-steroidal anti-inflammatories, and where possible stopping warfarin.

Near patient haemostatic assessment

The provision of timely biochemistry and haematology results can play a big role in the management of a surgical or bleeding patient. Timely and appropriate transfusion treatment where products are ordered and transfused based on real time results reduces unnecessary transfusion and aids clinical outcome. Instruments such as those in Figures 5.5 and 5.6 can be used to measure Hb and coagulation in the operating theatre.

Surgical and anaesthetic technique

The patient's position, body temperature, type of anaesthesia, surgical technique, and pain management can make a big difference to the amount of blood shed during the surgery.

Fibrin sealants

Fibrin sealants are topical biological adhesives which mimic the final stage of coagulation. These agents, made from human cryoprecipitate, convert fibrinogen to fibrin. The 'kit' consists of concentrated fibrinogen which is activated at the surgical bleeding site by adding thrombin and calcium chloride, and then sprayed onto the site of the bleed, ensuring local haemostasis.

Pre-operative autologous blood donation (PAD)

Although not now used in the UK, this is a system whereby a patient has a standard donation of blood collected every week for up to four weeks before a planned operation. The donations are labelled with the patient's details, tested in the same way as any donor blood and

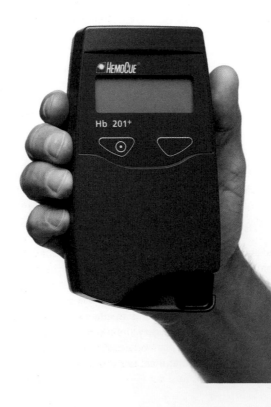

FIGURE 5.5
Picture of a hand-held 'HemoCue'® machine, used for quick haemoglobin assessment close to the patient. (© www.hemocue.com.)

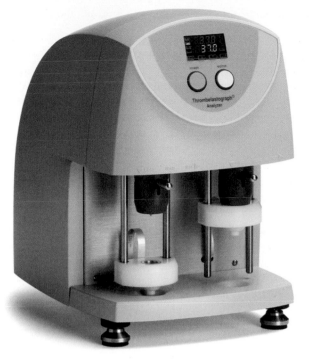

FIGURE 5.6
Picture of a TEG® 500
Thrombelastograph Analyser
(Haemonetics). (© www.
haemoscope.com.)

stored at 4–6°C. If the patient requires blood during or after their operation then these units can be transfused. Although this sounds an attractive proposition, in practice it was difficult to operate and its effect on the supply of allogeneic blood was minimal. It has therefore been abandoned except for patients who might have blood of a very rare phenotype and even for these their blood is usually collected on a regular basis and stored in the National Frozen Blood Bank.

Autologous salvage

Collecting the patient's own blood for return to them during the surgery has advantages in terms of the oxygen carrying capacity of the red cells, reduced risk of transfusion transmitted disease, alloimmunization, and immunosuppresion. There are a variety of ways of collecting the patient's own blood, some of which are outlined below. A combination of these techniques gives the biggest advantage in terms of reducing the need for allogenic transfusion.

Acute normovolaemic haemodilution (ANH) This is collection of the patient's whole blood immediately prior to anaesthesia/surgery, followed by infusion of colloid or crystalloid. Moderate isovolaemia means that the patient bleeds a lower haemoglobin/haematatcrit during the surgery. In patients with normal cardiac function the decrease in blood viscosity means that oxygen delivery is well maintained. The collected units are kept by the patient at room temperature and are re-infused towards the end of the procedure when blood loss is minimal. It has the advantage that no testing is required and the risk of bacterial contamination and/or the wrong blood being given back to the patient is reduced. This technique is considered to complement intra-operative salvage as the units collected have functional clotting factors and platelets. Acute normovolaemic haemodilution can be considered in patients without cardiac impairment, where the surgery is likely to result in significant loss (greater than 20% of the patient's blood volume) and the patient's starting haemoglobin is above 100 g/l. Some Jehovah's Witnesses patients may accept ANH, particularly if the collection and re-administration sets can be set up as a continuous loop, but this would be a matter of personal choice.

Intra-operative salvage (IOS) This system is useful in reducing or eliminating the need to use donor red cells. It is the process whereby shed blood lost during surgery is mixed with anticoagulant and collected into a reservoir. The patient's collected blood is then processed and returned to the patient. The decision to use IOS will be based on a number of factors, including the risk of the patient bleeding, the anticipated blood loss, the site of the surgical field and whether IOS is acceptable to the patient. This technique is usually used in surgical procedures where the blood loss is expected to be greater than 1 litre. Patients with religious beliefs where treatment cannot include the transfusion of donor blood (for example Jehovah's Witnesses) may often accept IOS. It should not be used in circumstances where the patient's shed blood may be contaminated, such as where there is a risk of bowel contents, infection, gastric or pancreatic secretions, or any pharmacological substances entering the system and being re-infused into the patient. In patients undergoing surgery for malignant disease, in obstetrics, or in patients with sickle cell disease careful consideration needs to be given due to the potential risk of malignant cells, foetal contaminants/aminotic fluid being re-infused, or causing a sickle cell crisis. It also must be remembered that where massive bleeding occurs the re-infused product does not contain any clotting factors or platelets. See Figure 5.7.

Post-operative salvage (POS) This is a relatively simple adaptation of existing wound drains. The wound drains are attached to a reservoir and the blood is collected directly into a blood bag within a closed system. When over 400 ml is collected, the bag can be detached from the system and the blood re-infused. This system is useful in patients where there is anticipated, clean post-operative blood loss. The system is of particular use in orthopaedic surgery traditionally for knee replacements. Collected blood must be reinfused within six hours of collection. Contraindications with this system are similar to IOS, such as a contaminated collection site, untrained staff using the system, patients with sickle cell disease, malignancy, and the potential risk of re-infusing activated white blood cells. See Figure 5.8.

Pharmacological approaches to reduce blood loss

Erythropoietin (EPO) Under normal conditions the production of red cells matches the natural loss. This process (erythropoiesis) is regulated by erythropoietin, a natural hormone produced by the kidney. An artificially made EPO (originally used in patients with renal failure) has been used in some patients to increase red cell production, usually either prior to or after surgery.

Intravenous iron (iv Fe) Serious iron deficiency, or where the patient is not responding, or is intolerant to oral iron, may be treated with intravenous iron solutions. Intravenous solutions are often used in combination with EPO to maximize an increase in the haemoglobin.

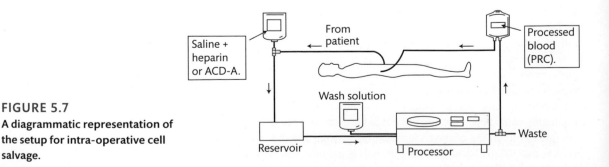

FIGURE 5.7
A diagrammatic representation of the setup for intra-operative cell salvage.

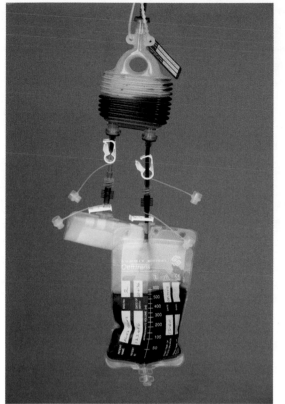

FIGURE 5.8
An example of post-operative salvage, where blood shed after the operation is collected into a blood bag for reinfusion. Picture of CellTrans™ Summit Medical.

Recombinant Factor VIIa Recombinant Factor VIIa works by activating coagulation and platelet adhesion. The product is normally used for the treatment of severe haemophilia. However, recombinant Factor VIIa has been used successfully to control bleeding in patients with life-threatening haemorrhage but, at the time of writing, it is unlicensed for such use. The major concern with using this product is that it can cause thrombosis.

Desmopressin (DDAVP) This drug can promote haemostasis by improving platelet function and release of coagulation factors. It may reduce the need for transfusion although it may have a limited effect if the patient has already lost a significant amount of blood.

Lysine analogues (tranexamic acid)/anti-fibrinolytics These act by attaching to plasminogen and inhibiting the activation of fibrinolysis.

Key points

Various blood conservation strategies are available for a bleeding or surgical patient and these include autologous blood salvage, such as acute normovolaemic haemodilution (ANH), intra-operative salvage (IOS), and post-operative salvage (POS).

SELF-CHECK 5.4

Name four contraindications when considering using intra-operative cell salvage.

5.8 Case history examples

The following case histories have been included as examples of poor practice. Some are based on examples cited in SHOT reports and others have been adapted from real cases from the author's place of work. They have been included to allow the reader to think about where things go wrong.

Inappropriate use of red cells

A pre-dialysis full blood count (FBC) result on a 20-year-old female patient attending for routine renal dialysis due to kidney failure showed her haemoglobin (Hb) was 43 g/l and her haematocrit 13.1%. No comment was made on the results and the patient received two units of red cells. At the following dialysis session two days later, the pre-dialysis FBC results showed an Hb 112 g/l and HCT 29.5%. Review of previous results showed that this young patient's HCT usually ran between 24 and 28%. It was likely that the FBC sample showing an Hb of 43 g/l was diluted, probably being taken from the same arm used for a saline drip. This example shows the need to review previous results before making a decision about transfusion and not basing that decision on just one result.

Timely transfusion and good communication

A 47-year-old male, with a history of non-Hodgkin's lymphoma, presented in the accident and emergency department. Initial bloods showed his haemoglobin as 37 g/l, a reticulocyte count 12.8%, his DAT was positive, and the blood film and blood group serology suggested warm type AIHA (see Chapter 7). It was suspected that the patient had suffered a CVA (stroke) and due to the profound anaemia four units of red cells were requested. Over five hours later the patient had still not received any blood. On investigation it was established that the laboratory had referred the sample to the reference laboratory as they were not able to find compatible blood and were waiting for that 'compatible' blood to arrive. Given the clinical condition of the patient and the need for an immediate transfusion, this was one instance when 'least incompatible', ABO, Rh, and Kell matched units should have been issued, rather than waiting for lengthy investigations to have been completed.

Importance of correctly calculating the dose

A 110 kg, 56-year-old male patient was brought into the accident and emergency department with liver failure and suffering from acute melaena. He had a history of alcohol and drug abuse. His haemoglobin was 79 g/l, platelet count was 90 g/l, PT 21 seconds, APTT 48 seconds, and fibrinogen 0.6. A request for two units of red cells and one unit of cryoprecipitate was made by the attending clinicians and issued by the laboratory. Whilst the request for cryoprecipitate (fibrinogen of <1) was appropriate, the amount requested, particularly in a man of this size, would not have been sufficient.

A four-year-old, 12 kg female patient with neuroblastoma and persistent thrombocytopenia was due to receive chemotherapy. One adult dose of platelets was requested, issued and all of the pack was transfused. The platelet pack contained 310 ml, which was twice the volume required by someone of that weight.

Calculating the amount or volume of a blood component that the patient should receive is very important. Larger patients require large volumes, and smaller patients will require smaller volumes. This is true of all blood components. As well as wasting resources and exposing the patient to unnecessary risks, consideration must be given to maintaining normovolaemia as overtransfusion and undertransfusion can be detrimental to the patient.

Examples of overtransfusion (adapted from data taken from the SHOT reports)

An 80-year-old female patient, with expressive dysphasia, had been to theatre for repair of a fractured neck of femur. Her pre-operative Hb was 95 g/l and there had been little intra-operative blood loss. Eight hours following surgery the patient was noted to be restless, hypotensive, and tachycardic; a repeat full blood count gave an Hb result of 39 g/l. A junior doctor diagnosed hypovolaemia and prescribed six units of red cells, all of which were administered over a 16-hour period. The post-transfusion Hb was 182 g/l; the patient subsequently died from cardiac failure. Investigation revealed that the pre-transfusion sample had been taken from an arm that had an intravenous infusion of saline running and that it was in fact diluted. Again, previous results should have been considered rather than basing the decision on just one result.

 CHAPTER SUMMARY

- Having considered the basic composition and function of blood, particularly the red cells and platelets, it is clear why these blood components are needed for transfusion: red cells to maintain or increase the oxygen carrying capacity of the blood, and platelets to prevent bleeding.

- Other clotting factors can be replaced either by using fresh frozen plasma (FFP) or cryoprecipitate which is rich in fibrinogen and Factor VIII.

- However, transfusion is not without risks, which have to be considered before deciding to transfuse.

- Allogeneic, or donor, blood can, in some surgical operations, be replaced by autologous blood salvaging techniques, such as by collecting blood from the patient either before or during the operation and reinfusing it afterwards.

- There are also some pharmacological approaches to reducing blood loss.

- Blood can be a life-saver but it is not a panacea.

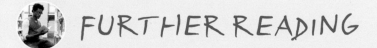 FURTHER READING

- **Contreras M (ed.)** *ABC of Transfusion*, **3rd edition. BMJ Books, London, 1998.**

- **Maniatis A, Linden PV, & Hardy J-F (eds)** *Alternatives to Blood Transfusion in Transfusion Medicine*, **2nd edition. Wiley-Blackwell, Oxford, 2010.**

- **McClelland DBL (ed.)** *Handbook of Transfusion Medicine*, **4th edition. The Stationery Office, Norwich, 2007.**

- **Murphy M & Pamphilon D (eds)** *Practical Transfusion Medicine* **Wiley-Blackwell, Oxford, 2009.**

- **Thomas D, Thompson J, & Ridler B, (eds)** *A Manual for Blood Conservation* **TFM Publishing, Shrewsbury, 2005.**

Blood transfusion is highly regulated with both statutory regulations and professional guidelines. These are constantly being reviewed and for the most up-to-date versions visit the following websites:

- **BCSH Guidelines covering many aspects of blood banking and transfusion: www. bcshguidelines.com.**

- *Handbook of Transfusion Medicine, Guidelines for the Blood Transfusion Services in the United Kingdom*. **Other guidelines, useful information and links: www. transfusionguidelines.org.uk.**

- **MHRA guidance for reporting incidents (SABRE): www.mhra.gov.uk/ Safetyinformation/Reportingsafetyproblems/Blood/index.htm.**

- **Serious Hazards Of Transfusion (SHOT) annual reports: www.shotuk.org.**

- **Network for Advancement of Transfusion Alternatives (NATA): www.nataonline.com.**

- **NHS Blood and Transplant (NHSBT) Blood Matters is a regular publication with up-to-the-minute articles on all aspects of transfusion and transplantation: www. hospital.blood.co.uk/communication/blood_matters/index.asp.**

- **Blood Stocks Management Scheme, monitors the usage of blood and components in hospitals: www.bloodstocks.co.uk.**

- **British Blood Transfusion Society (BBTS) has information and links to other relevant professional bodies: www.bbts.org.uk.**

Answers to the questions in this chapter are provided on the book's Online Resource Centre.

 Go to www.oxfordtextbooks.co.uk/orc/knight

Compatibility Testing and Adverse Effects

Carol Cantwell and Tony Davies

Learning objectives

After studying this chapter you should be able to:

- Describe the process of compatibility testing and how it applies to each type of blood component.
- Describe the various crossmatch methods used in laboratories to determine compatibility.
- Describe and explain when and why each crossmatch method may and may not be used.
- Describe how blood is issued in an emergency.
- Outline the national guidelines regarding pre-transfusion compatibility testing.
- Describe what constitutes an adverse reaction.
- Outline the role the laboratory has in the investigation of an adverse reaction.
- List the actions that might be taken by the laboratory in the event of an adverse reaction occurring.
- Distinguish between the Serious Hazards Of Transfusion (SHOT) reporting scheme and the incident reporting requirements of the Medicines and Healthcare products Regulatory Agency (MHRA).

Introduction

This chapter builds on the knowledge gained from previous chapters and shows how those procedures form a vital part of the process of providing safe blood for the patient. You will learn that compatibility testing is not just one test but a multi-factorial process, starting when the patient has their sample collected and completed when the blood is transfused. Within the laboratory, the process starts with sample acceptance and finishes with the issue of the appropriate red cell, plasma, or cellular product. The safety of the overall process relies on the combined input of many different staff groups.

Unfortunately, even when the compatibility testing process has been performed correctly adverse reactions to transfusion can occur and these can vary in severity from mild to life threatening. However, we can learn by properly investigating these events and collating data on a national basis; this was the basis for setting up the UK Serious Hazards Of Transfusion (SHOT) a haemovigilance system.

In this chapter we refer to a number of UK regulations, guidelines, and recommendations, but these will not necessarily apply in other countries where other regulations might be in place.

6.1 Compatibility testing (serological and non-serological)

Compatibility testing within the laboratory covers the processes by which donor red cells, plasma, or cellular components are either tested or checked to ensure that incompatible red cells, plasma, or cellular components are not issued or released from the laboratory for transfusion to patients.

Compatibility testing is performed using serological and non-serological methods. The purpose of compatibility testing is to minimize the possibility that the component selected will harm the patient, and that when the component is transfused it will have an acceptable survival *in vivo* so as to deliver the desired clinical outcomes. The transfusion of an incompatible blood component may decrease the survival of the transfused red cells or indeed cause a reaction so severe that it can lead to the death of the patient.

Blood transfusion laboratories may use a variety of methods to determine compatibility between donor blood components and a potential recipient. The methods should be compliant with the UK British Committee for Standards in Haematology (BCSH) guidelines for compatibility testing and validated for use within your laboratory. See Figure 6.1.

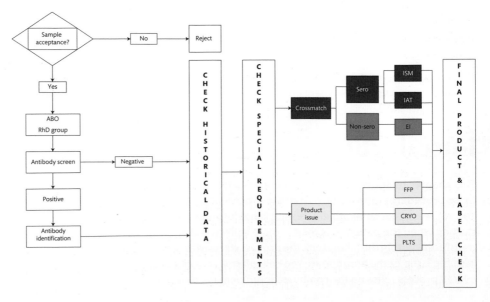

FIGURE 6.1

Blood and blood component compatibility process overview.

Sample acceptance

The integrity of the request and the sample is usually the responsibility of the clinical staff or the phlebotomy team. It is important that blood samples are taken and labelled according to BCSH guidelines and that a system of positive patient identification is used wherever possible. The biggest risk areas affecting the process of compatibility testing are clerical, documentation, or identification failures. In recognition of this fact the UK National Patient Safety Agency state that all staff involved in the transfusion process should be subject to appropriate and regular competency assessment.

All laboratories should have a sample acceptance policy that is known to the users of pathology services. Upon receipt into the laboratory the sample information and request information are checked and compared to ensure that they both contain the following matching minimum data:

- Last (family) name

- First name

- Date of birth

- NHS number/hospital number/accident and emergency number (A&E)/major incident number

The sample must be identified by at least four independent data items to confirm from whom the sample has been taken. The list above shows the national minimum requirements. However, in areas such as Wales where a large percentage of the population have the same family name additional data items are also required.

The person who performs the venepuncture should label the sample. It should also be dated and signed by that person. Samples that do not meet the laboratory's minimum standards should not be processed but dealt with as stated in the individual laboratory's protocol.

In some situations such as trauma calls from A&E, unconscious or confused patients, or during a major incident, the patient's identity may not be known and the sample cannot be labelled with the patient's demographics as described above. However, there must be at least one unique identifier, which may be either, the hospital number, A&E number, or the major incident number. In addition to this, the gender of the patient should be identified on the sample label. An indication of the patient's age is also helpful as this may help with the decision making regarding red cell selection, e.g. K negative for females of childbearing potential. The sample should be labelled by the person who performed the venepuncture and also be dated and signed by that person.

In pre-transfusion testing, the importance of careful checking of samples and requests cannot be over-emphasised.

Age of sample

The sample used for grouping, antibody screening, and crossmatching of red cells should represent as closely as possible the patient's current immunological status. Once an individual has been exposed to foreign red cell antigens they may start to produce antibodies against these antigens. A red cell transfusion is a source of foreign antigens. However, it is not only a red cell transfusion that can cause such an exposure but any transfusion of a product that contains cellular components such as platelets or granulocytes. This exposure can change the patient's immunological status, thus invalidating any previous antibody screen results for subsequent red cell selection. Appropriate timing of samples taken for grouping and antibody screening and crossmatching is therefore critical.

During pregnancy, foetal red cells may be found in small numbers in the maternal circulation. The foetal red cells may differ antigenically from the mother if they express antigens of paternal origin that the mother does not possess. These foreign antigens may stimulate an immune response in the mother. This is why after three days the antibody screen on samples from pregnant women is not considered representative of the woman's current immune status.

The BCSH guidelines advise on the timing of samples in relation to transfusion of red cell components. Each laboratory will have their own documented protocol, based on these guidelines on this subject.

Confirmatory samples

As discussed earlier, the biggest risk with regard to receiving a blood transfusion is that the the wrong patient has been bled. This could lead to a patient receiving blood that has been issued on the basis of the wrong patient's blood results which could lead to an ABO-incompatible unit of blood being transfused. To minimize the risk of this type of error going undetected, it is recommended that before any routine transfusion the laboratory has tested two blood samples on the patient collected at different intervals.

Key points

It is very important that any sample for compatibility testing is taken from the correct patient and correctly labelled at the bedside. When the sample and request form are received in the laboratory they are checked to ensure they meet stringent requirements to ensure errors have not been made.

SELF-CHECK 6.1

Why are pregnant women considered as a special group with regard to the timing of sample collection prior to transfusion?

ABO and D grouping and antibody screening

Pre-transfusion samples are grouped for ABO and D, and also screened for the presence of atypical red cell antibodies using two or three antibody-screening cells by an indirect antiglobulin technique. Patients who have been tested previously within the laboratory have the results of their ABO and D group compared against previous testing results as a further safeguard against sample/patient identification errors. This checking is usually carried out automatically by the transfusion laboratory's information management system (LIMS), and staff are alerted to any discrepancies.

The red cells selected for antibody screening are homozygous for all the major clinically significant red cell antigens, so that even weak antibodies are likely to be detected. If the antibody screening test is positive, further tests will be needed in order to identify the specificity and clinical significance of the antibody or antibodies present. Unless there is an emergency requirement for red cells, the results of the group and the antibody screen and antibody identification must be obtained before blood can be issued. For antibodies that are considered to be clinically significant, for example anti-E, -Fy[a], -K, -S, and -Jk[a], red cell units that have been tested and found negative for the corresponding antigen are selected and cross-matched by IAT (see below). For non-clinically significant antibodies, for example anti-Le[a], random ABO and D compatible units, which have not been specifically antigen typed are crossmatched by IAT.

ABO and RhD group selection of red cells

Whatever crossmatch technique is used the same rules apply regarding ABO blood group selection. It is best to use the same ABO group as the patient. However, this is not always possible. Table 6.1 shows the ABO groups that should be selected in order of preference. When supplies of D negative units are limited, D positive units may be selected for D negative recipients. However, D positive red cells should not be issued to D negative females under 50 years or patients who have or are known historically to have anti-D.

Although group O blood components can be given to those of other ABO groups this practice is avoided if possible as there are limited supplies of group O blood. If group O blood is used, provided it is in additive solution it does not need to be negative for high titre haemagglutinins (see later for full description) as the volume of residual plasma is too small to cause significant haemolysis.

Special requirements

An increasing number of patients have special requirements for the components they require. The following section is not a list of all the possible special requirements and you should always refer to local standard operating procedure (SOPs) or the current BCSH guidelines regarding indications for special requirements.

There are some special requirements that are indicated by the patient demographic. For example, the UK Department of Health requires that children born after 1996, who require FFP should receive pathogen-reduced FFP of non-UK origin, such as methylene blue treated FFP. However, other special requirements can only be known if the requesting clinician provides such relevant clinical information to the laboratory. Special requirements, such as those of irradiated or CMV-negative components, should be indicated on the request form.

Once these special requirements have been notified to the laboratory and recorded on the LIMS, it should bring these, and any demographically mandated requirements, to the attention of the laboratory staff automatically. Ideally, rules should prevent allocation of products that don't meet these special requirements. However, where the LIMS has this rules-based prevention there should be a facility for exceptional issue to override a rule by the use of controlled log-in, passwords, or some other security method. Other non-mandatory but advisable requirements, for example K negative red cell products for women of childbearing age, may be highlighted by the LIMS rules system.

TABLE 6.1 Selection of red cells according to donor and recipient ABO blood group.

Recipient's group	O	A	B	AB
First choice	O	A	B	AB
Second choice	–	O	O	A or B
Third choice	–	–	–	O

Electronic issue

Electronic issue is a *non-serological* method for selecting compatible blood. There is no serological testing performed between the donor red cells and the patient's serum/plasma. Electronic issue is the term given to the issue of red cells by the LIMS comparison of the patient's current ABO D grouping and antibody screen results with both the patient's historical results and the ABO and D group of the donor red cell units.

As the name suggests, this method can only be applied where the process of initial testing is automated and coupled with the electronic transfer of non-manually manipulated results from the analyser to the LIMS. This technique cannot be used if the patient has clinically significant atypical red cell antibodies detected in either the current sample or in an historical sample. This method relies on the principle that any clinically significant antibodies will be detected by the antibody screen and by checking the historical data in the LIMS system.

UK NEQAS found that the use of routine electronic issue in blood transfusion laboratories has increased from 10% in 2002 to 46% in 2009. Undoubtedly, the use of electronic issue is on the increase as more laboratories meet the guideline requirements for electronic issue. There are a number of patient categories where the process of electronic issue is not recommended and a full IAT serological crossmatch should be performed. These patient categories are summarized below:

- Patients who have a positive antibody screen.
- Patients with clinically significant antibodies, whether or not these antibodies are demonstrable in the current sample.
- Patients who have a group manually entered in LIMS.
- Patients where any of the results have been manually manipulated.
- Patients who have received an ABO incompatible solid organ transplant in the past three months due to the possible presence of passenger lymphocytes. Any IgG anti-A or anti-B produced by the passenger lymphocytes will not be detected in the antibody screen.

Advantages

- Simple technique.
- Improved turnaround time for issue of red cells in comparison to IAT technique.
- Decreased reagent and staff costs.

Disadvantages

- As this is a non-serological technique any errors in the ABO, RhD, or antibody screening that would lead to an incompatibility between donor and recipient will not be detected.
- Requirement for automation.
- Requirement for interface between automation and the LIMS.

SELF-CHECK 6.3

What is the potential problem with performing the ABO and RhD testing on the same sample twice and then issuing blood where there is no historical transfusion record for the patient?

Foetal and neonatal K negative crossmatch

Foetal, or intra-uterine, transfusions are only carried out in specialized hospitals where there are very specific procedures for determining compatibility. Neonatal transfusions occur in many more hospitals. The neonatal period is generally defined for transfusion purposes as from birth to four months, as infants rarely produce antibodies until after four months. Antibodies present in the foetus or neonate originate from the mother and it is these antibodies that can affect the compatibility of the foetal or neonatal transfusion. It is therefore appropriate to undertake pre-transfusion testing on samples from both the mother and the neonate, but occasionally this is not possible.

The mother's sample should be tested for:

- ABO and D group
- Atypical red cell antibodies
- Antibody identification if the antibody screen is positive

The neonate's sample should be tested for:

- ABO and D group
- DAT: if positive use monospecific antiglobulin reagents
- The presence of atypical red cell antibodies if no maternal sample available

The blood should be selected by reviewing the results of the above maternal and foetal investigations and should be compatible with the neonate's own ABO and D group. It must also be compatible with any ABO or atypical red cell antibody present in the maternal (neonatal if maternal plasma was not tested) plasma. Generally most hospitals use only group O blood for neonatal transfusions. If the DAT on the neonate is positive, or the mother has a positive antibody screen, blood should be crossmatched by IAT.

If the neonate requires further small volume transfusions then no further serological testing is required until the neonate is more than four months old. After four months of age, because the infant is now capable of producing red cell antibodies, pre-transfusion compatibility testing is the same as for adults.

Emergency issue (including use of emergency group OD negative red cells)

There are life-threatening occasions where red cells are required prior to the completion of all the pre-transfusion and compatibility tests. These occasions are determined by the medical team in charge of the patient not by the laboratory staff. Each transfusion laboratory should have an SOP for this situation based on the BCSH guidelines. In the case of such an emergency, group O, K negative blood may be issued before a blood sample is obtained or tested. If the patient is a female under 50 years then O D negative blood should be issued.

If red cells are to be issued for transfusion prior to completion of all the pre-transfusion tests then the patient's sample should be ABO and D grouped. A reverse group and a repeat cell group (using a different aliquot of the same sample) or an immediate spin crossmatch must be performed before the issue of ABO matched blood. The antibody screen should be performed as soon as possible and if it is negative then it is not necessary to perform a retrospective crossmatch. If time allows keep aliquots of the donor units should the patient's plasma be found to contain an atypical red cell antibody, so that these aliquots can be tested for the relevant antigen that the patient may have an antibody against.

In an emergency situation it is vital that efficient communication is established between the laboratory and the patient's medical team.

Key points

Before blood can be issued for transfusion to a patient it must be crossmatched. The technique used depends on the results of the pre-transfusion testing. If the patient has been grouped twice and there are no atypical antibodies present now or in the past, electronic issue can be used, but otherwise a full serological crossmatch using an IAT is performed.

6.2 Selection of plasma products

HT negative status

In the UK all donations irrespective of the group are tested for high titre anti-A and anti-B and units found to be negative are labelled as 'HT negative'. However, there is no guarantee that these products will not have the ability to cause ABO-related haemolysis, they are just less likely to do so.

Plasma from a non-HT negative donor is capable of causing acute haemolysis if transfused to an ABO-incompatible recipient. This is particularly important in large volume transfusions, transfusions to neonates and children, and transfusion of plasma-rich components such as FFP and platelets.

Fresh frozen plasma, cryoprecipitate, and cryoprecipitate-depleted plasma

Fresh frozen plasma (FFP) and cryoprecipitate (cryo) are plasma products. Compatibility is determined on the basis of the donor and the recipient's ABO group and not by a crossmatch technique. The D status of the recipient is irrelevant as there are only small amounts of red cell stroma present in the product. Red cell stroma is less immunogenic that intact red cells, therefore even in D negative females of childbearing potential D positive FFP, cryo, or cryoprecipitate-depleted plasma can be safely issued.

It is best to use the same ABO group of FFP as the patient. However, this is not always possible. In an emergency situation where the patient's group is not yet known AB FFP can be issued, but this should just be used in an emergency as group AB FFP is in reasonably short supply. Table 6.2 shows the ABO groups that should be selected in order of preference.

When transfusing neonates and children it must be remembered that they have a small blood volume, so even though a small volume is to be transfused in absolute terms this may constitute a large volume transfusion to the child in relative terms. Transfusion of plasma that contains antibodies to their red cells may cause passive immune haemolysis. For infants and neonates, plasma should be free of clinically significant irregular blood group antibodies.

SELF-CHECK 6.4

Why is it preferable to use group A FFP for group B patients and vice versa where ABO-identical FFP is not available?

TABLE 6.2 Selection of FFP according to donor and recipient ABO blood group.

Recipient's group	O	A	B	AB
First choice	O	A	B	AB
Second choice	A	AB	AB	A* HT neg
Third choice	B	B* HT neg	A* HT neg	B* HT neg
Fourth choice	AB	—	—	—

Group O FFP must only be given to group O recipients.
*HT neg—components which test negatively for 'high titre' anti-A,B should be selected. Only suitable for emergency use in adults.
Methylene blue treated FFP (MBFFP) is used instead of standard FFP for patients born after 1 January 1996.

6.3 Selection of cellular components

Platelets

Platelets are a cellular component suspended in plasma. Compatibility is determined on the basis of the donor and the recipient's ABO and D group and not by a crossmatch technique. It is best to use the same ABO and D group of platelets as the patient. However, this is not always possible and in an emergency situation, ABO non-identical units may be given. ABO antigens are expressed on platelets so the recipient's ABO antibodies may react with ABO incompatible platelets which may then have a reduced survival *in vivo*, for example group A recipient transfused with group B platelets would result in the recipient's anti-B reacting with the B antigen on the platelets.

However, using group O platelets for non-O patients should be avoided as much as possible because the donor's anti-A,B will react with the recipients A and or B antigens causing varying degrees of haemolysis. Should this scenario arise, the degree of haemolysis should be mitigated by the use of group O HT negative platelets. Table 6.3 shows the ABO groups that should be selected in order of preference.

TABLE 6.3 Selection of platelets according to donor and recipient ABO blood group.

Recipient's group	O	A	AB
First choice	O	A	AB (only by prior notice)
Second choice	B	B HT neg	A HT neg or B HT neg
Third choice	A	O HT neg	O HT neg

Only units marked as negative for high titre anti-A,B antibodies should be transfused into ABO non-identical but ABO compatible recipients, for example O into A, B, or AB, A into AB, or B into AB. Measurement of high titre antibodies is, however, a guide only, and caution should be observed if large volumes of group O platelets are transfused to non-group O recipients (particularly infants and children) as clinically significant haemolysis may ensue. The use of group O platelets for non-O patients should be avoided as much as possible for this reason.

Human lymphocyte antigen (HLA) matched platelets may, by necessity, be a different ABO group to the patient and only units marked as negative for high titre anti-A,B antibodies (HT neg) should be transfused into ABO non-identical recipients.

Platelet concentrates contain small numbers of red cells. Therefore, D negative platelet concentrates should be given to D negative patients where possible, particularly to females less than 50 years.

Buffy coats/granulocytes

Buffy coats and granulocytes are only transfused in specialized hospitals and usually only to patients with overwhelming infections. They are a cellular component containing red cells and compatibility is determined on the basis of the donor and the recipient's ABO and RhD group and crossmatching. It is best to use the same ABO and RhD group of buffy coats/granulocytes as the patient.

CASE STUDY 6.1 *Group O platelets to a group A patient*

- Three-year-old female with acute lymphoblastic leukaemia (ALL).
- Given one adult therapeutic dose (ATD) of group O apheresis platelets as no group. A available.
- Became unwell.
- Bilirubin rose from 40 umol/l to 102 umol/l.
- Hb fell from 10.2 g/dl to 8.2 g/dl.
- Fully recovered.
- Donation tested positive for 'high titre' anti-A.

6.4 Visual inspection and labelling of the units

The final stage of the compatibility process is the visual examination and labelling of the pack(s). Before any unit is issued it should be checked for the following:

- Leaks at the port or the seams
- Haemolysis in the plasma, if a red cell unit
- Discolouration, if a red cell unit
- Large clots, if a red cell unit
- Turbidity or clumping of the contents if FFP, cryo, or platelets
- It is vitally important to carefully examine all platelet packs as any abnormal appearance may indicate bacterial contamination

If any of the above defects are detected the units should not be issued but returned to the blood service for investigation. After all of the previous checks have been completed the unit(s) are ready to be labelled. The label should be securely attached to the pack and any previous labels should be removed. A compatibility report may additionally be issued by the transfusion laboratory. Any group substitutions or special requirements should be highlighted on this report. The labelled unit(s) and compatibility form, if used, should then be placed in the appropriate storage facility pending collection or return to stock if not required.

6.5 Traceability of blood components

The Blood Safety and Quality Regulations (BSQR) of 2005 require a record to be kept of storage conditions and movements of any blood component, from the time of the original donation, from processing at the supplying blood centre, testing in the hospital laboratory, to the component being transfused or discarded, for whatever reason. Under the terms of the Regulations, hospital transfusion laboratories are required to maintain an accurate record of the final fate of any component that they have issued to patients, transferred to another location, or discarded. Many hospitals are now investing in electronic systems that will track units from the time of receipt in the transfusion laboratory right through to administration at the patient's bedside. Records should also be kept in the patient's notes of the transfusion process and any untoward outcomes, such as a transfusion reaction.

> ### Key points
>
> For components other than red cells and buffy coats a crossmatch is not needed. FFP and cryo are issued on the basis of the ABO group of the donor and the recipient, but they are issued on the basis of the ABO group alone for FFP and cryo. For platelets and buffy coats the RhD group should also be considered.

6.6 Adverse effects of transfusion

As with any medical intervention, blood component transfusion has the potential for both benefit and risk to the patient, and the decision to transfuse in the first place must balance the benefits against the potential risks. Transmission of viral and other infections through transfusion may make the headlines, but the actual risk estimates for the UK in 2010, as reported by the Health Protection Agency, are very small:

- Hepatitis B   1 in 670,000
- HIV   1 in 5 million
- Hepatitis C   1 in 82 million
- HTLV-I   1 in 17 million

Although the risk of getting vCJD is probably very low with a single blood transfusion, the risk of any infection will increase with additional blood transfusions. Within the UK there have been just a handful of cases where patients are known to have become infected with vCJD from a blood transfusion.

Since 1996, there have been 34 cases of transfusion-transmitted bacterial infection reported, of which eight recipients died due to the transfusion. The majority of these cases (28) relate to platelet units, which are particularly prone to bacterial contamination due to the need to store them at 22°C.

Despite careful testing of the donation and the compatibility testing blood components may initiate a reaction when transfused. Non-infectious adverse reactions can be conveniently divided into immune or non-immune, and into immediate or delayed, as shown in Table 6.4.

Adverse reactions can occur due to human procedural error at any stage within the transfusion process and complications may even be due to a necessary constituent of the blood component, such as the citrate in the anticoagulant solution. Transfusion reactions can be classified as follows:

- **Febrile non-haemolytic reactions (FNHTRs)** are relatively common in blood transfusion and are defined as a 1°C or greater temperature rise with or without chills, and sometimes hypotension. They are thought to be caused by HLA or lymphocytotoxic antibodies, or cytokines released from white cells on storage, and so are much less common now that all blood components are leucodepleted before issue. Most symptoms are relatively mild and benign, and transfusion may usually continue if the patient's temperature resolves with antipyretics such as paracetamol.

- **Allergic (or urticarial) reactions** are as commonly reported as FNHTRs and are caused by histamine release when the patient recognizes an allergen in the donor plasma (or vice versa). This causes swelling and raised red welts that may be intensely itchy, and are treated with antihistamine. The majority of allergic reactions are mild and not life threatening, but they may occasionally be severe and may necessitate the provision of plasma-deficient blood components to minimize the risk of reaction.

- **Acute haemolytic reactions** most commonly occur very soon after the transfusion of incompatible red cells. The cells are rapidly destroyed, releasing free haemoglobin and red cell stroma into the circulation. Signs and symptoms can occur within minutes of starting a transfusion, and ABO-incompatible transfusions may be life threatening, causing shock, acute renal failure, and disseminated intravascular coagulation (DIC).

- **Delayed haemolytic reactions** are most often the result of an anamnestic response in a patient who has been previously sensitized against a particular antigen by transfusion, pregnancy, or transplant, and in whom antibody is not detectable during pre-transfusion

TABLE 6.4 Immune and non-immune adverse transfusion reactions.

Immune-mediated adverse events	
Immediate	Delayed
Febrile, non-haemolytic transfusion reaction Acute haemolytic transfusion reaction Allergic reaction Anaphylactic reaction Transfusion-related acute lung injury (TRALI)	Delayed haemolytic transfusion reaction Alloimmunization Post-transfusion purpura Transfusion-associated graft versus host disease (TA-GVHD) Immunosuppression
Non-immune-mediated adverse events	
Immediate	Delayed
Transfusion-associated circulatory overload (TACO) Physical damage to red cells Dilution of coagulation factors and platelets	Iron overload Air embolism

testing. Clinical signs and symptoms are relatively mild compared to acute haemolytic reactions, and any unexplained post-transfusion decreases in haemoglobin in the absence of bleeding should be investigated as a possible DHTR.

- **Transfusion-associated circulatory overload (TACO)** is most frequently caused by the transfusion of too much volume at too fast a rate, leading to congestive heart failure and pulmonary oedema. Patients at particular risk of TACO include young children, elderly patients, patients with cardiac disease, and patients with chronic normovolaemic anaemia.

- **Transfusion-related acute lung injury (TRALI)** is characterized by chills, cough, fever, cyanosis, hypotension, and increasing respiratory distress during, or within six hours of transfusion of volumes of blood components unlikely to cause circulatory overload (as in TACO, above). The most likely mechanism for TRALI is the presence of leucocyte antibodies in the plasma of the blood component, initiating complement-mediated cell damage in the pulmonary capillary network.

- **Iron overload** is a longer term complication of red cell transfusion, also known as 'transfusion haemosiderosis', and patients who are chronically dependent on transfusion therapy are particularly at risk. Accumulated iron begins to affect the function of the heart, liver, and endocrine glands, leading to symptoms including muscle weakness, fatigue, weight loss, jaundice, anaemia, cardiac arrhythmias, and mild diabetes. Removal of accumulated tissue iron stores without lowering haemoglobin levels is achieved by the use of various chelating agents, but another strategy could be to use the freshest possible blood for this type of patient, thus reducing the frequency of transfusion and the donor exposure over their lifetime.

- **Immunosuppression** is a non-specific effect that reduces the activity of the recipient's immune system soon after transfusion of blood components. This may actually be beneficial to the patient, in that transfusion prior to renal transplantation has been shown to result in better graft survival. Alternatively, other studies have shown an increase in post-operative infections in patients who have been transfused.

- **Post-transfusion purpura (PTP)** is an acute episode of thrombocytopenia typically occurring between 5 and 12 days following transfusion of red cells or platelets, associated with the presence in the patient of alloantibodies directed against the HPA (human platelet antigen) systems. The platelet count can drop from normal to below $10 \times 10^9/l$ within 24 hours or less, leading to haemorrhage. Platelet transfusion is not usually indicated unless bleeding is severe, and high dose IVIG is the treatment of choice.

- **Platelet refractoriness** is a failure to achieve a sustained increase in platelet count following a platelet transfusion. In many cases refractoriness may be due to 'non-immune' factors such as platelet consumption due to coagulation defects, increased sequestration of platelets in the spleen, following surgery, or where there is bacterial sepsis. Where there is immune destruction of platelets, it is usually due to the action of HLA class I antibodies, and in such cases satisfactory platelet increments may be achieved by the provision of HLA-selected donations. Less frequently, antibodies directed against human platelet antigens (HPA) may be involved, and it may be necessary to provide HPA-compatible platelet donations in order to achieve satisfactory increments.

- **Transfusion-associated graft versus host disease (TA-GVHD)** is a rare but life-threatening complication of transfusion or bone marrow transplantation caused by engraftment and clonal expansion of viable donor lymphocytes in a susceptible host. Characterized by fever, rash, liver dysfunction, diarrhoea, pancytopenia, and bone marrow hypoplasia occurring less than 30 days after transfusion, mortality has been estimated at greater than 80% and death is generally due to infection or haemorrhage as a result of the bone marrow aplasia. Patients at risk of TA-GVHD, such as those receiving treatment with purine analogues or with congenital immunodeficiency, should be transfused with irradiated cellular components.

- **Anaphylactic reactions** are immediate immune-mediated reactions in which there are systemic symptoms including hypotension, loss of consciousness, shock and, less commonly, death. Around 1 in 700 of the general population are IgA-deficient, half of whom have anti-IgA antibodies, but despite this apparent large risk group, anaphylactic reactions occur relatively infrequently. They are, however, much more likely with plasma-rich products such as FFP or platelets than with red cell transfusions.

Key points

There are a number of causes of adverse transfusion reactions that can be broadly classified as immune or non-immune, and immediate or delayed.

SELF-CHECK 6.5

What are the most common adverse transfusion reactions and how are they caused?

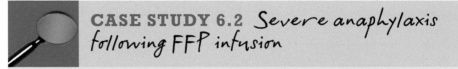

CASE STUDY 6.2 *Severe anaphylaxis following FFP infusion*

- Seventy-five-year-old required FFP for post-operative bleeding.
- Developed anaphylactic reaction with rash, dyspnoea, and hypotension.
- Required CPR.
- Condition improved after treatment over the next 2 ½ hours.

6.7 Monitoring the patient during transfusion

The 2009 BCSH guideline for the administration of blood and blood components and the management of transfused patients, requires hospitals to have a policy for the care and monitoring of patients receiving transfusions. This policy should define the staff responsible for the monitoring of the patient during transfusion, the information to be given to the patient about possible adverse effects of transfusion, and the recording of specific observations during the transfusion:

- Patients should be readily observable by members of the clinical staff while being transfused.
- The start and finish times of the infusion of each unit should be clearly indicated on observation charts.
- Vital signs (temperature, pulse, blood pressure, and respiration rate) should be measured and recorded before the start of each unit of blood or blood component, and at the end of each transfusion episode.
- Temperature and pulse should be measured 15 minutes after the start of each unit of blood or blood component.

Further observations during the transfusion are at the discretion of each clinical area, and need only be taken should the patient become unwell or show signs of a transfusion reaction. Unconscious or anaesthetized patients are more difficult to monitor for signs of transfusion reactions, so should have formal observations taken more often, again at the discretion of the clinical area.

Adverse reactions to transfusion of blood components range from brief episodes of fever to life-threatening haemolysis. The challenge for clinicians lies in recognition of these reactions, especially since the early signs and symptoms, such as fever and chills, may indicate either relatively benign febrile reactions or potentially fatal intravascular haemolysis due to ABO incompatibility.

Making an accurate assessment of an adverse event involves taking a clear history, and recording of temperature, pulse rate, blood pressure, respiratory rate, and oxygen saturation. Few symptoms and signs are entirely diagnostic of a particular type of reaction, but accurate recording will help build a picture of what may be going on, as exemplified with the following examples:

- Mild febrile or allergic reactions which result in a temperature rise of less than 1.5°C above pre-transfusion baseline, rigors, or an urticarial rash are relatively common and rarely need investigation, as long as the patient is more regularly monitored during the transfusion to ensure their condition does not worsen. A greater rise in temperature may indicate a more serious reaction.

- An increase in pulse rate (tachycardia) could be an indication that more serious problems are developing.

- A sudden drop in blood pressure (hypotension) may be seen in bacterial sepsis, acute haemolytic transfusion reactions, anaphylaxis, transfusion-related acute lung injury (TRALI), or citrate toxicity.

- Shortness of breath, excessively rapid breathing and hypoxia may occur as a result of circulatory overload, TRALI, bacterial contamination, anaphylaxis, and acute intravascular haemolysis.

- Swelling (oedema) of the lips, tongue, and airways may be associated with anaphylaxis, whereas swelling of the lower limbs could indicate circulatory overload.

- Chest pain or tightness may occur in circulatory overload, TRALI, and anaphylaxis, while back pain and pain at the infusion site may indicate acute intravascular haemolysis.

- Cramps and muscle pains, along with tingling in the fingers or lips, may be associated with citrate toxicity.

CASE STUDY 6.3 *Inappropriate transfusion of FFP for warfarin reversal results in anaphylaxis*

- Seventy-five-year-old given three units of FFP to reverse warfarin prior to amputation.
- Developed severe anaphylactic reaction, with rash, dyspnoea, and angioedema.
- Admitted to ICU.
- Improved over next two hours.

6.8 Investigation of transfusion reactions

In the event of an acute transfusion reaction being suspected, the transfusion should be immediately discontinued and the IV line maintained for fluid resuscitation if necessary. The patient should be clinically evaluated, monitored and given immediate supportive care as appropriate. The bedside check of the patient identification wristband and pack labelling should be repeated to ensure that an administration error has not occurred and the units should be returned to the transfusion laboratory for investigation. If the patient has received more than one unit of red cells or other components, then all the packs are suspect, not just the one that happened to be infusing at the time the patient's symptoms were noted.

It is important to inform the hospital transfusion team (consultant haematologist, transfusion laboratory manager, and transfusion practitioner) as soon as possible after a suspected reaction, so that appropriate actions and investigations can be carried out. Good communication between the clinical area and the laboratory is essential to ensure effective investigation of suspected adverse reactions to transfusion.

For the laboratory investigation to proceed it is important to obtain a post-transfusion sample for grouping and a direct antiglobulin test, DAT, as well as a sample for a repeat full blood count. In addition to the grouping sample, which is usually anticoagulated to facilitate testing by automated analysers, it is also useful to take a clotted sample. Complement-fixing antibodies such as anti-Jk^a are better detected in serum than in plasma, where the anticoagulant typically celates calcium ions necessary for complement function. It is also of value to examine the first urine passed by the patient following the suspected reaction, as the presence of a dark tinge (haemoglobinuria or bilirubinuria) may indicate a haemolytic process. This may be confirmed by dipstick testing on the ward.

Laboratories should have a standard operating procedure based on current national guidelines for investigating a case of a suspected transfusion reaction, but in general the transfusion laboratory should:

- Check for any clerical, collection, or administration errors that may have occurred.
- Check for signs of visible haemolysis in samples and component packs.
- Investigate any possible serological incompatibility as soon as possible after stopping the transfusion.

The transfusion laboratory must first exclude the possibility of an administrative error, including the possibility that a patient received a component intended for a different recipient. If the investigation implicates a patient identification, issuing, or collection error, then the possibility that other patients are also at risk due to a component mismatch or sample labelling error must be considered and addressed.

It may be decided to ask for fresh samples on all patients received in the laboratory at approximately the same time as, or from the same location as, the suspect sample, and to quarantine all blood components issued at approximately the same time, in order to ensure that blood grouping results are correct, and that components have been correctly labelled.

- Visual inspection of the patient's plasma after transfusion and comparison with a pre-transfusion sample is a sensitive method to detect intravascular haemolysis, as destruction of as little as 5 ml of transfused red cells will produce a reddish tinge indicative of haemoglobinaemia.

- Care must be taken in gross examination, however, as poor sample collection technique, as well as myoglobinaemia seen in severe trauma, burns, or muscle injury may also cause red-tinged plasma unrelated to intravascular haemolysis.

- Icteric (dark yellow/brown) plasma caused by hyperbilirubinaemia may indicate a haemolytic process that has been going on for some hours, or may be a sign of coincidental liver disease.

- The presence of clots, discolouration, or significant haemolysis in the component pack could be consistent with bacterial contamination, and if this is suspected then the local blood service that supplied the component must be notified as soon as possible so that they may quarantine other components from the same donor.

- The DAT has been reported to be positive in 90% of haemolytic transfusion reactions. Where it is negative, it may be that all incompatible cells have already been destroyed and cleared, with associated signs of haemoglobinaemia or haemoglobinuria.

- A DAT should be performed on both the post-transfusion sample and the pre-transfusion sample, if available, for comparison. Where the DAT is positive, elution of antibody from post-transfusion red cells may aid identification, or confirm specificities of antibody detected in plasma or serum.

- Where an acute haemolytic reaction is suspected, the patient's blood group and antibody screen should be retested with both the pre- and post-transfusion samples to ensure that they are the same blood group, and that a weak antibody has not been missed during pre-transfusion screening. If using a serum sample for antibody screening, it is important to use an polyspecific antiglobulin reagent containing anti-C3, as many test systems designed for anticoagulated samples use only anti-IgG.

- Compatibility testing should be repeated using both the pre-transfusion and post-transfusion samples to ensure that all results were correct and to detect any antibody that may now be apparent post-transfusion.

- Where a delayed haemolytic reaction is suspected, it is extremely unlikely that the implicated blood packs will still be available, so a repeat crossmatch with pre- and post-transfusion samples will not be possible. In these cases, it is important to test a post-transfusion sample for the presence of atypical antibodies and perform a DAT. Sometimes it may not be possible to determine the clinical significance of a red cell antibody, or there may be clinical evidence of a haemolytic reaction in the absence of conclusive serology. More specialized tests such as red cell survival studies may be useful in these cases.

- Where an immune antibody has been implicated in a reaction to red cells, it is useful to perform a red cell phenotype on both the pre-transfusion sample and the implicated unit, if still available, to confirm absence of the corresponding antigen in the patient, and its presence in the unit.

- A post-transfusion full blood count may be useful to establish baseline parameters, and it is also possible to identify agglutinated red cells on a film.

- A coagulation screen is useful in monitoring the development of a coagulopathy in either acute haemolysis or infection.

- If bacterial contamination is suspected, then cultures for bacteria and fungi should be performed on both the patient and the implicated component pack(s). The pack(s) should be returned to the laboratory as soon as possible, with giving sets *in situ*, and should be forwarded as soon as practically possible to the blood service for further testing.

- Renal function tests and urinary output are useful measures of the onset of renal impairment and other metabolic disorders. Raised bilirubin, lactate dehydrogenase (LDH), and haptoglobin levels are useful markers of haemolysis, and a low level of ionized calcium is consistent with citrate toxicity.

- In the case of anaphylactic reactions, samples may need to be sent to reference laboratories to test for platelet antibodies, HLA antibodies, or for IgA deficiency and anti-IgA antibodies.

Careful records should be kept of all investigations performed and also of those performed by a reference laboratory as it may be necessary to report the results to SHOT or the MHRA, as detailed in the next section.

Key points

In the event of an acute transfusion reaction being suspected, the transfusion should be immediately discontinued and an investigation initiated. Checks should be made to ensure the correct component is being given to the correct patient. Laboratory testing includes repeating the compatibility testing on a pre-transfusion sample if available and with a freshly collected post-transfusion sample.

SELF-CHECK 6.6

What are the initial laboratory tests to be carried out if a haemolytic transfusion reaction is suspected?

6.9 Haemovigilance in the UK

Haemovigilance is defined as the systematic surveillance of adverse reactions and adverse events related to transfusion, and is aimed at improving safety throughout the transfusion chain from donor to patient. Across the European Union, there is a legal requirement to submit data on Serious Adverse Reactions (SAR) and Serious Adverse Events (SAE) to the EU Commission, under the terms of the European Union Directive 2002/98/EC and Commission Directive 2005/61/EC. These directives have been transposed into UK law as the Blood Safety and Quality Regulations (BSQR).

Serious adverse reaction (SAR)
'An unintended response in a donor or in a patient that is associated with the collection or transfusion of blood or blood components that is fatal, life threatening, disabling, or incapacitating, or which results in, or prolongs, hospitalization or morbidity'.

Serious adverse event (SAE)
'Any untoward occurrence associated with the collection, testing, processing, storage and distribution of blood or blood components that might lead to death or life-threatening, disabling, or incapacitating conditions for patients, or which results in, or prolongs hospitalization or morbidity'.

- **A serious adverse reaction (SAR)** is defined within the regulations as; 'An unintended response in a donor or in a patient that is associated with the collection or transfusion of blood or blood components that is fatal, life threatening, disabling, or incapacitating, or which results in, or prolongs, hospitalization or morbidity'.

- **A serious adverse event (SAE)** is defined as: 'Any untoward occurrence associated with the collection, testing, processing, storage, and distribution of blood or blood components that might lead to death or life-threatening, disabling, or incapacitating conditions for patients, or which results in, or prolongs hospitalization or morbidity'.

Within the UK, the Medicines and Healthcare products Regulatory Agency (MHRA) has been appointed as the 'competent authority' to oversee the regulations on behalf of the Secretary of State. In its regulatory role, the MHRA emphasis is on the quality management systems (QMS) in place in blood establishments and hospital transfusion laboratories, and its legislative remit extends to the point where the transfusion laboratory responsibility ends. The MHRA has to provide total numbers of reactions and events on an annual basis to the EU Commission. To make the reporting of adverse reactions and events more streamlined, the

MHRA have developed a web-based reporting portal, called SABRE (Serious Adverse Blood Reactions and Events).

Hospitals notify and confirm incidents that have occurred, and provide the MHRA with evidence that the incidents have been discussed within risk management structures and that 'corrective and preventative actions' (CAPA) have been put in place to lessen the likelihood of recurrence. This web portal is also used to submit reports to the Serious Hazards Of Transfusion (SHOT) scheme (see below), and hospitals can print a summary of reports submitted to use as evidence of participation for compliance with NHSLA (NHS Litigation Authority) standards.

The Serious Hazards Of Transfusion (SHOT) confidential reporting scheme was launched in 1996 following growing concern amongst UK transfusion specialists, haematologists, and other clinicians that there was little information on the safety of the transfusion process. It collects a wider scope of data than that of the MHRA, extending into the professional and clinical areas of transfusion practice, as well as the part of the transfusion process under the control of the hospital laboratory or blood establishment. SHOT is a professionally led, confidential, voluntary organization that aims to collect anonymized reports from across the UK on adverse events related to transfusion of blood and blood components (red cells, platelets, fresh frozen plasma, cryoprecipitate, granulocytes), and more recently anti-D immunoglobulin and cell salvage.

All cases reported to SHOT are subject to expert scrutiny, to ensure that the data reported is accurate and comprehensive. An annual report and a separate summary leaflet have been published each year by SHOT since 1998 (based on 1996/7 data) in which several general and specific recommendations are made with the aim of improving transfusion safety. Recommendations are targeted at all relevant professional groups, from the four UK Chief Medical Officers, through to each and every member of hospital staff involved in transfusion, as there is the opportunity for everyone to influence the safety of the process.

SHOT findings are used to:

- Aid the production of national clinical and laboratory guidelines for the use of blood.
- Improve standards of hospital transfusion practice.
- Educate users on the hazards of transfusion and their prevention.
- Inform policy within the four UK transfusion services and via the EU Commission.
- Identify new trends in adverse events and stimulate research.

What is reportable?

- Serious adverse reactions are reportable to both the MHRA and to SHOT, regardless of where in the transfusion process the error originated.
- Serious adverse events are reportable to the MHRA if they fall within the responsibility of the blood establishment or hospital transfusion laboratory quality system. Adverse events involving clinical staff, or involving a blood product such as anti-D immunoglobulin, are not reportable to the MHRA, but should be reported to SHOT.

More reported incidents fall into the incorrect blood component transfused (IBCT) category than any other. This includes all reported episodes where a patient was transfused with a blood component or plasma product that did not meet the appropriate requirements or which was intended for another patient. Incorrect blood component transfused also includes inappropriate or unnecessary transfusions: cases where the intended transfusion is carried out, and the component itself is suitable both for transfusion and for the patient, but where the decision making is faulty. Handling and storage errors are cases of transfusion of a

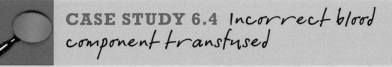

CASE STUDY 6.4 *Incorrect blood component transfused*

- A unit of group A RhD positive blood was correctly checked and collected from the blood bank by a healthcare assistant.
- The blood was taken to the ward and handed to a staff nurse.
- The 'bedside' check was completed in the treatment room but unfortunately the nurse then connected the unit to the wrong patient, who was group O RhD positive.
- The patient suffered an acute haemolytic reaction, requiring supportive therapy and prolonged hospital stay, but made a full recovery.

correct component to the intended patient, but where handling or storage errors may have rendered the component less safe for transfusion.

There have been some important trends in reporting since 1996. These include:

- A decrease in the number of ABO incompatible transfusions erroneously administered from a high in 1997–1998 of 41 ABO incompatible transfusions to a low of 8 ABO incompatible transfusions in 2006.
- The number of cases in which blood of the wrong group was transfused to a patient, or where blood was transfused that was intended for another patient has actually not increased over the years, fluctuating between 16–80 cases per year. Initiatives which may have had an impact on the incidents of ABO incompatibility and wrong blood include *Better Blood Transfusion* and the role of hospital transfusion practitioners, the NPSA (National Patient Safety Agency) Safer Practice Notice 14 'Right Blood Right Patient' and data from the National Comparative Audit.
- Mortality and morbidity: overall mortality rates have dropped, with only one case of mortality definitely related to transfusion in both 2007 and 2008. Episodes of major morbidity have also gradually reduced.
- The incidence of TRALI peaked in 2003 with 36 cases, but reached an all-time low in 2006 with just 10 cases but 17 were reported in 2008. This trend coincided with the introduction of male only plasma for FFP and for suspension of pooled platelets, where possible, in an attempt to reduce the number of TRALI cases.
- The incidence of TTI has also tailed off from 14 proven cases in 1996–1997 down to just 2 cases in 2006 and 6 in 2008. This is due to the cumulative effect of new generations of microbiological testing, as well as initiatives to reduce bacterial contamination such as improved cleaning of the donor arm and diversion of the first 20 ml of blood at donation.
- Transfusion-associated graft versus host disease (TA-GVHD) has reduced in incidence from four cases in 1996–1997 to one case in 2000–2001 with no cases in the subsequent years. This is likely to be the direct effect of universal leucodepletion which was commenced in the UK in November 1999. However, it should be noted that one of the cases occurred post leucodepletion and that therefore leucodepletion cannot be considered as eliminating all risk of TA-GVHD.
- The incidence of ATR remained steady over the ten-year period until 2006–2007 when the number of cases increased. This is likely to be a direct result of the influence of the

CASE STUDY 6.5 Severe allergic reaction leading to cardiac arrest after platelet transfusion

- Fifty-six-year-old given a dose of pooled platelets pre-operatively.
- Developed a rash and became hypotensive under anaesthetic, followed by cardiac arrest.
- Successfully resuscitated.
- Vital signs returned to normal after 30 minutes with treatment.
- Decided to use washed platelets in future.

blood safety and quality regulations which require that all serious transfusion reactions are reported.

- The incidence of delayed haemolytic transfusion reactions has not significantly altered over the ten-year reporting period.
- There has been an increase in the number of handling and storage errors reported that may also have been influenced by the BSQR 2005.
- Inappropriate and unnecessary transfusions have also increased in the last few years. This may be the effect of increased awareness of this as a major risk for patients.

The figures show that SHOT has been working effectively as a haemovigilance system; although it has seen an increased rate of reporting over the years the rate of the most severe category

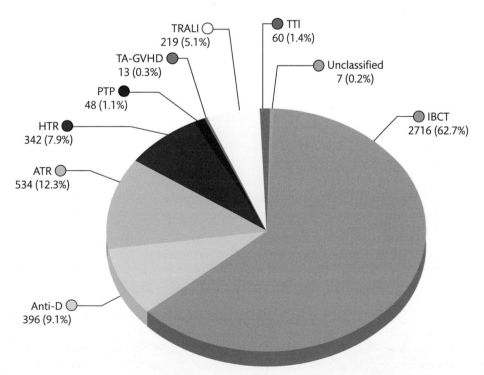

FIGURE 6.2
Cumulative number of cases reported to SHOT 1996–2007 (before 2006 the HTR category was referred to as delayed haemolytic transfusion reactions).

of adverse events and reactions is dropping. This shows that there is increased awareness of safety issues for patients and an improved culture of reporting. Although the advent of the BSQR may have been a slight setback, overall reporting to the haemovigilance systems, SHOT, and MHRA, has increased, and SHOT anticipates an increase in reporting of true SHOT incidents in the coming years as the value of haemovigilance becomes more and more apparent, and the web-based reporting systems enhance access for users. See Figure 6.2.

Key points

Haemovigilance is the systematic surveillance of adverse transfusion reactions and events, and collating data on these to improve safety throughout the transfusion chain from donor to patient.

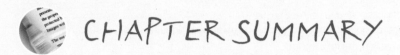

CHAPTER SUMMARY

- Compatibility testing ensures that the correct blood component is selected for a patient and that the correct tests have been performed and compared with any historical results for that patient.

- Pre-transfusion testing consists of ABO and D grouping plus an antibody screen.

- In the absence of atypical antibodies then an immediate spin crossmatch can be used, or the blood issued electronically.

- If an antibody is present then blood that is antigen compatible should be crossmatched by IAT.

- Even if the compatibility procedures have not identified any incompatibility then the recipient may have an adverse reaction when transfused; this could be immune or non-immune, immediate, or delayed.

- Laboratory investigation of suspected reactions includes re-testing pre-transfusion and post-transfusion samples plus further tests, depending on the nature of the reaction.

- Reactions can be classified as either a serious adverse reaction (SAR) or a serious adverse event (SAE).

- Serious adverse reactions are reportable to both the MHRA (SABRE) and to SHOT, regardless of where in the transfusion process the error originated. Serious Adverse Events are reportable to the MHRA.

- Since SHOT started collecting data in 1996 the overall trend has been towards safer transfusions, with fewer cases of death directly associated with transfusion and an increased awareness of the pitfalls of the transfusion process.

- The aim is: right blood to the right patient at the right time.

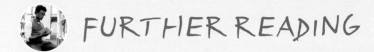

FURTHER READING

For the most up-to-date versions of statutory regulations and professional guidelines visit the following websites:

- **BCSH Guidelines for compatibility procedures in blood transfusion laboratories: www.bcshguidelines.com.**

- **Handbook of Transfusion Medicine: www.transfusionguidelines.org.uk.**

- **MHRA guidance for reporting incidents (SABRE): www.mhra.gov.uk/Safety-information/Reportingsafetyproblems/Blood/index.htm.**

- **Serious Hazards Of Transfusion (SHOT) annual reports: www.shotuk.org.**

- **Blood Stocks Management Scheme, monitors the usage of blood and components in hospitals: www.bloodstocks.co.uk.**

- **NHS Blood and Transplant (NHSBT) Blood Matters is a regular publication with up to the minute articles on all aspects of transfusion and transplantation: www.hospital.blood.co.uk/communication/blood_matters/index.asp.**

- **British Blood Transfusion Society (BBTS) has information and links to other relevant professional bodies: www.bbts.org.uk.**

Answers to the questions in this chapter are provided on the book's Online Resource Centre.

 Go to www.oxfordtextbooks.co.uk/orc/knight

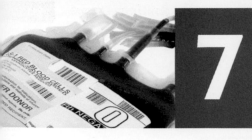

7

Immune Red Cell Destruction

Robin Knight

Learning objectives

After studying this chapter you should be able to:

- Describe the difference between intravascular and extravascular haemolysis.
- Describe the role of antibodies and complement in red cell destruction.
- Outline the clinical significance of red cell antibodies.
- Describe the use of the direct antiglobulin test.
- Outline the causes of haemolytic transfusion reactions.
- Outline the types of autoimmune haemolytic anaemias and the problems associated with finding compatible blood.
- Describe the causes and investigation of haemolytic disease of the foetus/newborn.

Introduction

In this chapter we will look at how and why red cells are destroyed in the body, *in vivo*, by antibodies. This can happen in the following situations, and each will be considered after some general information about red cell mediated haemolysis.

- Transfused red cells destroyed by an antibody the individual has produced—a haemolytic transfusion reaction.
- Patient's red cells destroyed by antibody in transfused plasma, for example anti-A/B in group O platelets given to group A patient.
- An individual's red cells being destroyed by an autoantibody they have produced—autoimmune haemolytic anaemia (AIHA).

- An individual's red cells destroyed by an antibody derived from donor lymphocytes in a transplant, or transplanted donor red cells being destroyed by an antibody from/ in the recipient.
- Foetal red cells destroyed by a maternal antibody—haemolytic disease of the foetus/ newborn (HDN).

7.1 What is immune (antibody mediated) red cell destruction?

The result of an interaction between an antigen on the red cell and an antibody can be the destruction of that red cell, but it is not the antibody itself that causes that destruction, rather it acts as a trigger for other mechanisms, such as the complement pathway **or** macrophages **in the liver or spleen.** The role of antigens, antibodies, and their interaction with the complement system and macrophages was considered in Chapter 1. In summary, antibodies binding to their appropriate antigen on a red cell can lead to the destruction of that cell by one of two ways **intravascular lysis** or **extravascular lysis**.

Antibodies, usually IgM, which activate the complement pathway and lyse the red cells within the circulation (intravascular haemolysis) are mainly anti-A, anti-B, and particularly anti-A,B. Most deaths resulting from the transfusion of incompatible blood are associated with these strongly *lytic* antibodies. Most IgG antibodies, however, bring about red cell destruction outside the circulation (extravascular haemolysis). The IgG antibody molecules on the cell surface are recognized by macrophages, mainly in the spleen, and it is these cells that remove the antibody-coated cells from the circulation.

The binding of both IgM and IgG antibodies can lead to various immune mediators being activated, such as C3a and C5a, and it is these that cause most of the symptoms associated with increased red cell destruction. The clinical signs and symptoms that might be seen in a haemolytic transfusion reaction include some, or all of the following:

- Fever (>1°C rise in temperature)
- Flushing of the face
- Chest pain
- Lumbar back pain
- Hypotension (low blood pressure)
- Nausea

If the cell destruction is very brisk, such as in an ABO incompatible transfusion, other clinical symptoms might include:

- Haemoglobinuria (Hb in the urine)
- Anuria—renal damage (not passing urine)
- Unexplained bleeding, such as disseminated intravascular coagulation (DIC)

The anaphylactic and chemotactic action of the complement fragments, C3a and C5a, and the pro-inflammatory cytokines are the main effectors of these symptoms. C3a causes the constriction of gut and bronchial smooth muscles that results in the classical symptoms of a

Intravascular lysis
Cells being lysed within the circulation by antibodies that activate the complement pathway, especially anti-A and anti-B.

Extravascular lysis
Immune mediated cell removal that takes place outside the circulation in the liver or spleen.

haemolytic reaction of chest and lumbar back pain. C3a can also lead to tachycardia by constricting the blood flow to the heart. C5a is chemotactic for phagocytes and neutrophils as well as stimulating the pro-inflammatory cytokines, Interleukin-1 (IL-1), IL-6, IL-8, and tumour necrosis factor α (TNF α).

Rapid intravascular red cell destruction, due to ABO incompatibility, for example, rapidly stimulates the release of high levels of TNF α, followed by a more sustained production of interleukins (principally IL-1) and monocyte chemoattractant protein -1 (MCP-1). By acting to release histamine from basophils, and activation of T and B lymphocytes, these molecules produce the effects of fever, hypotension, and shock.

IgG antibodies, that lead to extravascular lysis, also stimulate the release of IL-8, IL-1, and IL-6, but again in a sustained manner, with elevated levels still being detectable 24 hours after the original stimulus. IL-1 leads to a raised body temperature (fever) and hypotension, whereas IL-6 will activate T cells and induce B cells to become antibody-producing plasma cells. These cytokines can also activate the fibrinolytic pathway, which might lead to DIC or cause the renal circulation to be reduced. If this is not treated quickly, it can lead to renal failure, one of the commonest sequelae of haemolytic transfusion reactions.

If blood samples were taken soon after a haemolytic episode and analysed in the laboratory the findings might include:

- Fall in Hb
- Fall in haptoglobins (Hp)
- Presence of spherocytes
- Raised reticulocyte count
- Rise in bilirubin
- Rise in serum lactate dehydrogenase (LDH)

These results are easily explained. As red cells are destroyed or removed from the circulation quicker than they can be replaced, then the Hb level falls. Haemoglobin released into the circulation from the red cells binds with Hp, which carry it to the liver, where it is broken down with the globin chains forming bilirubin, hence the increased levels of bilirubin. Raised levels of the liver enzyme LDH are often associated with haemolysis. Spherocytes are formed when IgG-coated cells bind to macrophages in the spleen, but instead of being fully ingested, the macrophage only removes a section of the cell membrane. The cell is then released back into the circulation as a spherocyte, but with a greatly reduced half-life. If lysis is very brisk, such as in intravascular destruction, the Hb might be found free in the plasma or urine. Once bound to albumin, it appears as the distinctively brown-coloured methaemalbumin.

Key points

When antibodies combine with antigens *in vivo*, they can activate complement and cytokines that, in turn, lead to the symptoms seen in haemolytic reactions.

SELF-CHECK 7.1

What is meant by 'intravascular' and 'extravascular' haemolysis?

7.2 Clinical significance of red cell antibodies

Do all antibodies cause red cell destruction? The simple answer is 'no', but all have that potential if the right conditions exist. In general, an antibody, if capable of causing red cell destruction *in vivo*, is considered to be clinically significant. There are a number of factors which contribute to the destructive potential of an antibody, including:

- Immunoglobulin class (IgM or IgG)
- IgG sub-class
- Complement activation
- Activity at 37°C
- Blood group antigen specificity
- Number of antigen sites per cell
- Number of antibodies bound per cell
- Equilibrium constant of antibody
- Presence of 'blood group substances' (antigens) in plasma
- Activity of the recipient's reticulo-endothelium system (RES)

As a general rule, antibodies that are reactive at 37°C and are detectable by an antiglobulin test are considered to be 'clinically significant'. Those that fail to react at 37°C are considered to be clinically insignificant, but, as with any biological system, there are exceptions.

The specificity of an **alloantibody** (e.g. is it anti-D or anti-K?) is the main indicator as to its potential significance, and this is based on reports in the literature of these antibodies having caused *in vivo* cell destruction, either HDN or transfusion reactions. Therefore, antibodies to most of the major blood group antigens within the Rh, Kell, Duffy, and Kidd blood group systems and the Ss antigens are considered significant. Antibodies that react at temperatures below 37°C to Lewis, P, and N antigens, for example, are not significant. There are, of course, some antibodies that fall outside this clear definition, the most notable being anti-M; some examples react by IAT, others do not.

> **Alloantibody**
> An antibody that reacts with a foreign antigen, usually stimulated by red cells that have been transfused or as the result of a foetal-maternal haemorrhage.

Most IgM naturally acquired, T cell independent, antibodies react only by direct saline agglutination techniques in the cold—some might react at 'room temperature', but few react above 30°C. The major exception being the ABO antibodies and anti-H, as found in O_h phenotype individuals.

Therefore, most **clinically significant antibodies** are IgG, but they do not usually cause intravascular haemolysis. However, there are four subclasses of IgG, 1–4, and only IgG1 and IgG3 are recognized by splenic macrophages, leading to extravascular red cell removal. Although most antibody specificities are composed of a mixture of all four IgG subclasses, IgG 1 and 3 predominating, some antibodies are composed of just IgG2 and/or 4, therefore they are not clinically significant.

> **Clinically significant antibody**
> An antibody capable of causing red cell destruction *in vivo*.

The rate of cell destruction is dependent on the number of antibodies bound to each cell, and this in turn, is influenced by the number of antigens available on the red cell surface to which the antibodies can bind, and how well those antibodies do bind (the equilibrium constant). There is evidence that 100 IgG3 antibody molecules per red cell can lead to the recognition and removal of that cell by macrophages, whereas it takes 1,000 IgG1 molecules per cell to produce the same degree of cell destruction.

Some antigens found on red cells are also found in the plasma, for example Lewis, or, as is the case with Chido and Rodgers antigens, associated with complement C4. If these are present in the plasma of blood being transfused to someone with the corresponding antibody, then that antibody will preferentially bind to the non-red cell antigens. There will then be little or no antibody bound to the transfused cells, which will then not be destroyed.

As most IgG-coated cells are removed by the spleen, then in a patient who has an enlarged spleen, the cell destruction can be increased above normal. But if the patient has a defective spleen, or it has been surgically removed (splenectomy), then the major site for the removal of IgG-coated cells is absent, and they will have a longer survival time.

Sometimes knowing just the specificity of the antibody, or mixture of antibodies, and that it reacts by IAT, is not sufficient to tell if it will be significant *in vivo*. Therefore, one or all of the following additional investigations can be performed:

- Determining the antibody's IgG sub-class by using specific antiglobulin reagents
- A titre to find the antibody potency
- The thermal range over which the antibody reacts (e.g. does it react at 37°C?)
- Cellular assays, using macrophages *in vitro*, to assess if the antibody will be recognized by macrophages *in vivo*
- *In vivo* cell survival by injecting a small volume of red cells that have been labelled with Cr^{51}, and measuring how long these cells remain in the circulation

Key points

Although most antibodies have the potential to cause red cell destruction, those that do not react at 37°C by the antigolbulin test are unlikely to be clinically significant.

Antibodies reactive at 37°C that are unlikely to be clinically significant

As stated above, the general rule is that red cell antibodies that do not react *in vitro* at 37°C are regarded as clinically insignificant, as they do not lead to increased red cell destruction *in vivo*. But, is the converse true—are all antibodies that react at 37°C significant? Clinical experience (supported by many publications) has shown that several alloantibodies reactive at 37°C do not cause haemolysis of serologically incompatible cells *in vivo*.

IgG antibodies that react with epitopes on the C4 component of complement are not uncommon, and are usually anti-Ch1 ('anti-Chido') or anti-Rg1 ('anti-Rodgers'). These antibodies can be neutralized by using inert, ABO compatible plasma. The termed neutralized is slightly misleading, as it is not the antibody itself that is neutralized, but its apparent activity against red cells is *inhibited*. As stated above, an antibody will more readily react with a non-cell bound antigen; in this case the C4 molecule that is abundant in plasma. Red cells take up C4 in a non-specific manner, especially those stored *in vitro*. One way of assigning the specificity is using red cells coated with C4, which will react strongly with these antibodies. Inhibition, or neutralization, is a simple method for ensuring other alloantibodies present are detected and identified, and for crossmatching to be undertaken.

The CR1 (complement receptor 1, or CD35) protein on the red cell surface carries the Knops blood group antigens. The antibodies usually exhibit so-called *high titre, low avidity*, or HTLA, characteristics, as the antibodies react weakly, but when the serum is titrated they are active at quite high dilutions. Although the antibodies are invariably IgG, reacting by IAT, they are clinically insignificant.

Some patients' serum contains antibodies that react with the small number of HLA class 1 antigens present on all normal red cells; these were often referred to as Bg antibodies. Although a specificity can sometimes be assigned, usually these antibodies react with most panel cells, but they, too, are clinically insignificant.

The common feature of these IgG IAT reacting, but clinically insignificant antibodies, is that they react with the red cells of almost all individuals; therefore, they 'get in the way' when investigating a blood sample for the presence of antibodies that are clinically significant. A variety of methods, such as inhibition with inert serum, or treating the cells with dithiothreitol (DTT) can be used to eliminate their reactivity.

Antibodies that react only by an enzyme technique are generally considered to be clinically insignificant for transfusion purposes and indeed, some examples of anti-E have been shown to be non-red cell immune or naturally-acquired. However, developing Rh antibodies are often first detected by enzyme techniques, and examples have been reported where such antibodies have increased in strength, become reactive by IAT and have caused HDN. But for routine antibody screening, the use of enzyme techniques is not recommended in the UK.

Key points

Not all antibodies that react in the IAT at 37°C are clinically significant; knowing the specificity of the antibody will help decide which are likely to be significant.

SELF-CHECK 7.2

Why are some antibodies not considered to be clinically significant?

Direct antiglobulin test

If a case of immune red cell destruction is suspected, then the test most widely used is the direct antiglobulin test (DAT). In this test, the red cells from the person being investigated are tested *directly*, without having to incubate cells and plasma as in the indirect antiglobulin test, with antiglobulin reagents to see if the cells are coated with antibody, IgG, IgM, or IgA, and/or complement (C3 or C4). Gel/column cards are available commercially for performing a DAT that include monospecific anti-IgG, anti-C3c, anti-C3d, anti-IgA, and anti-IgM reagents. By using these, all the key players in red cell destruction are covered. However, a positive DAT, in itself, is not diagnostic of an increased rate of red cell destruction *in vivo*, as there also has to be other evidence, such as a low Hb, raised reticulocyte count, reduced Hp, raised bilirubin, and/or raised LDH.

7.3 **Haemolytic transfusion reactions**

Despite all the pre-transfusion tests that are performed to detect antibodies in the recipient's blood and to select compatible blood, some patients have a reaction to their transfusion, which can be haemolytic. Patients being transfused should be closely monitored for temperature, pulse, and blood pressure, and if there are any significant changes to any of these, then a reaction should be suspected. See Chapter 6 for a more detailed account.

A patient might react to transfused blood almost as soon as the drip has started—an immediate reaction, or the onset of the reaction might be delayed for some hours, or days, after the transfusion—a delayed reaction. Immediate reactions are usually caused by ABO incompatibility, such as wrongly giving group A red cells to a group O individual. There are also cases reported of these reactions occurring when group O platelets are given to a group A or B patient, where the platelet preparation contains high titre anti-A/B. ABO incompatible transfusion reactions are usually accompanied by the classical symptoms, as detailed above, fever, lumbar pain, etc. Once suspected or recognized, the transfusion must be stopped and replaced by a saline drip to help maintain kidney function. Further blood transfusion must not be given until the cause of the reaction is known.

Delayed reactions are often not noticed until 5–8 days after the transfusion has been given, when a fall in Hb is noted. Usually, there are no other signs to alert medical or nursing staff, although sometimes fever is reported. In these cases, an antibody stimulated by a previous sensitizing episode, a pregnancy or transfusion, is present at the time of the transfusion, but at low levels, not detectable in the pre-transfusion testing. A secondary immune response follows the transfusion and, as the antibody level increases, the incompatible red cells become coated with antibody and are removed from the circulation. Red cells thus coated will give a positive DAT, but as the transfused cells disappear, the DAT becomes negative and antibody appears in the plasma. Whilst the DAT is positive, but before there is free antibody in the plasma, it is usually possible to make an eluate (remove antibody from the cell surface) to test to find its specificity. Should the patient need a transfusion at this time, it is essential that the red cells transfused are compatible with the antibody causing the haemolysis, the antibody eluted from the red cells.

Reports sent to the UK Haemovigilance Scheme, SHOT, show that anti-Jk[a] is associated with delayed haemolytic transfusion reactions (DHTR) in 75% of cases; other antibodies implicated include anti-c.

Clinical correlation

Hyperhaemolysis
Characterized by marked reticulocytopenia (a significant decrease from the patient's usual absolute reticulocyte level) hyperbilirubinemla, and haemoglobinuria.

Hyperhaemolysis is a rare complication of transfusion, which has been mainly reported in patients with sickle cell disease (SCD). It has also been referred to as the sickle cell haemolytic transfusion reaction syndrome. It is characterized by the destruction of both the transfused, usually serologically compatible red cells and those of the recipient. This condition is marked by the post-transfusion Hb falling to below that found pre-transfusion, together with a low reticulocyte count. The DAT is usually negative and no red cell antibodies incompatible with the units transfused are found. Further transfusion can exacerbate the haemolysis or even be fatal; therefore, it is important that this condition is recognized early and treatment with steroids and/or intravenous immunoglobulin (IVIG) started as soon as possible.

The exact mechanism for hyperhaemolysis is not known, but two have been postulated:

- Bystander lysis, in which an antibody, not necessarily a red cell antibody, but possibly HLA, activates complement, which attaches to both the transfused and the recipient's own cells, leading to their destruction.

- Hyperactive macrophages, in which both donor and recipient red cells are destroyed by these cells.

Key points

Haemolytic transfusion reactions can happen immediately blood is transfused, usually because of ABO incompatibility, or might be delayed and not noticed for several days, as is the case with most incompatible IgG antibodies.

SELF-CHECK 7.3

Define the terms 'immediate' and 'delayed' transfusion reactions, and give examples of both.

7.4 **Autoimmune haemolytic anaemias**

Some patients produce **autoantibodies**, directed against their own red cells, which can lead to an increased rate of cell destruction—an autoimmune haemolytic anaemia (AIHA). These differ from red cell alloantibodies, produced as a result of transfusion and/or pregnancy, which do not destroy the individual's own cells, only those of a different blood group. Although the autoantibodies do react with antigens on the patient's own red cells, the actual specificity of the antibody, or the exact antigen involved, is often difficult to determine. These autoantibodies not only react with the patient's own cells, but also the red cells of most other people, thus presenting a dilemma when trying to find compatible blood for transfusion.

Autoantibodies
Antibodies directed against antigens on one's own cells, which can lead to an increased rate of cell destruction as in autoimmune haemolytic anaemia.

Autoimmune haemolytic anaemia is a relatively rare condition, usually found secondary to other clinical disorders, especially haematological malignancies. Patients with AIHA may present on admission with a very low Hb, sometimes <5 g/dl, and require an immediate transfusion to maintain their Hb until other treatment has time to suppress the increased rate of red cell destruction. A positive DAT helps with the diagnosis of these cases, but, as stated above, is not diagnostic on its own, as other indicators of increased red cell destruction should be present. Autoimmune haemolytic anaemias can be divided into four categories; see Table 7.1:

- Warm AIHA
- Cold AIHA
- Paroxysmal cold haemoglobinuria (PCH)
- Drug induced/associated

Autoantibody immune cell destruction is not confined to red cells, both autoimmune and drug-associated immune destruction of platelets can also occur.

Warm AIHA

Warm AIHA is the most common, so called, because it is caused by an IgG autoantibody that reacts more readily at 37°C, than at lower temperatures. Sometimes, the C3 component of complement is also present on the patient's red cells. Therefore, the DAT is positive with anti-IgG and sometimes anti-C3 as well. If the red cells are coated with IgG, destruction takes place in the spleen, but if complement has been activated there might be some more rapid cell destruction in the liver.

In some cases IgM or IgA antibodies may be found in addition to IgG, and very rarely IgA might be present on its own. It is only by using a monospecific anti-IgA reagent that these

TABLE 7.1 Immunoglobulins and complement (C3) on red cells in cases of autoimmune and drug-related haemolytic anaemias.

AIHA type	IgG	C3	IgA	Notes
Warm AIHA	+	+	(+)	IgA sometimes present
Warm AIHA	+	+	(+)	IgA sometimes present
Warm AIHA	−	+	−	In 10% of cases
Warm AIHA; IgA	−	−	+	Rare
Cold haemagglutinin disease	−	+	−	High titre cold reacting antibody
PCH	−	+	−	D-L antibody (gG anti-P)
Drug adsorption	+	(+)	−	e.g. penicillin
Drug immune complex	−	+	−	e.g. phenacetin
Drug independent	+	(+)	−	e.g. methyldopa
Non-immune adsorption	(+)	−	(+)	e.g. cephalosporins

(+) may be present

cases are recognized. There have been cases reported where a patient has clinical AIHA, but the DAT has been negative. On further full investigation with monospecific antiglobulin reagents, many of these have been shown to have IgA on the cell surface, but in others it is assumed that either low-affinity autoantibodies are involved, or there are low levels of IgG1 or IgG3 that are not detectable by the standard DAT.

The DAT has been reported positive (IgG and/or C3) in some patients with *Plasmodium falciparum* malaria. It is not clear to what extent red cell destruction is exacerbated when the DAT is positive, but there is evidence that mean Hb levels are lower in patients with a positive DAT than those without, and more transfusions are needed.

The autoantibodies found in the plasma of patients with warm AIHA usually react with all red cells tested, but sometimes less strongly with some cells than others. These are likely to have an Rh-related specificity, with autoanti-e or 'e-like' being most commonly encountered. Although autoantibodies will probably lead to a decrease in the lifespan of any transfused red cells, because they react with antigens found on most red cells, any alloantibodies present are more significant, as these could cause the rapid removal of incompatible transfused cells. In addition to the adverse effects of the ensuing transfusion reaction, this might also exacerbate the underlying destruction of the cells coated with the autoantibody.

Although some cases of warm AIHA are *idiopathic*, occurring without any obvious underlying cause, most cases of positive DATs now seen in the UK are related to haematological malignancies. In a series of cases referred to an immunohaematology reference laboratory, only 5% were idiopathic AIHA, 16% were associated with cases of malignancy, and 10% specifically with myelodysplastic syndromes (MDS). With an increasing number of people being treated for these conditions, the number of positive DAT cases is increasing. Also, many of these patients, presenting with a positive DAT and with 'warm reactive' autoantibodies present, have been transfused. Figures show that about 75% of DAT positive cases referred to reference laboratories have had transfusions, and about 40–50% have alloantibodies present. The investigation and provision of blood for these patients is considered below.

Positive DAT without cell destruction

A number of patients and blood donors have a positive DAT, with no evidence of increased cell destruction; for donors the figures vary from 1 in 3,000 to 1 in 15,000. The reason for the apparent lack of clinical significance might be that the cells are coated with IgG4 molecules that do not initiate cell destruction.

Some patients with raised IgG levels can also have a weak positive DAT, presumably due to non-specific uptake of their IgG onto their red cells. The use of the therapeutic immunoglobulin preparations, anti-lymphocyte and anti-thymocyte globulins, can also result in a transient positive DAT, as the immunoglobulins 'stick' to the red cells in a non-specific manner.

Key points

IgG antibodies are usually involved in warm-type autoimmune haemolytic anaemia, which can be idiopathic or, more likely, secondary to another disease such as malignancy.

Cold AIHA

The antibodies associated with cold AIHA are not usually detected on the cells by the DAT, but C3 is present, indicating that an antigen:antibody reaction has taken place. These cases are rare and caused by a cold-reacting IgM autoantibody, often anti-I or anti-i.

These antibodies are usually considered to be cold-reacting and clinically insignificant, as they do not react at body temperature. However, after some infections, such as glandular fever or mycoplamsa pneumonia, the level of antibody can increase, and also its *thermal range* or *amplitude*, so it might become active at 30°C. These antibodies could then react with the patient's own cells in the peripheral capillaries, such as the fingertips, where the blood might be at 30°C rather than 37°C. At these lower temperatures, the antibody binds to the antigen and initiates the complement cascade. As the blood returns to the warmer parts of the body the antibody elutes from the cells but, as the complement cascade has been started, it might in extreme cases, go to completion, resulting in intravascular lysis or rapid lysis of the C3b-coated cells in the liver. When this happens, the patient can present with haemoglobinuria after exposure to the cold. In less extreme cases, the complement cascade is halted at the C3 stage and C3d is found on the red cells that probably have a near normal half-life in the circulation.

In some disease states, such as lymphoma, the malignant cells might form a single clone, producing an antibody with anti-I specificity. As the antibody all comes from that single clone, each molecule will be identical—a monoclonal antibody. In some patients, the abnormal immunoglobulin produced might not have antibody specificity, but can be produced in such large quantities that the total IgM levels rise so high that the patient suffers from effects of the raised plasma viscosity, affecting their circulation.

Mixed cold and warm AIHA has been reported but is rare.

Paroxysmal cold haemoglobinuria (PCH)

Paroxysmal cold haemoglobinuria is usually categorized as a cold-AIHA, but is unlike AIHA caused by IgM antibodies. The causative antibody in PCH is bi-phasic, IgG, usually with anti-P specificity; the so-called Donath-Landsteiner antibody. The antibody reacts in the cold and activates complement in the warm, leading to haemolysis and haemoglobinuria. The Donath-Landsteiner (D-L) test is used to detect these antibodies. In this, group O cells and the serum under test are first incubated at 0°C then at 37°C, with a control incubated just at 37°C. In a positive test, lysis in seen in the tube incubated at both temperatures, but not in the one incubated just at 37°C. As complement has to be present in the test system, an indirect D-L test, adding fresh inert serum as a source of complement, is the method of choice.

Although classically associated with syphilis, this condition is now almost always seen in children, and is often associated with a viral infection. Although it is self-limiting, that is, resolves after a few days, some patients do present with acute haemolysis that requires transfusion. Although some patients tolerate P positive blood, for others it is necessary to transfuse rare P negative units, if the P+ cells are quickly destroyed.

Key points

IgM cold-reacting antibodies, with an increased thermal range/amplitude, are associated with cold autoimmune haemolytic anaemia, unlike PCH, which is caused by a bi-phasic IgG antibody.

SELF-CHECK 7.4

How do the antibodies that cause warm and cold autoimmune haemolytic anaemia cause red cell destruction?

Drug induced or associated AIHA

Over one hundred drugs have been reported that are capable of binding to red cells and initiating an immune antibody response. The exact mechanism is not known; however, it is likely that the drug, or its metabolite, interacts in some way with parts of the cell membrane, and antibodies are stimulated that can react with the drug itself, to drug plus membrane components, or to the cell membrane.

There are four possible mechanisms; the first two are drug dependent, the third is drug independent. It is possible that a drug might 'work' by more than one of these mechanisms.

- *Drug-adsorption*: the antibodies react mainly against the drug coating the cell, rather than the cell itself. The DAT in these cases is usually positive with anti-IgG and sometimes also with anti-C3. The drugs mainly involved are the penicillins; haemolysis develops slowly, but can be life threatening.

- *Immune complex*: the formation of drug–antibody immune complexes attached to the cell surface can result in acute haemolysis with haemoglobinuria and renal failure. Severe haemolytic episodes can recur, even with small doses of the drug. The DAT is usually positive with anti-C3, but with some drugs that seem to complex poorly with cells, IgM or IgG can be detected. The antibody only reacts with drug-coated cells. Some of the newer cephalosporins have been implicated with this mechanism.

- *Drug independent autoantibodies*: in some instances, the drug stimulates the production of an antibody that reacts with the red cell membrane, not the drug itself. This type cannot be distinguished from warm AIHA, as the cells react with anti-IgG, and in some cases anti-C3. The serum and eluate also react with normal red cells without the drug having to be present. This type was more common when methyldopa was widely used as a drug to treat hypertension.

- *Non-immunological protein adsorption*: some cephalosporin drugs can alter the cell membrane causing non-specific uptake of proteins, including IgG and IgM, which are detectable by the DAT. It is not clear if these cells have a shortened lifespan.

As cases of drug associated AIHA are rare in the UK, investigation of these is usually performed by a small number of specialist reference laboratories.

Key points

In some patients, red cell destruction can be caused by a drug which, in combination with red cells, can lead to the production of an autoantibody.

Investigation and crossmatching patients with autoantibodies

Transfusions should be avoided in these cases if other treatments can be employed. However, a transfusion is sometimes required to correct a low Hb where the patient has symptoms of the anaemia.

Grouping cells that have a positive DAT due to IgG can be performed using IgM blood typing sera, but those that require an IAT cannot be used, as the cells would react with the AHG regardless. Where possible, in addition to the standard ABO and D type, these patients should be typed, at least once, for Rh C, c, E, e, and K antigens.

If the antibody screen is negative, blood should be selected and crossmatched in the normal manner. If, however, the antibody screening tests are positive, then additional tests need to be employed to exclude the presence of alloantibodies, which may also be present with, and masked by, unbound autoantibody, free in the patient's serum.

It is important to identify these alloantibodies, as they are more significant when selecting blood for transfusion than the autoantibodies. Specialist techniques involve adsorption of the autoantibodies onto either the patient's own red cells—autoadsorption—or selected reagent cells—allo-adsorption. The latter is used if the patient has been transfused within the past three months, or there are insufficient patient cells available for auto-adsorption. The serum usually has to be adsorbed at least three times, with fresh cells to remove the auto-antibodies. It is then tested by standard methods to detect and identify any alloantibodies present. Selection of blood for transfusion is based on the findings of these tests and the patient's phenotype, and adsorbed serum might have to be used for the crossmatch. Blood tested in this way is issued as being 'suitable for' rather than 'compatible'.

Making and testing an eluate is only performed if the patient has recently been transfused, received a transplant, or if there is unexplained increased destruction of transfused red cells, as this might be due to a haemolytic transfusion reaction, rather than the underlying AIHA, or it could be a combination of the two. Elution removes antibody bound to the cell so that its specificity can be determined and its significance assessed. If the antibody appears to be an allo, rather than autoantibody, then any red cells transfused must be compatible with the alloantibody.

The practice of selecting units of blood for patients with a positive DAT and a positive antibody screen as 'the least incompatible', by virtue of reaction strength with un-adsorbed plasma in the crossmatch, is a procedure that should not be used unless blood is required urgently before these tests can be completed. Autoantibodies in the patient's serum can mask alloantibodies, and it is these alloantibodies that cause rapid destruction of transfused red cells that might exacerbate, rather than help, the patient's condition.

In cold AIHAs it is normally sufficient to perform all tests, including ABO and D typing, strictly at 37°C, to avoid agglutination of the cells by the cold reacting IgM autoantibody. If the autoantibody is very strong, it might be necessary to adsorb the antibody onto the patient's own cells that have first been washed several times with saline at 37°C to remove the bound antibody. Rabbit red cells, or cell stroma, can also be used to adsorb some cold reacting antibodies, or the IgM antibody agglutinating activity can be destroyed by the use of DTT.

> ## Key points
>
> **The presence and specificity of alloantibodies is more important than autoantibodies when selecting blood for transfusion to patients.**

7.5 Haemolysis post-transplantation bone marrow/stem cell transplant

In stem cell or bone marrow transplants although the donor and recipient are HLA matched, they may be of different ABO and Rh blood groups, and this can cause problems post-transplant. *Minor mismatches*, where the donor is group O, but the patient is group A, B, or AB can result in the production of antibodies to the recipient's red cells, that is, anti-A and/or anti-B. In *major mismatches*, as in an A donor and O recipient, the converse situation arises: the recipient can produce antibodies (anti-B) to the donor cells.

If haemolysis occurs in ABO minor mismatches, it is usually 5–15 days post-transplant, often with an abrupt onset, a rapidly falling Hb, and possible renal failure as a result of the cell destruction. Anti-A or anti-B are thought to be produced by lymphocytes transfused with the bone marrow, so-called passenger lymphocytes. The haemolysis subsides as the patient's remaining incompatible red cells are destroyed and replaced with those of donor origin. During the haemolytic episode, the DAT may be positive and the causative antibody eluted from the patient's red cells. When investigating such cases, the eluate should always be tested, by IAT, with A or B cells, depending on the group of the recipient. Likewise, an IAT crossmatch must be performed post-transplant, even if no antibodies are detected in the antibody screen, so that IgG anti-A/B, if present, will be detected.

In major ABO mismatches, the recipient's ABO antibodies could destroy the donor's red cells. This might lead to the delay in the engraftment of the donor red cells or, as erythropoiesis increases, the residual antibodies might haemolyse these cells. In these cases, the haemolysis is not usually noted until several weeks after the transplant; times of 30–100 days have been reported. The DAT is usually positive, with IgG anti-A/B being eluted from the red cells. Depleting the marrow of red cells, or reducing the patient's antibody levels can reduce the likelihood of this lysis occurring. Although ABO antibodies are most commonly implicated, other antibodies, Rh, Kidd, and Lewis, have been reported after both stem cell and solid organ transplants; the antibodies are usually donor-derived from passenger lymphocytes.

With an increasing demand for kidney transplants, more patients are being transplanted with an *ABO incompatible* organ. To prevent rejection by ABO antibodies, the patient is prepared by a course of plasmapheresis to reduce their levels of anti-A and anti-B. In some institutions, instead of just removing the patient's antibody containing plasma and replacing it, their plasma is passed through a column that contains A and B antigens on a matrix, so that the antibody binds to the antigen, effectively removing it from the circulation. Antibody levels are assessed in the laboratory before and after each session, and the transplant undertaken when the antibody level reaches a very low level. However, the antibody is quickly replaced, often rebounding to a higher level than there was before the conditioning started.

Transfusion post-bone marrow/stem cell transplant

As a general rule, post-transplant, group O red cells are transfused to all patients, irrespective of their ABO, until all of the following criteria are fulfilled:

- No mixed-field reactions are seen when ABO grouping the patients red cells.
- Anti-A/B is no longer detectable by standard 'saline' reverse grouping and by IAT, using A_1 and B cells.
- The DAT is negative with polyspecific AHG.

When these criteria are fulfilled, then the patient's ABO blood group can be altered in their records, and further red cell transfusions are with the blood of the *donor's* group.

Where *RhD major incompatibility* exists, for example the donor is D positive, the recipient D negative, give RhD negative blood until D positive cells are detectable, then give D positive blood. Where *RhD minor incompatibility* exists, for example the donor is D negative, the recipient D positive, then transfuse D negative blood indefinitely.

Key points

When haemopoeitic stem cells are transplanted, there might be an immune antibody reaction between the recipient and donor cells leading to red cell destruction.

7.6 Haemolytic disease of the newborn or foetus (HDN)

Another form of red cell destruction is caused by an antibody in a pregnant woman's bloodstream that can cross the placenta and lead to the destruction of the foetal red cells—haemolytic disease of the foetus. In the past, this condition was not often recognized until the baby had been born, hence it is referred to commonly as haemolytic disease of the newborn—HDN.

Haemolytic disease of the newborn occurs when a maternal IgG antibody, stimulated either by a transfusion or previous pregnancy, crosses the placenta and destroys the incompatible foetal red cells, leading to the foetus becoming anaemic. As the foetus will inherit blood group genes from each parent, some of the blood group antigens will be different from the mother's, for example the mother could be D negative and the foetus and father D positive.

The anaemia caused by these antibodies destroying the foetal red cells might be so severe that, unless transfused *in utero*, the foetus will die of the effects of anaemia or, if less severe, will need to be treated once delivered. Most IgG antibodies have been implicated in causing HDN, often causing only mild disease, but the Rh antibodies anti-D and anti-c, and anti-K are known to cause severe disease, depending on their concentration. Antibodies that are IgM, IgG2, or IgG4 are not transported across the placenta, so it is only IgG1 and IgG3 antibodies that can cause foetal cell destruction. Haemolytic disease of the newborn is not usually found in first pregnancies, as the stimulation is mainly from foetal red cells entering the mother's circulation at delivery, but if she has been transfused, and produced an antibody prior to the first pregnancy, then HDN could result. Whereas anti-D and anti-c antibodies are usually the result of stimulation by pregnancy, anti-K, and probably anti-E, antibodies are usually the result of transfusion.

There is a correlation, although not that good, between the antibody level and the severity of disease: the more antibody in the maternal blood, the more will be transported across the placenta and the greater the potential for destruction of the foetal red cells. However, not all red cell antigens are well developed in the foetus. For example, the H antigen (the precursor of the A and B antigens) is very weakly expressed on foetal red cells, so although the IgG anti-H in an O_h mother might cross the placenta, very little will be bound and, consequently, there will be little or no increased red cell destruction.

Not all IgG antibodies cause HDN, for example anti-In[b] is normally an IgG antibody that can cause a haemolytic transfusion reaction but, because the In antigens are associated with CD 44, which is found on cells on the placenta and other organs, the effect of any antibody in the foetal circulation on its red cells is small. The red cells might have a positive DAT, showing antibody present, but haemolysis does not seem to occur.

As the foetal RES develops, it can remove IgG-coated red cells, but it is mainly the mother's liver that deals with the resultant bilirubin, as the foetal liver has not developed the enzymes to conjugate the bilirubin and excrete it. Whilst *in utero* this is not a problem, but once born, any unconjugated bilirubin that cannot be excreted builds up in the newborn's circulation. When the albumin in the blood has become saturated with bilirubin, it is deposited in cells in the basal ganglia of the brain and can cause brain damage, such as deafness—a condition known as kernicterus.

In cases where there is evidence of severe haemolysis in the foetus and a low Hb, then a small volume of compatible blood can be transfused into the foetus, via its umbilical vein, whilst *in utero*. Once it is born, the newborn might require an immediate exchange transfusion if its Hb is low, or an exchange a few hours later, if the bilirubin produced from the antibody-coated cells being destroyed approaches the danger zone of 300 mmol/l or more. Other treatment might be a simple top-up transfusion if the Hb falls in the first few days of life, or phototherapy to reduce jaundice.

In utero
Literally within the uterus.

Key points

If the mother has an IgG antibody stimulated by a previous pregnancy or transfusion, it can cause the destruction of the foetal red cells if they carry an incompatible antigen gene inherited from the father. The destruction can be severe enough to cause death *in utero* or anaemia of the newborn infant.

BOX 7.1 *Factors affecting the destruction of foetal red cells in utero, by a maternal antibody*

- Strength of antibody (titre; quantification value)
- Antigen sites/development on foetal red cells (some antigens are poorly expressed on foetal cells, e.g. H)
- Antigens on cell other than RBCS (e.g. In^b antigen is also found on cells in the placenta)
- Maturity of foetal RES

Anti-D prophylaxis

Anti-D Ig prophylaxis is the name given to one of the most successful preventative medicine interventions of the past 50 years. Immunoglobulin G anti-D is given, by injection, to prevent D negative women producing allo anti-D. Despite its widespread use in the UK, anti-D is still the most common cause of HDN, followed by anti-c and anti-K. However, the absolute numbers of pregnancies affected has dropped dramatically over this time. In the early 1960s, 10% of perinatal deaths (150 per 100,000 births) were HDN-related, fewer than 100 are now reported in the UK each year (see Figure 7.1).

Foetal red cells can leak into the mother's circulation, especially during the third trimester of the pregnancy and more commonly at birth when the placenta detaches itself from the uterus. If the mother is, for example, D negative and the baby D positive, the baby's cells could stimulate her to produce anti-D: but by giving a dose of passive anti-D immunoglobulin, this antibody stimulation can be suppressed. The exact mechanism for this antibody-mediated

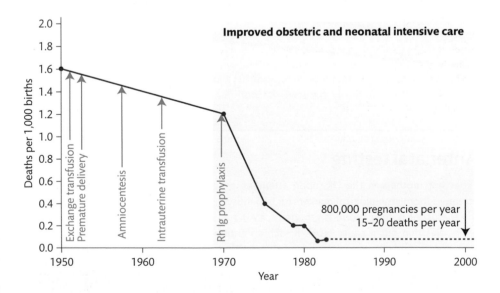

FIGURE 7.1
Effect of changes in clinical practice to the rate of perinatal deaths per 1,000 births due to anti-D HDN.

immune suppression is not fully understood, but the passive anti-D binds to the D positive foetal cells that are then cleared from the mother's circulation by the spleen before they have a chance to stimulate B cells to produce antibodies. Sufficient anti-D has to be administered so that each D positive cell is coated by about 500 antibody molecules to ensure its rapid removal from the circulation. There is evidence that the effects of this anti-D-mediated immune suppression are long-lasting, because fewer individuals who have received anti-D immunoglobulin respond to D positive cells for up to 16 months afterwards. Also the severity of any HDN in subsequent pregnancies is seen to be reduced.

Where possible, the anti-D dose should be administered within 72 hours of the birth or potential sensitizing event, but it seems to be effective if given within five days. Before anti-D immunoglobulin is given after either trauma during the pregnancy or the birth of the baby, the mother's blood should be tested to see if there are any foetal red cells present and, if so, how many. A Kleihauer is the usual screening test performed, with flow cytometry being used to estimate the number of foetal cells (hence the size) of the haemorrhage from the foetus to the mother: the foetal-maternal haemorrhage (FMH). The dose of anti-D required to remove all these cells from the circulation is then calculated.

Anti-D immunoglobulin is given after the birth of a D positive baby to a D negative woman, and also after any trauma during pregnancy that might cause a bleed from the foetus into the maternal circulation. Also, it is now routinely offered to all D negative women during the last trimester (third) of the pregnancy, when the risk of an FMH is high. This is called RAADP, routine antenatal anti-D prophylaxis.

One significant disadvantage of RAADP is that all D negative women can receive the anti-D injections, although 65% will be carrying a D negative foetus and not therefore, be in danger of producing anti-D. Plans are in place to be able to process a sample of the mother's plasma to extract the very small amounts of foetal DNA that are present. This DNA can then be analysed by PCR techniques to determine the foetal Rh genotype. If the foetus is found to be D negative, the mother will not need anti-D immunoglobulin, saving the mother an unnecessary injection. Foetal genotyping from a maternal sample can be used for genotyping for other blood groups, such as K, and also for HPA (platelet antigens); see Chapter 8.

Key points

The use of anti-D immunoglobulin to suppress allo anti-D production in RhD negative mothers has dramatically reduced the number of cases of HDN, and associated deaths.

Antenatal testing

Expectant mothers in the UK, upon attending an antenatal clinic, will have their blood screened for microbiological markers for hepatitis B, HIV, and syphilis, all of which can affect the foetus. Also, their blood is grouped for ABO and D and screened for the presence of antibodies that might cause HDN. If such an antibody is found, then, at regular intervals throughout the pregnancy, the level of that antibody is assessed. In the UK, Rh antibodies, anti-D, and anti-c, are quantified against a British standard, using a *continuous flow analyser*, that measures the amount of agglutination the antibody causes, compared to the standard run at the same time. The result is then expressed in IU/ml.

The level of other antibodies known to cause HDN, such as anti-K, anti-E, and anti-Fy^a, are measured by titration: testing serial dilutions of the plasma with red cells carrying the corresponding antigens with a (presumed) heterozygous expression, by IAT. The titre is the greatest dilution at which a reaction is found. The higher the titre, the more antibody is present. For example, if the last positive reaction is found with the plasma diluted 1 in 64, the titre is 64.

Evidence gathered over many years has led to some general criteria for the risk of HDN occurring when an antibody is present. The greater the amount of antibody the greater the risk of HDN; a titre of 32 or greater for antibodies other than anti-D and anti-c is considered to be significant. The significance of levels of anti-D and anti-c are given in Table 7.2.

If a pregnancy falls into the high-risk category, the mother-to-be is referred to a specialist centre, where they can assess the foetus by using Doppler techniques and, if there are signs of anaemia due to increased red cell destruction, an *in utero* transfusion (IUT) can be given to prevent foetal death.

At one time, anti-D immunoglobulin was only given after the delivery of a D positive baby, but it is now widely administered during the last trimester (third) of pregnancy. Therefore, it is more likely to be detected in antibody screening later in the pregnancy. It is impossible to differentiate between passive (prophylactic) and immune anti-D at low levels. Therefore, the level of the anti-D and the history of anti-D administration, must be taken into account when trying to decide if the antibody is a newly formed immune antibody that could affect the foetus, or just the injected anti-D immunoglobulin.

High levels of maternal IgG anti-A/B can cause ABO HDN, but this is rarely as severe as HDN caused by Rh antibodies, and if treatment is required, phototherapy post-delivery is usually sufficient. If transfusion is needed, it is normally just a top-up; an exchange transfusion is rarely needed. The diagnosis of ABO HDN in the newborn is based on both clinical and laboratory findings, such as a high IgG anti-A/B titre, anti-A/B eluted from the infant's red cells, and evidence of anaemia. Titres of IgG anti-A/B during pregnancy give a very poor indication of eventual disease severity.

On occasions, if there has not been any antenatal care, for example, a baby might be born with unexpected and unexplained anaemia and/or jaundice. There may be non-serological causes, but serological investigations would be required if the DAT was positive. The mother and baby's ABO and D groups should be determined and her plasma should be screened for antibodies and, if positive, the specificity of the antibody determined. An eluate made from the infant's red cells should also be tested against a panel of cells, if there is sufficient, plus A and/or B cells, if the mother is of a different ABO group to the baby. This is to test for IgG anti-A/B that might be causing the anaemia—ABO HDN. In rare cases, although HDN is highly suspected, no antibodies can be detected in routine testing and an antibody directed against a low frequency antigen might be implicated. In such cases, the infant's serum and/or eluate should be tested against the father's red cells, as it is from him that an antigen

TABLE 7.2 Level of antibody and the risk of HDN.

HDN risk	Anti-D IU/ml	Anti-c IU/ml	Other antibodies
Unlikely—small	<4	<7.5	Titre <32
Moderate	4–15	7.5–20	
High	>15	>20	Titre >32

gene, incompatible with the mother's antigens, would have been inherited. Many of the low-frequency red cell antigens have been discovered this way and, doubtless, more will be in future.

Key points

Pregnant women are ABO RhD grouped and tested for the presence of alloantibodies that might cause HDN and, if found, the pregnancy is closely monitored.

SELF-CHECK 7.5

How do maternal antibodies bring about destruction of foetal red cells?

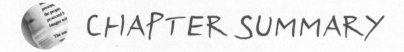

CHAPTER SUMMARY

- Despite, or perhaps because of, advances in clinical practice, immune-mediated red cell destruction still has to be considered in transfusion, transplantation, and pregnancy.

- All red cell antibodies have that potential to cause cell destruction if the right conditions exist. In general, an antibody capable of causing red cell destruction *in vivo* reacts at 37°C by the indirect antiglobulin test, and is considered to be *clinically significant*.

- Some patients produce *autoantibodies*, directed against their own red cells, which can lead to an increased rate of cell destruction—an autoimmune haemolytic anaemia (AIHA).

- As the population gets older, more people are treated for malignancies, and the number of patients with autoantibodies is increasing.

- Laboratory tests are employed pre-transfusion and transplant, and products selected, to try to prevent *in vivo* cell destruction, but an increasing number of stem cell and solid organ transplants are being given that are knowingly ABO and/or D incompatible and, of course, not typed for other red cell antigens.

- The use of anti-D immunoglobulin to suppress anti-D production in D negative women has greatly reduced the number of babies suffering from HDN, but other IgG antibodies can, and do, cause HDN, hence the continuing need to detect and monitor them during pregnancy.

- Although these problems are recognized and better understood, they have not been fully resolved, and so the need to investigate red cell antibodies, both allo and auto, will remain.

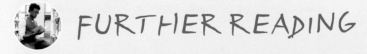

FURTHER READING

- **British Committee for Standards in Haematology. Guidelines for compatibility procedures in blood transfusion laboratories** *Transfusion Medicine*, **14 (2004), 59–73.**

- Daniels G, Poole J, de Silva M, Callaghan T, MacLennan S & Smith N. The clinical significance of red cell antibodies. *Transfusion Medicine*, 12 (2002), 287–95.

- Do HLA antibodies cause hemolytic transfusion reactions? Editorial in *Transfusion*, 43 (2003), 687–90.

- Hemolysis associated with transplantation. Editorial in *Transfusion*, 38 (1998), 224–8.

- Posters about HDN are available for download from www.transfusionguidelines. org. Follow 'National Blood transfusion Committee' then 'Transfusion Awareness'.

Answers to the questions in this chapter are provided on the book's Online Resource Centre.

 Go to www.oxfordtextbooks.co.uk/orc/knight

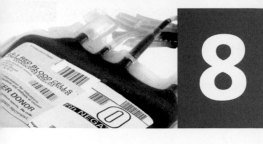

8

Human Leucocyte Antigens and Their Clinical Significance

Colin Brown

Learning objectives

By the end of this chapter you should be able to:

- Describe the HLA system.
- Outline the role of the HLA system in transplantation and transfusion.
- Explain the principles of matching for haemopoietic stem cell transplantation, solid organ transplantation, and platelet transfusion.
- Outline the common methods and technology for HLA typing and antibody testing used in the HLA laboratory.

Introduction

Humans have a highly developed immune system that can distinguish self from non-self proteins and the principle molecules enabling this function are coded for by genes found in a region of the genome on the short arm of chromosome 6, known as the *Major Histocompatibility Complex* or MHC. In fact many species have an MHC, even fish.

This ability to recognize cells from another individual of the same species or different species as foreign is a major barrier to transplantation and can cause some serious hazards of transfusion.

In this chapter you will learn about the human leucocyte antigens (HLA) the genes of which are found within the MHC and how the detection and matching of the genes and gene products has contributed to the success of transplantation and the study of human disease.

8.1 A brief history of transplantation

- In 600 BC, Hindu surgeon Sushrutha experimented with *autologous* (see Box 8.1) skin grafting.

- In 1778 John Hunter first used the term 'transplant' when describing his work in transplanting ovaries and testis in animals.

- The nineteenth century saw a number of workers experimenting with autologous skin grafts.

- In 1910 Carrel and Guthrie developed methods for joining blood vessels together called 'anastomosis' that allowed many experiments on grafting kidneys, which all failed.

- In the 1930s Snell discovered the dominant histocompatibility locus in mice, the H-2.

- In 1933 the first kidney transplant in humans was performed by the Russian surgeon, Voronoy, but this transplant failed as the kidney was harvested approximately six hours after the donor had died.

- In 1937 Gorer developed the concept of self and non-self following the observation that antigens on tissue cells are genetically determined and are involved in the destruction of foreign grafts.

- In the 1940s Medawar worked on the immunological problems of rejection when observing the problems associated with treating burn victims and injuries sustained as a result of the Second World War.

- In 1966 Kelly and Lillehei transplanted a kidney and pancreas into a patient suffering from end stage diabetic nephropathy.

- In 1967 Dr Christian Barnard carried out the first human heart transplant.

BOX 8.1 Types of transplant

Autologous: the patient receives their own cell/tissues.

Syngeneic: the patient receives cells/tissue from a genetically identical donor, that is, an identical (monozygotic) twin.

Allogeneic: the patient receives cells/tissues from a non-identical donor of the same species.

Xenogeneic: the patient receives cell/tissues from a donor of a different species.

8.2 Human leucocyte antigens

The discovery of human leucocyte antigens

It was George Snell who showed that genetic differences were involved in the response to transplanted tissue. Snell bred **congenic** mice to discover the locus that was intimately involved in tumour graft rejection and named it 'H' for histocompatibility. Peter Gorer independently discovered an agglutinating antibody associated with rejection of tumour grafts and named it as the antigen II. It was later established that the antigen II was coded for by a gene located at the H locus described by Snell. The term H-2 was used to describe the murine MHC.

Congenic
Organisms produced as the result of specific inbreeding in an experimental setting so that they only differ in one gene locus.

In the late 1950s three groups, in France, the USA, and the Netherlands were instrumental in the discovery of the human MHC. Jean Dausset (France) who identified a leucocyte agglutinating antibody in transfused patients recognizing an antigen he termed 'MAC'. This antigen was found in 60% of the French population and was subsequently found to be HLA-A2. Rose Payne (USA) found similar leucocyte agglutinating antibodies in the sera of multiparous women, and noted the pattern of reactivity of the sera with leucocytes of the newborn infant and their fathers and concluded that the offspring had inherited a paternal 'leucocyte factor'. Jon van Rood (the Netherlands) reported a systematic analysis of the reactivity of sera from patients that had undergone febrile transfusion reactions as well as sera from pregnant women. Van Rood described the recognition of different leucocyte groups using panels of sera and speculated on the possible use in forensic medicine and bone marrow transplantation.

Human leucocyte antigen gene location

The genes that code for HLA molecules are found within the MHC, which can be divided into two regions based on the structure and function of their products: the class I region where HLA-A, B and C gene are located, class II which contains the HLA-DR, DQ, and DP genes. There is also a class III region which does not contain any HLA genes, but genes encoding complement factors (C3 and factor B), tumour necrosis factor (TNF) alpha, heat shock proteins (HSP), and other genes involved in immune function. See Figure 8.1.

SELF-CHECK 8.1

What is the major histocompatibility complex and what is its function?

Human leucocyte antigen class I molecules

Human leucocyte antigen class I gene products consist of 45 kilodalton (kD) glycopeptides folded into three extracellular domains called alpha 1, 2, and 3, a transmembrane region and

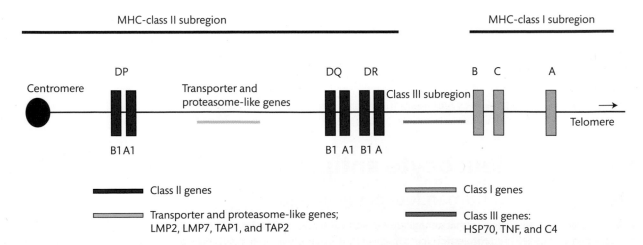

FIGURE 8.1

Map of the human major histocompatibility complex. The human MHC span a region of approximately 8 Mb on the short arm of chromosome 6. This region of the genome is gene rich, containing 224 genes many of immune function and over half are predicted to be expressed. The MHC class I and II sub-regions contain the genes that code for HLA molecules.

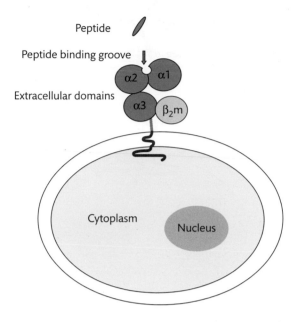

FIGURE 8.2

Human leucocyte antigen class I molecule. The HLA class I molecule comprises a membrane bound heavy chain of ~45kDa, folded into 3 extra-cellular domains α1-3, a transmembrane region, a cytoplasmic tail and a water soluble light chain known as β2-microglobulin. The peptide binding groove is formed by the α1 and α2 domains and β2-microglobulin non-covalently associated with the α3 domain.

a cytoplasmic tail; it is often called the class I heavy chain. The alpha 3 domain is non-covalently associated with beta 2 microglobulin, a ubiquitous plasma protein that is a product of a gene not within the MHC but on chromosome 15, and is also known as the light chain. The alpha 1 and alpha 2 domains of the heavy chain are folded to form a peptide binding cleft. The antigenic differences or polymorphisms of HLA-A, B, and C molecules are as a result amino acid sequence variations in this region of the heavy chain. See Figure 8.2.

BOX 8.2 *Determining the structure of the human leucocyte antigen class I molecule*

The structure of the HLA class I molecule was first visualized using X-ray crystallography (Bjorkman 1987) and was a landmark discovery in the history of HLA. The peptide binding cleft was shown to consist of a beta pleated sheet at its base and the sides were alpha helices. The size of the groove showed it was capable of binding peptides consisting of between eight and ten amino acids.

Human leucocyte antigen class II molecules

Human leucocyte antigen class II molecules consist of two chains, alpha and beta, and the genes coding for both chains are located within the MHC. The alpha chain is a 31-34 kD glycoprotein non-covalently associated with a 26-29 kD beta chain, and both chains have a transmembrane region and a cytoplasmic tail. Both the alpha and beta chain are polymorphic in HLA-DQ and DP molecules but only the beta chain contributes to polymorphism in HLA-DR molecules. Human leucocyte antigens polymorphism will be discussed in more detail later in this chapter. See Figure 8.3.

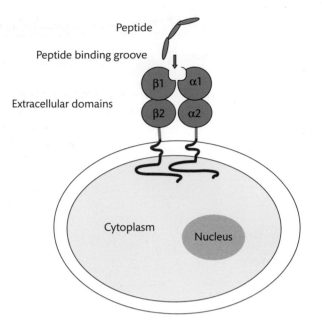

FIGURE 8.3

Human leucocyte antigen class II molecule. The HLA class II molecule comprises an α and β chain, both have two extracellular domains α1, α2 and β1, β2 respectively, a transmembrane region and a cytoplasmic tail. The α1 and β1 domains form the peptide binding groove for HLA-DR, DQ and DP molecules.

Human leucocyte antigen expression

Human leucocyte antigen class I and II molecules can be distinguished by their distribution on different cell types. Human leucocyte antigen class I molecules are expressed on nearly all nucleated cells and platelets and are also found in a soluble form in plasma, where they can be adsorbed onto erythrocytes that do not normally express HLA molecules.

Human leucocyte antigen class II molecules have a more restricted distribution and are found on macrophages, dendritic cells, B-lymphocytes, Langerhans' cells, and thymic epithelium or so-called 'professional' antigen-presenting cells.

Antigen processing and presentation

The main function of HLA molecules is the presentation of foreign molecules, in the form of peptides, to the immune system. In this way, T lymphocytes, cells of the adaptive immune response, can be activated.

Cytosol
The aqueous component of the cytoplasm in an intact cell.

Proteasome
An intracellular proteolytic complex that degrades cytosolic and nuclear proteins.

Endosome
A membrane bound intracellular compartment providing an environment for material to be sorted before degradation by the lysosome.

Pathogens that reside inside cells, such as viruses, can be recognized by HLA class I molecules. Viral proteins found in the **cytosol** are degraded by intracellular structures known as **proteasomes**, some of the genes of which are located within the MHC. The peptides produced by this degradation are between eight and ten amino acids in length, just the right length to be loaded into the peptide binding groove of HLA class I molecules. However, the viral peptide will only bind if that particular HLA class I molecule has the correct binding groove for the viral peptide. These newly formed HLA class I molecules containing antigenic peptide are transported to the cell's surface via the Golgi apparatus and present their peptides to predominately CD8 positive (cytotoxic) T lymphocytes.

Pathogens that reside outside the cell, such as bacteria, can be taken up by phagocytosis or pinocytosis and degraded in the **endosome** normally by acid digestion. The peptides produced are of varying length and are loaded into the peptide binding groove of an appropriately complementary HLA class II molecule. These newly-formed HLA class II molecules are transported to the cell's surface via the Golgi apparatus and present their peptides to predominately CD4 positive (helper) T lymphocytes.

This explains the biological role of HLA molecules and how they allow the immune system to recognize pathogens located inside or outside the cell. If an individual's HLA molecules are unable to bind to peptides derived from a pathogen, it can lead to infection and/or disease.

In normal circumstances, pregnancy, where the mother is exposed to the HLA molecules of the foetus inherited from the father, is the only natural situation when an individual would be exposed to another individual's HLA. However, transplantation and transfusion exposes the recipient to foreign (non-self) HLA which can cause powerful immune responses.

SELF-CHECK 8.2

What are the main functions of HLA class I and HLA class II antigens?

Key points

HLA genes are found within the MHC locus. This is divided into two regions, the class I region (HLA-A, B, and C genes) and class II (HLA-DR, DQ, and DP genes). Human leucocyte antigen class I molecules are expressed on nearly all nucleated cells and platelets, whereas HLA class II molecules have a more restricted distribution, being found on antigen-presenting cells.

Human leucocyte antigen nomenclature

The different antigens of the HLA system were defined using antibodies from patients who had received multiple transfusions or pregnancies. Throughout the world, different laboratories used local names to define the reactivity of their HLA **antisera**. It was through collaboration at international histocompatibility workshops that a universal system of naming the different antigens was established. As a new antigen was found it was numbered sequentially, that is, the first three antigens to be named were A locus specificities A1, A2, A3, followed by B locus specificities. New antigens that had not been officially named by the workshop nomenclature committee were distinguished by a 'w', for example Aw74, Cw3. The 'w' was removed following confirmation by the international workshop. However, the 'w' was retained for HLA-C locus antigens to prevent confusion with complement factors, particularly those whose genes are found within the MHC. Human leucocyte antigen Bw4 and Bw6 were found to be **public epitopes** on certain HLA-B locus antigens so they have kept their 'w'.

Antisera
Blood serum containing polyclonal antibodies.

Human leucocyte antigen class II molecules were originally defined using cellular assays, the most commonly used was the *mixed lymphocyte culture* (MLC). When lymphocytes from two individuals are mixed in culture they can respond by the production of **cytotoxic** T lymphocytes directed against the determinant recognized as foreign. These were termed HLA-D. It was later shown that MLC reactivity could also be influenced by cell surface molecules that could be detected by antibody. These determinants were found on B lymphocytes but not T lymphocytes and named HLA-D related or HLA-DR molecules.

Public epitopes
A region of an antigen shared by many different antigens that is recognized by antibodies, B cells, or T cells.

Cytotoxic
The ability to kill cells either by loss of membrane integrity, necrosis, or programmed cell death, apoptosis.

The naming of new HLA class II loci followed a different convention, going backwards through the alphabet. We now have HLA-DQ, DP, DO, and DM. There was originally an HLA-DN gene but this was later shown to be a sub-unit of HLA-DO.

The application of DNA-based techniques in the late 1980s and early 1990s to HLA typing resulted in the definition of HLA polymorphism at the molecular level. Antibodies can detect differences at the protein level but molecular techniques allow the detection of nucleotide differences.

Human leucocyte antigen nomenclature has developed over the last 40 years to account for the high degree of polymorphism that can be detected using DNA-based techniques. The latest change to HLA nomenclature occurred in April 2010, and using HLA-DRB1*13 as an example an explanation is shown in Table 8.1.

There are some alleles that end with a letter of the alphabet. This letter indicates some additional characteristics of the molecule:

A   Aberrant expression

C   Cytoplasmic expression only

L   Low expression levels

N   Null allele, no cell surface expression

S   Secreted, this molecule is only present in a soluble form

TABLE 8.1 HLA Nomenclature.

HLA	HLA region
HLA-DR	Identifies the HLA locus.
HLA-DR13	A serologically-defined antigen.
HLA-DRB1*	Identifies the HLA locus and gene, the asterisk indicates the HLA allele(s) have been defined using DNA-based techniques.
HLA-DRB1*13	A group of HLA alleles with a common DRB1*13 sequence, termed **first field resolution**, that is, this is the field before the first colon.
HLA-DRB1*13:01	A specific HLA allele, termed **second field resolution** as the numerals appear in the second field between the first and the second colon.
HLA-DRB1*13:01N	A **null allele**; there is no cell surface expression of the DRB1*13 gene product.
HLA-DRB1*13:01:02	An allele that differs by a synonymous (silent or non-coding) mutation.
HLA-DRB1*13:01:01:02	An allele that contains a mutation outside the coding region.
HLA-DRB1*13:01:01:02N	A null allele which contains a mutation outside the coding region.

When describing serologically-defined specificities, they are not preceded by *.
Thus the serological HLA type of HLA-A1, B8, Cw7, DR3, and DQ2 would be reported as HLA-A*01, B*08, C*07, DRB1*03, DQB1*02 if typed using DNA techniques.

First field resolution
This is how a low resolution HLA type is described because the numerals describing the HLA molecule are in the first field before the colon, for example HLA-DRB1*12.

Second field resolution
This is how a high resolution or allele level HLA type is described because the second field after the first colon is populated, for example HLA-DRB1*12:01.

Null allele
A mutant gene that does not function like the normal gene. Many null HLA alleles lack cell surface expression and cannot present peptides to the immune system.

How many human leucocyte and alleles?—polymorphism

The number of serologically defined HLA molecules has remained constant for many years. However, the number of HLA alleles that have been described has increased rapidly and the statistics from October 2011 (www.ebi.ac.uk/imgt/hla/) are shown in Table 8.2.

The reason for this extensive polymorphism is apparent when we consider that the role of HLA is to present peptides from pathogens to the immune system. Human leucocyte antigen polymorphism is pathogen driven and HLA class I and II molecules have evolved to present peptides from a wide variety of pathogens. At a population level, it is important that there are many different HLA alleles to make it more likely that there will be individuals able to respond to a novel pathogen and maintain the survival of the species.

At an individual level HLA polymorphism is achieved by the following three factors:

1. Multiple loci—if we just consider the HLA loci important in transplantation (HLA-A, B, C, DRB1, DQB1, and DPB1), there are six different loci, increasing the potential number of peptides that can be bound by HLA molecules.

2. Multiple alleles—at each loci there are many different alleles so there is a low probability of two unrelated individuals having the same HLA type.

3. Co-dominant expression—each individual will inherit a set of HLA alleles on one chromosome from each parent and both sets will be expressed.

Studies of HLA polymorphism in different populations show that some HLA types are found almost exclusively in some populations, whilst other HLA types are found throughout the world (Table 8.3).

Key points

The extensive polymorphism of the HLA system enables peptides from pathogens to be presented to the immune system. The HLA nomenclature is agreed internationally and reflects the known HLA polymorphism at a molecular level.

TABLE 8.2 **The number of human leucocyte antigen alleles and serological and cellular human leucocyte antigen specificities.**

HLA Locus	Antigens/specificities	Alleles
A	28	1,729
B	60	2,329
C	10	1,291
DRB1	21	1,051
DQB1	9	160
DPB1	6	150

TABLE 8.3 Examples of HLA types and distribution.

HLA-A*02	Throughout the world
HLA-A*01	European Caucasoid
HLA-A*25	European Caucasoid
HLA-A*36	Black African
HLA-A*36	Black African
HLA-A*43	Black African
HLA-A*08	European Caucasoid
HLA-B*54	Japanese
HLA-B*42	Black African
HLA-B*46	Chinese and Japanese
HLA-DRB1*03:02	Black African
HLA-DRB1*10	Indian/Middle Eastern

8.3 The detection and definition of human leucocyte antigens, alleles, and antibodies

Serological human leucocyte antigen typing

The first HLA typing methods were serologically based and relied on the detection of cell surface HLA molecules on lymphocytes isolated from peripheral blood (or spleen or lymph nodes in the case of deceased donors). Human leucocyte antigen typing laboratories maintained panels of well characterized HLA antisera obtained from multiparous women, patients immunized by transplantation or transfusions and in some cases healthy donors given planned immunizations of HLA typed lymphocytes. The principle of the typing technique, termed the lymphocytoxicity test (LCT) or complement-dependent cytotoxicity (CDC), has remained the same since the mid-1960s when Terasaki and McClelland pioneered the use of a microtitre plate format: the Terasaki plate (see Method box).

Serological typing had its limitations, which include:

- It requires viable cells that are sufficiently robust to withstand the LCT.
- Patients with low numbers of lymphocytes due to their disease or disease treatment may not be able to provide sufficient lymphocytes for typing.
- B lymphocytes are required for HLA class II typing, which constitute only 15% of peripheral blood cells and an additional B cell isolation method was required.

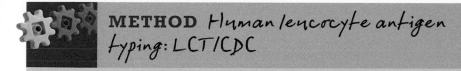

METHOD Human leucocyte antigen typing: LCT/CDC

Each Terasaki plate contains 60 different antisera, including negative and positive controls and at least two plates (120 different sera) are used to obtain a basic HLA type.

In the standard LCT 1 ul of lymphocytes is added to 1 ul of antiserum already plated on the Terasaki plate, incubated for 30 minutes to allow antibody–antigen interaction to occur. Then 5 ul of rabbit complement is added to each well and the plate is incubated for a further 60 minutes before the reaction is stopped and the plate read. Where there has been specific binding of complement-fixing antibodies to the cells used in the test, the integrity of the membrane is disrupted, allowing the entry of dyes that allow the detection of dead cells. One of the most commonly used dyes is a mixture of acridine orange and ethidium bromide. Acridine orange is taken into the cytoplasm of live cells and, under UV light from a fluorescence microscope, these cells appear green. Ethidium bromide (EB) cannot cross the intact cell membrane, but when the cell membrane is disrupted, EB will enter the cell and intercalate with DNA and these cells appear red under UV light.

- Good quality typing required large panels of well characterized antisera, which are expensive to maintain as only about 15% of multiparous women produce HLA antibodies and a small proportion of these are useful typing sera.

Serological typing is still used as many commercial companies produce HLA typing trays and utilized monoclonal antibodies directed against different HLA specificities. Serological typing is also used in combination with typing using DNA-based techniques, to detect null alleles, where the gene for the allele is present but the protein is not expressed on the cell surface. The presence or absence of cell surface expression can have functional consequences, provoking alloreactions which are important when considering clinical transplantation.

DNA-based human leucocyte antigen typing

One of the main drivers for the introduction of DNA-based HLA typing was the limitations of serological HLA class II typing. DNA-based typing for HLA class II molecules was introduced before HLA class I typing.

Initially, the techniques involved treating DNA with restriction enzymes, which cut the DNA sequence at specific sites and the resulting fragments were of different sizes depending upon the HLA type, and visualized on a gel, usually involving radioactive markers. However, this technique was laborious and not sensitive enough for a highly polymorphic system such as HLA. The introduction of polymerase chain reaction (PCR) technology revolutionized HLA typing and currently the methods used by HLA typing laboratories all involve PCR.

1. *Sequence Specific Primer* (PCR-SSP): this approach requires the design of short sequences of DNA or primers specific for particular HLA allele or groups of alleles that can serve as templates for DNA synthesis when that particular allele is present. Patient or donor DNA, plus the building blocks for DNA synthesis, are added to a panel of primers, usually in a 96 well format, that cover all of the major HLA alleles groups, sufficient to obtain a basic HLA type. Each primer pair is tested for DNA amplification by performing agarose gel

electrophoresis on the reaction mixture. If DNA amplification has occurred the product has a specific band on the gel of a specific molecular weight. The HLA type is determined by analysis of the reactivity with the panel of specific primers. Sequence Specific Primer is a rapid technique as the plates of primers can be stored frozen or freeze dried and be ready for immediate use, so this technique is commonly used for patient typing or situations where results are required rapidly, such as deceased donor typing. The resolution of PCR-SSP for rapid typing is usually first field or low to medium level (see Box 8.3), which is not satisfactory for stem cell transplantation but useful for solid organ transplants or matching for platelet transfusion.

2. *Sequence Specific Oligonucleotide Probes* (PCR-SSOP): this approach to HLA typing requires the design of strands of DNA that bind in the region of the HLA allele that is specific for that allele or allele group. The probe can be labelled with a fluorescent or radioactive tag so that specific binding can be detected. The patient or donor DNA to be HLA typed undergoes PCR amplification but the primers are not specific for a particular HLA allele group; they are usually HLA locus-specific. Originally, PCR-SSOP for HLA typing required DNA to be separated into its single strands, immobilized on suitable membrane, and reacted sequentially with probes of different specificity. Probes with the complementary sequence of the DNA under investigation would bind and be detected via its fluorescent tag. Since the late 1990s, the PCR-SSOP has been modified so that the probes are immobilized on nylon membranes or fluorescently labelled microbeads. The PCR amplification involves the incorporation of **biotin** into the amplicons so that it can be detected with a **streptavidin** coupled label, such as **phycoerythrin (PE)**. The HLA type is determined by analysis of the reactivity with the panel of specific probes. The resolution of typing by PCR-SSOP can be varied by the number of probes used and medium-to-high resolution typing can be obtained using this approach. Sequence Specific Oligonucleotide Probes is not normally suited to rapid typing as required for deceased donor testing, but is well suited to typing large numbers of individuals, as required for donor registry typing.

3. *Sequence Based Typing* (PCR-SBT): this is currently the gold standard of HLA typing that can give allelic level typing but is more costly and time consuming than PCR-SSP or PCR-SSOP. The SBT approach to HLA typing involves determining the nucleotide sequence of the HLA alleles of an individual. However, to save time and cost, the sequencing is usually restricted to the region of greatest polymorphism, the peptide binding cleft, in HLA class I genes. Exons 2 and 3 code for this region of the molecule. In HLA class II molecules, exon 2 codes for the peptide binding cleft.

Biotin

A water soluble B complex vitamin, necessary for the growth of cell, production of fatty acids, and metabolism of protein and fat. It is used in the laboratory because it interacts strongly with streptavidin. Thus molecules labelled with biotin can be detected with streptavidin conjugated to a reporter molecule.

Streptavidin

A bacterial protein purified from *Streptomyces avidinii* that has a high affinity for biotin.

Phycoerythrin (PE)

A red protein found in red algae and cyanobacteria. It is used as a fluorescent label for antibodies used in the laboratory for the detection of specific markers on cell surfaces, in the cytoplasm, or on DNA, by utilizing its ability to absorb blue green light and emit orange-yellow light (475 ± 10 nm).

Key points

The first HLA typing methods were serological detection of cell surface HLA molecules on lymphocytes. This has been largely replaced by DNA-based HLA typing using methods such as Sequence Specific Primer (PCR-SSP), Sequence Specific Oligonucleotide Probes (PCR-SSOP), and Sequence Based Typing (PCR-SBT).

Human leucocyte antigen antibody detection and definition

Human leucocyte antigen antibodies can be produced in response to pregnancy, blood transfusion, and transplantation. The route of immunization can affect the type of antibody that can be detected.

BOX 8.3 *Human leucocyte antigen typing resolution*

Low resolution typing; serological or antigen level typing HLA-DR12 or HLA-DRB1*12

Medium resolution typing; molecular typing that identifies a group or string of alleles belonging to the same antigenic group, for example HLA-DRB1*12:01/12:06/12:10/12:17

High resolution typing; molecular typing that identifies a single or group of alleles that share the same sequence of the peptide binding cleft that interacts with the T cell receptor, for example HLA-DRB1* 12:01/12:06/12:10/12:17

Allele level typing; molecular typing that identifies the specific HLA allele, for example HLA-DRB1*12:01

Human leucocyte antigen typing (LCT/CDC)

The LCT technique described for HLA typing is the same as was originally used for antibody screening but, in this process, the panel of well-characterized sera is replaced by a panel of HLA-typed donor lymphocytes, which is employed to detect antibody of unknown specificity. Many laboratories employ an extended incubation time to increase sensitivity, that is, 60 minutes for cells and serum followed by 120 minutes after the addition of complement. This extra time allows the detection of low affinity or low titre antibodies.

The procedure has remained popular because it is simple, reproducible, and relatively inexpensive, but cannot detect non-complement fixing antibodies that are also clinically significant, and is probably the least sensitive technique available. False positive reaction can occur when testing patients receiving antibody therapy such as anti-thymocyte globulin (ATG), or anti-CD3 therapy.

Enzyme-linked immunosorbent assay (ELISA)

In the ELISA technique, purified HLA antigen is immobilized on the surface of a 96 well plate. Patient serum or plasma is added to the plate and incubated to allow antibody–antigen binding to take place. Excess serum is washed off and an anti-human immunoglobulin conjugated to an enzyme, such as horseradish peroxidise, is added. This binds to any HLA antibody–antigen complex and when the enzyme substrate is added, the breakdown of the substrate is linked to a colour change which can be read in an ELISA reader.

The method of antigen preparation can determine whether the ELISA can be used for screening or antibody definition of specificity. Pooled antigen stripped from the surface of platelets or cells and purified, has been used to manufacture antibody screening kits but will only indicate the presence or absence of HLA-specific antibody. Antigen isolated from individual cell lines, but not pooled, has been one approach used to manufacture antibody specificity definition kits and mimics the cell panel approach used in the LCT technique.

Enzyme-linked immunosorbent assay is also a relatively simple technique, with an objective readout and is amenable to testing large batches of samples. This technique can indicate the presence of HLA-specific antibody as it is a not affected by non-HLA antibodies such as ATG. There is always the possibility with any technique that does not use antigen in its native form that the isolation, purification, and immobilization procedure may expose epitopes not normally seen in the native antigen.

Flow cytometry

The flow cytometry method uses the same principle of the LCT and ELISA methods; a panel of HLA typed lymphocytes or purified HLA molecules immobilized on beads is mixed with patient sera or plasma and incubated to allow antibody binding to take place. The detection of bound antibody is achieved using a fluorescently-labelled anti-human Ig antibody. The most common labels used are fluorocein and phycoerythrin (PE).

In the flow cytometer, the cell suspension is passed through a laser, which excites the fluorescent tag on the cell surface. The excited tag emits light at a specific wavelength governed by the fluorescent label used and is detected and measured by the machine.

Luminex

A new type of solid phase technique using Luminex technology has been the most widely used technique for both HLA-specific antibody detection and definition of specificity. In this system, fluorochrome-dyed polystyrene beads are coated with specific HLA antigens, which are then used to detect the antibodies in the serum or plasma. The precise ratio of these fluorochromes creates one hundred distinctly coloured beads, each of them coated with a different antigen. The beads are then incubated with the patient's serum and specific antibody bound to the beads is detected by the addition of a PE-conjugated antihuman IgG (Fc specific) antibody. The resulting positive or negative reactions are read using a Luminex analyser, which consists of two lasers. One laser can distinguish between up to one hundred different beads sets in a single tube, and the other detects PE label bound to the HLA antibody–antigen complex.

Antibody detection using Luminex is now widely used and it has been shown to be more sensitive than either CDC or ELISA, although the clinical benefit of this increased sensitivity is not yet clearly defined, particularly in the transplant setting.

Key points

Human leucocyte antigen antibodies can be produced in response to pregnancy, blood transfusion, and transplantation. Techniques for antibody screening and identification include the LCT technique, the ELISA technique using purified HLA antigen, flow cytometry using the same principle as the LCT and ELISA methods. A new type of solid phase technique using Luminex technology is now widely used.

8.4 Clinical significance of human leucocyte antigens in transplantation

The importance of the HLA system in transplantation was first seen in renal transplantation, where it was observed that graft survival was improved in transplants between siblings, when compared to unrelated stem cell or deceased solid organ donors. In solid transplants between parents and children where only one HLA haplotype is shared, graft survival was observed to be at a level between that seen in identical sibling and deceased donor transplants.

Data from all solid organ transplants in the UK is collated by NHSBT ODT (Organ Donation and Transplant). Internationally, bodies such as the Collaborative Transplant Study (CTS) based in Europe or the United Network for Organ Sharing (UNOS) in the USA have all shown the benefits of HLA-matching, through analysis of the outcome of thousands of transplants. Independently, many of these studies have shown a hierarchy in the effect of the different HLA loci on graft survival, where HLA-DR matching is shown to be the most beneficial when compared to HLA-A or B matching.

Solid organ transplantation

The importance of HLA in solid organ transplantation differs with the type of organs transplanted and is discussed later in the chapter. The immediate problem with transplanting an organ is the presence of pre-formed HLA and ABO blood group antibodies, which can cause the rapid rejection of the organ. Therefore, prior to transplantation every effort is made to detect and define donor-specific antibodies and, where possible, the HLA type of the donor and recipient is matched to limit graft rejection.

Types of rejection

Organ rejection can be categorized as hyperacute, acute, and chronic. *Hyperacute rejection* occurs when there is irreversible damage to the transplanted organ within minutes or hours due to the presence of preformed circulating antibodies, primarily directed against ABO blood group antigens or HLA class I antigens on the endothelial cells of the graft. Antibody–antigen interaction can result in the activation of the complement system, leading to cell lysis, but also to the formation of clots, leading to ischaemia and infarction of the graft. The incidence of hyperacute rejection can be limited by performing extensive characterization of the patient's pre-transplant serum to detect the presence of donor-specific antibodies, and performing a crossmatch with the patient's serum against donor lymphocytes. A positive crossmatch, due to donor specific IgG antibodies, would normally be a contraindication to transplantation for organs such as kidney and pancreas, but there are now methods to transplant organs in the presence of donor-specific antibodies. Human leucocyte antigen-specific antibody incompatible transplants (AiT) have been performed, but require the careful monitoring of antibody levels and specificity, in conjunction with a protocol to reduce antibody levels.

Acute rejection is primarily a cellular event where the mismatched HLA molecules on the graft serve as targets for cytotoxic T lymphocytes. Human leucocyte antigen molecules can be recognized by T cells directly or indirectly: direct allorecognition occurs when recipient T cells recognize peptides, derived from the graft and presented by donor antigen-presenting cells; indirect allorecognition involves the patient's own antigen-presenting cell processing and presenting peptides, derived from the kidney allograft, to alloreactive T lymphocytes.

Using kidney transplantation as an example, direct allorecognition occurs when donor antigen-presenting cells, such as dendritic cells, migrate from the graft to a local lymph node, where they stimulate alloreactive T cells. These T cells can mediate graft destruction if untreated.

Human leucocyte antigen-specific antibodies can also be associated with acute rejection as studies, which demonstrate plasma cells and T cells infiltrating the rejecting allograft have shown. The donor-specific antibodies are normally formed *de novo* following transplantation and can damage the graft via the activation of complement, or through antibody-dependent, cell-mediated cytotoxicity (ADCC), whereby the antibodies coat graft cells and immune effector cells cause graft damage via interaction with antibody Fc binding. Acute rejection usually occurs within the first three months following transplantation, but can occur within days, and can be limited by HLA-matching and the use of immunosuppressive drugs.

Chronic rejection can be caused by immunological and non-immunological factors and results in a slow deterioration in graft function, occurring months to years following transplantation. Both donor-specific antibody and T lymphocytes have been implicated in mediating this chronic deterioration in graft function. In kidney allografts, it is characterized by fibrous intimal thickening of the arteries, interstitial fibrosis, and atrophy of the renal tubules. Studies have also shown that an increased number and severity of acute rejection episodes is a risk factor for developing features of chronic rejection. Other non-immunological factors, which have been shown to be associated with chronic rejection, include how the organ is preserved and perfusion when the organ is harvested, recipient factors such as infection, hypertension and drug toxicity, donor age, and organ tissue quality.

SELF-CHECK 8.3

What is the importance of HLA typing in solid organ transplantation?

Renal transplant allocation

In the UK kidneys are normally allocated on the basis of blood group and HLA type, where priority is given to donor-recipient pairs showing no (0) mismatch at HLA-A, B and DRB1, that is, 000 mismatched. Paediatric patients are given first priority, then the level of sensitization is taken into account. Other factors considered in the allocation algorithm are: waiting time, HLA match and age combined, donor-recipient age difference, location of the patient relative to the donor, HLA-DRB1 and HLA-B homozygosity, and blood group match. These factors are considered to, where possible:

- Prevent a patient waiting for a transplant for many years.
- Avoid an 'old' kidney being grafted into a young recipient.
- Reduce **cold ischaemia time**, which has been shown to be a risk factor in graft survival, by keeping a short distance between where the organs are harvested to where they are implanted.

Cold ischaemia time
During transplantation this time begins when the organ is cooled with a cold perfusion solution after organs are harvested and ends after the tissue reaches physiological temperature during the implantation procedure.

Those patients that are HLA homozygous and, therefore, require a homozygous donor for a 000 mismatched graft are also given access to these very useful donors. Finally, although transplants should be blood group compatible, an effort is made to match blood group so that O group donors are given to O group patients, where possible.

CLINICAL CORRELATION

The HLA-matching scheme used in the allocation of kidneys in the UK initially takes into account polymorphism at the HLA-A,-B and DRB1 loci:

| 000 | No mismatch at HLA-A, B, or DR |
| 010 | One HLA-B mismatch |

100	One HLA-A mismatch
110	Two mismatches (1x HLA-A, 1xHLA-B)

Sensitization to HLA-A, B, C, DR, DQ, and DP is considered prior to crossmatching and transplantation.

Pancreas transplant allocation

Blood group matching is a priority for the pancreas allocation. A number of clinically-relevant patient, donor, and transplant-associated factors are used to award the patient points, resulting in an individual total points score (TPS). The number of points each patient has is used to rank them in terms of priority for transplantation. Matching at HLA-A, B, and DR, HLA sensitization, time waiting for a transplant list, and factors previously mentioned that are used for kidney allocation, all contribute to a patient's TPS.

Heart and lung transplant allocation

Retrospective studies have shown that HLA-matching, particularly for HLA-DRB1, has a beneficial effect on graft survival. However, there are a number of factors that prevent the prospective HLA-matching of hearts in the UK:

- Physical size of the heart compared to the recipient is important.
- Small donor pool.
- Relatively small patient waiting list.
- Short cold ischaemia time (hearts should be transplanted within four hours of harvesting).

Lung transplants have similar restrictions and organ allocation protocols that apply to heart transplantation. In some cases, the heart and lungs are transplanted as a block.

Liver transplant allocation

Livers are allocated on the basis of blood group compatibility and matching of O group donors for O group patients, where possible. Human leucocyte antigen matching plays no role in the allocation of livers for transplantation.

Cornea transplant matching

The eye is often described as an immunologically privileged site, being protected from the normal effects of the immune system. No HLA-matching is performed for first corneal transplants, but, if the graft is rejected, HLA sensitization is taken into account for subsequent grafts as vascularization has usually occurred, meaning the cornea is accessible to the recipient's cellular and humoral immune system.

Crossmatching

The presence of donor-specific HLA antibodies have been shown to be important in hyperacute, acute, and chronic rejection and it is recommended that, where possible, a pre-transplant crossmatch be performed prior to transplantation. The logistical issues associated with cardiothoracic transplantation (see heart and lung transplant allocation) means that it is not always possible to perform a pre-transplant crossmatch in the laboratory. Instead, a 'virtual crossmatch' is performed, whereby the HLA mismatch between the patient and donor and the

HLA antibody screening history of the patient is formally assessed to avoid pre-formed donor-specific antibodies. This practice is also applied to a well-defined category of renal patients, namely, patients who are not sensitized to HLA and have a full and current sensitization history.

The crossmatch test is designed to partially reproduce, *in vitro*, what will happen *in vivo* when the organ is transplanted, by 'bathing' donor cells in patient's serum. The LCT and/or flow cytometry techniques are most widely used for solid organ transplantation. Patient serum samples, selected to represent the sensitization history of the patient, are mixed with donor cells, from peripheral blood in live donors (or prior to organ retrieval for deceased donors) and lymph node or spleen cells from deceased donors. The T and B lymphocyte populations can be isolated prior to the LCT crossmatch or labelled with lineage-specific conjugated antibodies as part of the flow cytometric crossmatch, and the patient's own lymphocytes can be tested to allow detection of autoreactive antibodies, which can aid interpretation of the crossmatch results. The techniques used are the same as described previously for LCT and flow cytometry.

Interpretation of the crossmatch is usually performed in conjunction with information from the antibody screening history and sensitization events. T cell positive crossmatches could be due to HLA class I-specific antibodies or autoantibodies. B cell positive crossmatches can be due to the presence of HLA class II, but B cells also express high levels of HLA class I, which can detect antibody that are not detectable using T cells alone. Therefore, it is important to a have an accurate antibody profile of the patient prior to embarking on crossmatching as this may prevent unexplained positive crossmatches, which could potentially increase the cold ischaemia time of the organ whilst another recipient is found for the organ.

Key points

Organ rejection can be minimized by HLA typing, matching, and crossmatching.

Rejection can be categorized as:

Hyperacute, occurring within minutes or hours of the transplant.

Acute, usually occurring within days up to the first three months following transplantation.

Chronic, slow deterioration of graft function, occurring months to years following transplantation.

Haemopoietic stem cell transplantation

Haemopoietic stem cell transplantation (HSCT) is the treatment of choice for a variety of haematological malignancies, primary immunodeficiencies, inborn errors of metabolism, and bone marrow disorders. Haemopoietic stem cells for transplantation can be derived from bone marrow, peripheral blood, or umbilical cord blood, and the source of stem cell used can be dependent on the disorder to be treated, which also can influence the type of donor used, for example HLA matched or mismatched.

Studies in Western Europe show that most patients have a 30% chance of finding an HLA identical sibling donor. Figure 8.4 shows that patients with siblings have a 1 in 4 chance of being HLA identical and also shows the potential for the generation of new haplotypes due

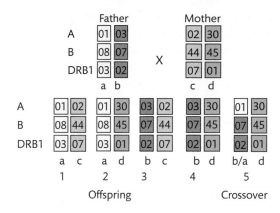

FIGURE 8.4

Human leucocyte antigen inheritance. Human leucocyte antigen genes are inherited en bloc and a set of genes on one chromosome are known as a haplotype. Each offspring inherit one paternal and one maternal haplotype, giving four possible haplotype combinations. However, there are rare occasions when there is reciprocal exchange of DNA between homologous chromosomes during meiosis or crossing over leading to a recombinant haplotype as seen in offspring 5.

to crossing over or recombination. The best outcomes for HSCT in terms of overall survival are seen in HLA identical sibling transplants as they may also be matched for products of non-HLA genes. If no suitable family donor is available a search for an unrelated donor is performed, first nationally, then, if no suitable match is found, internationally. See Figure 8.5.

In the UK the National Registries include: the British Bone Marrow Registry (BBMR) (part of NHSBT), which recruits blood donors in England, Scotland, and Northern Ireland; the Anthony Nolan Trust, which is a charity that recruits donors throughout the UK; and the Welsh Bone Marrow Registry, which only recruit donors from Wales. Bone Marrow Donors Worldwide (BMDW) facilitates donor searches throughout the world by holding data of over 17 million donors from 64 HSC Registries in 44 countries and 44 cord blood banks in 26 countries. More registries and cord banks are added every year.

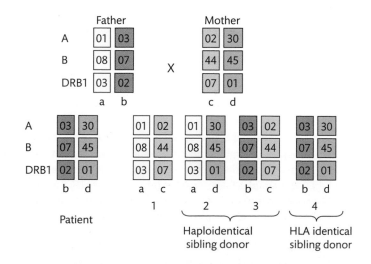

FIGURE 8.5

Human leucocyte antigen matching. An HLA identical sibling is the ideal donor as they share the same haplotypes inherited from their parents. Haploidentical transplants can be between parents or siblings that share one haplotype with the patient, in this example, siblings 2 and 3 and the parent share one HLA haplotype with the patient.

The HLA matching requirements for adult unrelated stem transplantation are more stringent than those used for solid organ transplantation or platelet transfusions. Haemopoietic stem cell transplantation involves transfusing **immunocompetent** cells into an immunosuppressed recipient. Any HLA mismatches could be recognized as foreign by the donor lymphocytes and lead to graft versus host disease (GVHD), which can be fatal. Most centres would aim to match for both alleles at the five loci (HLA-A, B, C, DRB1, and DQB1), so they describe a fully-matched donor as a 10 out of 10 match, and would aim to achieve at least a 9 out of 10 match. Human leucocyte antigen-DP is taken into account by some transplant centres where there is a choice between equally matched donors. Since HLA-DP is not in **linkage disequilibrium** with HLA-DR, it is often mismatched, but this HLA mismatch on the patient's cells may also serve as a target for the graft versus leukaemia (GVL) effect.

The lymphocytes present in cord blood are more naive and not as immunocompetent as adult lymphocytes and this has been used in part to explain the lower incidence and milder severity of GVHD seen in cord blood transplants compared to adult stem cell transplants. The two main factors influencing the outcome of cord blood transplantation are HLA-matching and haemopoietic stem cell dose. The level of HLA-matching is not as stringent for cord blood transplantation and Eurocord studies show that up to two mismatches at the HLA-A or B loci can be tolerated, but the cell dose must be increased where mismatching takes place. The minimum matching requirements are high resolution for HLA-DRB1 and low-to-medium resolution for HLA-A and B. As more data become available, better outcomes are seen where high resolution typing is performed for HLA class I in addition to HLA class II.

Human leucocyte antigen mismatching can have a crucial effect on transplant outcome so it is important that the HLA laboratory performs the appropriate level of typing, and that the reports and advice are relevant for the type of transplant.

Other factors influencing donor selection for HSCT include:

CMV status:	they try to match the CMV status of the donor and recipient.
Age:	transplant outcomes are better with young donors <30 years old.
Male donors:	as male donors have both X and Y chromosomes their T cells do not see sex chromosome products as foreign, but T cells from female donors can recognize male HY minor histocompatibility antigens as foreign.

Post-transplantation chimerism testing

There are a number of ways to assess engraftment or disease re-occurrence following allogeneic HSCT. One of the most sensitive methods used by histocompatibility and immunogenetics laboratories employs the use of short tandem repeat (STR) markers with allele sizes that differ among individuals. The pre-transplant genotypes of the recipient and donors are established and samples taken from the recipient post-HSCT are tested to determine the presence of donor material. Where the recipient sample consists of 100% donor DNA, it is referred to as full donor chimerism, or mixed chimerism where both recipient and donor DNA are detected.

HSCT for malignant disease often involves myeloablative conditioning using total body irradiation and/or chemotherapy. In these cases, the aim is to achieve full donor chimerism as the presence of any recipient cells may potentially result in the malignancy returning. Mixed chimerism may be satisfactory if the haematological disorder does not require full donor chimerism. For example, in the case of some haemoglobinopathies or enzyme deficiencies, there may be a minimum number of donor cells required to produce enough cells carrying the corrected haemoglobin or enzyme to counteract the effects of the defect.

> **BOX 8.4** Human leucocyte antigen matching for haemopoietic stem cell transplantation
>
> Most adult unrelated stem cell transplant programmes match for: HLA-A, B, C, DRB1, and DQB1 and aim to achieve a 10/10 or 9/10 match using high resolution HLA typing.
>
> Cord blood transplant programmes also aim to match for the same HLA loci as adult stem cell programmes, but the minimum requirement is to match for: HLA-A, B, DRB1 and aim to achieve a 6/6, 5/6, or 4/6 match using high resolution typing for HLA-DRB1 and low to medium resolution for HLA-A and B.

8.5 Clinical significance of human leucocyte antigens in transfusion

Immunological refractoriness to random platelet transfusions

Many patients with haematological disorders and some cancers require transfusion support (red cells and platelets) due to the disease itself or the side effects of its treatment. A normal platelet count can range from 150×10^9/l to 400×10^9/l but, when the count falls below 30×10^9/l, there is a risk of bleeding. Patients with low levels of platelets are transfused with donor platelets until they regain the ability to produce their own platelets.

Both pooled or single donor platelets are leucodepleted and have the same average number of platelets. Therefore, stable patients transfused with either product should have a rise in platelet count of between 30 and 40×10^9/l. In approximately 30–50% of transfusion-dependent patients, there is not an adequate rise in platelet count following transfusion. These patients are described as *refractory* to random platelet transfusion. Platelet refractoriness is defined as the failure of the transfused patient to gain adequate platelet increments ($<10 \times 10^9$/l), one hour or up to 24 hours post-transfusion. The causes can be immune-related on non-immune.

Non-immune causes include:

- Old or badly stored platelets
- Sepsis
- Disseminated intravascular coagulation in the patient
- Drugs such as amphotericin B, ciprofloxacin

Immune causes include:

- Human leucocyte antigen class I specific antibodies
- Human platelet antigens (HPA) specific antibodies
- High titre ABO alloantibodies

Most cases of immunological refractoriness are due to HLA class I-specific antibodies, which will bind to transfused platelets that express the cognate HLA class molecules. Cells of the monocyte/macrophage system will, in turn, recognize the antibody complex via the Fc region and remove the platelets from circulation. Human platelet antigen antibody-mediated destruction follows the same mechanism. ABO-mismatched platelets transfused into alloimmunized patients can result in a 20% reduction in the platelet increments post-transfusion. Circulating immune complexes involving the ABO system have also been shown to decrease the survival of transfused platelets.

Laboratory investigation of refractory patients involves:

- Screening the patient's serum for the presence of HLA-specific antibodies
- Definition of HLA antibody specificity
- Human leucocyte antigen class I typing of patient and donors
- Provision of HLA selected platelets

Although platelets express HLA-class I, the expression of HLA-C is lower than HLA-A or HLA-B on cells and poorly expressed on platelets. Therefore, most laboratories only match for HLA A and B. In addition, HLA-B and C are closely co-located on the chromosome and, as such, usually inherited together, so matching for HLA-B can often result in matching for HLA-C.

The provision of HLA selected platelets is based on the HLA type of the patient and their HLA antibody profile using a panel of HLA typed donors. The matching system used for the provision of HLA selected platelets is different to that used for solid organ or haemopoietic stem cell transplantation. The NHSBT matching criteria are based on two grades of matches:

- 'A' grade, where there is no mismatch between donor and recipient.
- 'B' grade, where patient and donor are mismatched, with the number of mismatches denoting the type of B match, for example B1 for one mismatch, B2 for two mismatches, etc. Mismatching is carried out on the basis of the known **serological crossreactivity** that exists between different antigens of the HLA-A and B loci.

Serological crossreactivity

This is where antibodies react with a public epitope shared by different HLA molecules. These HLA molecules that share a public epitope are often described as Cross Reactive Groups (CREG), for example anti-HLA-B7 antibodies can crossreact with a shared epitope on HLA-B42, B55, and B56

BOX 8.5 Human leucocyte antigens matching for platelet transfusion

'A' grade match:

Patient:	HLA-A*01, A*02; B*08, B*44	
Donor 1:	HLA-A*01, A*02; B*08, B*44	No mismatch
Donor 2:	HLA-A*01, A*01; B*08, B*08	No mismatch

'B' grade match:

Patient:	HLA-A*01, A*02; B*08, B*44	
Donor 1:	HLA-A*01, A*11; B*08, B*44	B1 match (one mismatch)
Donor 2:	HLA-A*01, A*11; B*08, B*49	B2 match (two mismatches)

Key points

Platelet refractoriness is the failure to gain adequate platelet increments ($<10 \times 10^9/l$), one hour or up to 24 hours post-transfusion. The causes can be non-immune or immune due to HLA, HPA, or ABO antibodies.

Febrile non-haemolytic transfusion reactions (FNHTRs)

Febrile non-haemolytic transfusion reactions (FNHTRs) are some of the most common transfusion reactions and are characterized by fever, chills, and a rise in temperature of more than 1 or 2°C, occurring during or 30–60 minutes following the transfusion. Other symptoms, such as rigor, flushing, increased heart beat rate (tachycardia), nausea, and vomiting can also be present.

Febrile non-haemolytic transfusion reactions can be triggered by a variety of factors. Human leucocyte antigen or HNA antibodies, present in the recipient and reacting with white blood cells in the transfused product, have been shown to be the main immunological trigger of these reactions, and antibodies against white cells are found in 70% or more of patients who suffer from FNHTRs. In most cases, it is likely that the antibody–antigen complex may directly activate the cells to produce pyrogenic cytokines leading to the febrile reaction.

A number of studies have reported that the incidence of FNHTR is reduced when the white cells are removed from the transfused product by leucodepletion. The decreased number of leucocytes not only presents fewer targets for leucocyte-reactive antibodies, but also reduces the probability of sensitization in the non-sensitized patient.

Universal leucodepletion was introduced in England in October 1999, but cases of FNHTR have still been reported. It is likely that some of these reactions are due to an accumulation of cytokines released by the residual white cells in the stored blood component, especially in platelet concentrates.

Transfusion-related acute lung injury (TRALI)

Transfusion-related acute lung injury (TRALI) is a rare but life-threatening complication of blood transfusion where the patient experiences respiratory distress within 2–6 hours following a transfusion. Symptoms generally include fever, hypotension, chills, cyanosis, non-productive cough, dyspnoea, and sometimes severe hypoxia. Chest X-ray shows severe bilateral pulmonary oedema or perihilar and lung infiltration, without cardiac enlargement or involvement of the vessels.

The mechanism of action

Most cases of confirmed TRALI are associated with the presence of HLA class I or class II antibodies in the plasma of the transfused component, with specificities corresponding to the HLA antigen(s) present in the recipient. Granulocyte-specific antibodies, for example anti-HNA1, HNA-2, and HNA-3 have also been implicated. These antibodies are most commonly found in blood and blood components donated by women who have had multiple pregnancies.

Products that contain a significant proportion of plasma, such as whole blood, platelets and fresh frozen plasma (FFP), and even the small amount of plasma in red cells in optimal additive solution (e.g. SAGM), have been implicated in some TRALI reactions.

Transfusion-related acute lung injury cases have also been reported where no HLA or granulocyte antibodies have been detected. These reactions also appear to be mediated by a soluble lipid substance, which accumulates during the storage. Animal studies have shown that these soluble lipids are biologically active and can activate granulocytes to induce the release of anaphylatoxins, cytokines and chemokines, which promote neutrophil chemotaxis and aggregation in the lungs. The resulting reaction causes endothelial damage and increased pulmonary vascular permeability, resulting in fluid leakage into the alveoli and an accumulation of fluid in the lungs (oedema).

Look-back studies have shown that products from donors implicated in TRALI reactions have been transfused into other patients with no reported serious clinical consequences, suggesting that other factors, such as the predisposing clinical condition of the recipient, may influence the initiation of TRALI. These observations have led to the proposal of the 'two hit' hypothesis for the development of TRALI. The first hit involves the action of antibodies or soluble mediators and the second hit involves the influence of the clinical condition of the patient.

Treatment of TRALI includes intensive respiratory and circulatory support. In almost all cases, oxygen supplementation is necessary, although mechanical ventilation may not always be required. The majority of patients improve both clinically and physiologically within two or three days with adequate supportive care and, once recovered, there is no residual damage in these patients. Mortality still remains at 6%, however.

Transfusion-related acute lung injury reduction

The English National Blood Service and other Blood Services around the world have introduced changes in the manufacture of blood components, with the aim of reducing the incidence of TRALI. These measures take into account that HLA and granulocyte antibodies in blood components primarily originate from female donors who have been sensitized by pregnancy.

The TRALI reduction measures include:

- The production of FFP from donations collected from male donors.
- The use of male donor plasma to re-suspend pooled platelets.
- The preferential recruitment of male apheresis donors such that, from 2008, 80% of all apheresis platelets collected by NHSBT were from male donors.
- Human leucocyte antigen and HNA antibody screening of all new female apheresis donors added to the panel.

Transfusion-associated graft versus host disease (TA-GVHD)

Transfusion-associated graft versus host disease (TA-GVHD) is a rare but fatal adverse reaction to transfusion. Acute GVHD, usually associated with allogeneic haemopoietic stem cell transplantation, and TA-GVHD share similar features, but there are important differences. Both types of GVHD result from the presence of viable lymphocytes in the allograft or transfusion recognizing the host mismatched HLA molecules. These donor lymphocytes must be immunocompetent and share one HLA haplotype with the host; the donor is commonly HLA homozygous and is not recognized by the host as foreign.

Clinically, the GVHD reactions are similar, affecting the skin, liver, and gut, but TA-GVHD differs in that it occurs much sooner (normally 8–10 days following transfusion) and over 90% of TA-GVHD cases are fatal, whereas HSCT GVHD can be treated successfully.

The diagnosis of TA-GVHD mainly depends on finding evidence of donor-derived DNA in the blood and/or affected tissues of the recipient, known as detection of chimerism. Using DNA analysis allows a wider range of markers to be employed, including HLA genes or other genetic markers.

The chimerism test requires DNA to be extracted from recipient samples taken pre- and post-transfusion and from samples of the implicated donors. DNA can be extracted from skin (both affected and unaffected areas), hair follicles, or nail clippings. Post-mortem samples from the spleen or bone marrow, if available, can also be used as a source of DNA. If donor chimerism can be detected in the patient, it can be used to confirm the diagnosis of TA-GVHD.

As there is no effective treatment of TA-GVHD and the mortality rate is extremely high, a lot of effort is put into preventing its occurrence. Although the introduction of universal leucodepletion in the UK has been associated with a significant reduction in the number of reported cases of TA-GVHD, the residual lymphocyte numbers may still be enough to initiate TA-GVHD.

Irradiation of cellular blood components renders the donor lymphocytes non-viable and protects the recipient from potentially developing TA-GVHD. It is recommended that all cellular blood products for at risk patients should be irradiated with a minimum of 25 Gray (Gy), prior to transfusion. See Chapter 5 for more on irradiated blood components.

SELF-CHECK 8.4

What measures have Transfusion Services introduced to reduce the incidence of HLA-related adverse effects of transfusion?

Key points

Human leucocyte antigen antibody-mediated complications of transfusions include febrile non-haemolytic transfusion reactions, TRALI (caused by HLA antibodies present in the donor), and TA-GVHD (resulting from the presence of viable lymphocytes in the allograft or transfusion recognizing the host mismatched HLA molecules).

 CHAPTER SUMMARY

- The human leucocyte antigens play a pivotal role in the induction and regulation of immune responses as the main function of HLA molecules is the presentation of peptides derived from foreign molecules to T lymphocytes.

- A key feature of the HLA system is its extensive polymorphism, which is advantageous to humans in enabling responses to a wide variety of pathogens but presents a barrier to transplantation and some transfusions.

- The immunological complications of transplantation and transfusion such as allograft rejection, graft versus host disease, and platelet refractoriness can be limited by HLA matching, with a higher degree of HLA matching required for T cell mediated complications such as GVHD in HSCT, compared with antibody mediated complications such as immunological platelet refractoriness.

- The current technology used for the definition of HLA polymorphism is DNA-based molecular techniques, allowing the discrimination between different HLA alleles for HSCT or antigens for solid organ transplantation or platelet transfusion. The availability of purified single HLA molecules has revolutionized antibody detection and definition such that complex antibody reactivity can be defined in a single Luminex based test.

■ Advances in allele, antigen, and antibody definition is associated with some challenges in determining the clinical relevance of this increased sensitivity.

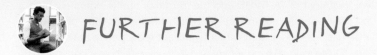# FURTHER READING

- Brown CJ & Navarrete CV. Clinical relevance of the HLA system in blood transfusion. *Vox Sanguinis*, 101 (2011), 93–105.

- Howell WM, Carter V, & Clark B. The HLA system: immunobiology, HLA typing, antibody screening and crossmatching techniques. *J Clin Pathol*, 63 (2010), 387–90.

- http://hla.alleles.org/antigens/recognised_serology.html.

- www.ebi.ac.uk/imgt/hla/stats.html.

- Opelz G & Döhler B. Effects of human leucocyte antigen compatibility of kidney graft survival: comparative analysis of two decades. *Transplantation*, 84 (2007), 137–43.

- Petersdorf EW. Optimal HLA matching in hematopoietic cell transplantation. *Curr Opin Immunol*, 20 (2008), 588–93.

- Tait BD, Hudson F, Cantwell L, et al. Review article: Luminex technology for HLA antibody detection in organ transplantation. *Nephrology (Carlton)*, 14 (2009), 247–54.

- Taylor C, Navarrete C, & Contreras M. Immunological complications of transfusion. In: A Maniatis, P Van der Linden, & JF Hardy (eds) *Alternatives to Blood Transfusion in Transfusion Medicine*, 2010.

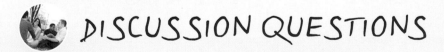# DISCUSSION QUESTIONS

8.1   Explain why HLA polymorphism is important to the human species.

8.2   Outline the methods available for HLA typing.

8.3   Outline the methods available for the detection of HLA antibodies.

8.4   What level of HLA matching is required for major solid organ and stem cell transplants?

Answers to the questions in this chapter are provided on the book's Online Resource Centre.

 Go to www.oxfordtextbooks.co.uk/orc/knight

9

Human Platelet Antigens (HPA) and Human Neutrophil Antigens (HNA) and Their Clinical Significance

Geoff Lucas

Learning objectives

By the end of this chapter you should be able to:

■ Describe the nomenclature of human platelet antigens (HPA) and human neutrophil antigens (HNA).

■ List the most important HPA and HNA.

■ Understand the principles, techniques and problems in detecting HPA and HNA and the associated antibodies.

■ Detail the most important clinical conditions in which platelet and granulocyte antibodies occur.

■ Have a detailed understanding of the clinical management and problems associated with the management of NAIT cases.

■ Describe the current interventions that are used to treat the other clinical conditions associated with HPA and HNA antibodies.

Introduction

In Chapter 2 you learned the range of different antigens that are found on red cells, the techniques used to identify them and the antibodies that arise to these antigens following transfusion, pregnancy or as the result of autoimmune disease. Subsequent chapters (3–7) explored the different facets of blood transfusion and the clinical disorders.

This chapter examines similar principles again but in the context of platelets and granulocytes as the affected cells. There are many common principles involved in the immunohaematology of red cells and the immunohaematology of platelets and granulocytes. Equally, there are some key differences which have resulted in different strategies for both typing and antibody detection and identification. Some differences arise from the nature of the cells, for example these cells are physiologically active and prone to aggregation *in vivo*; other differences occur because human platelet antigens (HPA) and human neutrophil antigens (HNA) occur on cells also expressing other common immunological targets, for example HLA class I, which are widely distributed antigens (see Chapter 8). The antigens uniquely expressed on platelets or neutrophils are implicated in immune-mediated thrombocytopenias and neutropenias respectively. Alloantibodies formed during pregnancy, following transfusion or bone marrow transplantation against HPA or against HNA may cause alloimmune thrombocytopenia or neutropenia respectively. Other antibodies against platelets and granulocytes can arise as part of an autoimmune process or as the result of an immune response following drug administration. The detection and determination of the specificity and nature of such antibodies is therefore of clinical significance in determining the appropriate clinical treatment for the patient.

Autoantibodies
Antibodies that react with 'self' antigens.

Alloantibodies
Antibodies that react with an inherited antigenic characteristic that is lacking in the recipient.

Isoantibodies
Antibodies that react with an antigen that is normally found in all individuals but which is lacking in the recipient.

Drug-dependent antibodies
Antibodies that react with a drug directly or with an antigenic structure created when the drug binds to a naturally occurring structure (referred to as haptenization).

9.1 Overview of platelet and granulocyte antigens

Antigens on human platelets and granulocytes can be categorized according to their biochemical nature into:

1. Carbohydrate antigens on glycolipids and glycoproteins:

    (a)   A, B, and O

    (b)   P and Le on platelets; I on granulocytes

2. Protein antigens:

    (a)   human leucocyte antigen (HLA) class I (A, B, and C)

    (b)   glycoprotein (GP) IIb/IIIa, GPIa/IIa, GPIb/IX/V, etc. on platelets

    (c)   FcγRIIIb (CD16), CD177, etc. on granulocytes

3. Hapten-induced antigens, for example those associated with the following drugs:

    (a)   quinine, quinidine

    (b)   penicillins and cephalosporins

    (c)   heparin

These antigens can be targeted by some or all of the following types of antibodies:

- **Autoantibodies**
- **Alloantibodies**
- **Isoantibodies**
- **Drug-dependent antibodies**

Many antigens on platelets and granulocytes are also found on other cells, for example. ABO and HLA class I (Table 9.1); other antigens, however, are largely, but not always exclusively, restricted to platelets and granulocytes and these are known as **human platelet antigens (HPA)** and **human neutrophil antigens (HNA)**. The genetic basis of most HPAs and HNAs has been resolved, allowing DNA-based typing of patient, donor, and foetus. Methods for high throughput DNA-based typing have dramatically improved the availability to HPA selected blood products in England and made clinical intervention with these products a reality.

> **Human platelet antigen (HPA)**
> The term given to allelic forms of platelet glycoproteins that give rise to an alloimmune response.
>
> **Human neutrophil antigen (HNA)**
> The term given to allelic forms of granulocyte glycoproteins that give rise to an alloimmune response.

TABLE 9.1 The distribution of major platelet and granulocyte glycoproteins amongst peripheral blood cells.

Antigens	Erythrocytes	Platelets	Neutrophils	B lymphocytes	T lymphocytes	Monocytes
A, B, H	+ ++	(+)/ + +	–	–	–	–
I	+ ++	+ +	+ +	–	–	–
Rh*	+ ++	–	–	–	–	–
K	+ ++	–	–	–	–	–
HLA class I	–/(+)	+ ++	+ +	+ ++	+ ++	+ ++
HLA class II	–	–	–/ + ++ §	+ ++	–/ + ++ §	+ ++
GPIIb/IIIa	–	+ ++	(+)'	–	–	–
GPIa/IIa	–	+ ++	–	–	+ +	–
GPIb/IX/V	–	+ ++	–	–	–	–
CD109	–	(+)/ + +§	–	–	–/ + +§	(+)
FcRIIIb (CD16b)	–	–	+ ++	–	–	–
CD177	–	–	+ ++ a	–	–	–
CTL2	–	+ (personal observations)	+ ++	++ (B and T lymphocytes not separated)		?
CD11b/18	–	–	+ +	–	–	+ +b
CD11a/18	–	–	+ +	+ +	+ +	+ +

++ + , ++ , + Indicates level of antigen expression in decreasing order (+) indicates weak expression. ? Indicates not known.

* Non-glycosylated.

§ On activated cells.

' GPIIIa(β_3) in association with an alternative α chain α_v.

a Expressed on a sub-population of neutrophils.

b Also expressed on natural killer cells.

Key points

Allo-, auto-, iso-, and drug-induced antigens may be found on platelets and neutrophils and are implicated in a range of immune cytopenias.

SELF-CHECK 9.1

What is the distinction between the following terms: white blood cells, granulocytes, and neutrophils?

Biallelic
The two alternative alleles of a gene.

Allele
One of two or more alternative forms of a gene that arise by mutation and are found at the same place on a chromosome.

Codominant
Relating to two alleles of a gene pair that are both fully expressed in a heterozygote.

Monoclonal antibody immobilization of platelet antigens (MAIPA) assay
An ELISA assay which uses monoclonal antibodies against platelet antigens as the basis of detection and identification of platelet specific antibodies.

Polymerase chain reaction (PCR)
An enzyme reaction utilizing Taq polymerase to amplify the copy number and hence enable detection of a genetic characteristic.

Single nucleotide polymorphism (SNP)
A single nucleotide substitution in the DNA reading frame that encodes a particular inherited characteristic.

Neonatal alloimmune thrombocytopenia (NAIT)
Thrombocytopenia in a neonate (or foetus) caused by the maternal foetal transfer of platelet specific antibodies recognizing either HPAs or platelet glycoproteins inherited by the foetus from the father but absent in the mother.

9.2 Human platelet antigens (HPA)

Inheritance and nomenclature

All the HPAs reported to date (with the exception of HPA-14) have been shown to be **biallelic**, with each **allele** being **codominant**. Historically, platelet-specific antigens were named by the authors first reporting the antigen, usually using an abbreviation of the name of the propositus in whom the alloantibody was first detected. Some systems were published simultaneously by different investigators and several names were assigned to the same antigen, for example Zw and Pl^A, and Zav, Br, Hc, were later found to be the same polymorphism, that is, HPA-1 and HPA-5 respectively. In 1990, the working party for platelet immunology within the International Society of Blood Transfusion (ISBT) agreed the HPA nomenclature for platelet-specific alloantigens and subsequently the international Platelet Nomenclature Committee has published guidelines for the naming of newly discovered platelet-specific alloantigens. In this nomenclature, each system is numbered consecutively (HPA-1, -2, -3, and so on) (Table 9.2) according to its date of discovery, with the major allele in each system being designated 'a' and the minor allele 'b'. Antigens are only included in a system if antibodies against the alloantigen encoded by both the major and minor alleles have been reported; if an antibody against only one allele has been reported, a 'w' (for workshop) is added after the antigen name, for example HPA-10bw (Metcalfe et al. 2003). Use of techniques such as immunoprecipitation of radioactive labelled platelet membrane proteins, the **monoclonal antibody-specific immobilization of platelet antigens (MAIPA) assay** and the **polymerase chain reaction (PCR)** have enabled the genetic and molecular basis of all HPAs to be elucidated (Figure 9.1 and Table 9.2). For all but one of the 21 HPAs, the difference between the two alleles is a **single nucleotide polymorphism (SNP)** which changes the amino acid in the corresponding protein (Table 9.2). Twelve of the HPAs are grouped into six HPA systems (HPA-1 to 5 and HPA-15) and for all of these, except HPA-3 and HPA-15, the minor allele frequency is ≤0.2 and consequently homozygosity for the minor allele is relatively rare.

Most of the 21 HPA polymorphisms were first discovered during the investigation of cases of **neonatal alloimmune thrombocytopenia (NAIT)**. The majority of the antigens are located on the IIIa sub-unit of the platelet glycoprotein GPIIb/IIIa (CD41/CD61), which is a high abundance (~1%) and physiologically important component of the platelet membrane as it is the main platelet receptor for fibrinogen and critical to the final phase of platelet aggregation. The other HPAs are located on the IIb sub-unit of GPIIb/IIIa, on GPIa/IIa (CD49b), on GPIb/IX/V, and CD109. Three of these receptor complexes are critical for haemostasis

TABLE 9.2 The human platelet antigen (HPA) systems.

HPA System	Antigen	Alternative names	Phenotype frequency* (%)	Glycoprotein	SNP	SNP rs number	Amino acid change
1	1a	Zw^a, Pl^{A1}	97.9	GPIIIa	T^{196}	rs5918	Leucine[33]
	1b	Zw^b, Pl^{A2}	28.8		C^{196}		Proline[33]
2	2a	Ko^b	>99.9	GPIbα	C^{524}	rs6065	Threonine[145]
	2b	Ko^a, Sib^a	13.2		T^{524}		Methionine[145]
3	3a	Bak^a, Lek^a	80.95	GPIIb	T^{2622}	rs5911	Isoleucine[843]
	3b	Bak^b	69.8		G^{2622}		Serine[843]
4	4a	Yuk^b, Pen^a	>99.9	GPIIIa	G^{526}	rs5917	Arginine[143]
	4b	Yuk^a, Pen^b	<0.1		A^{526}		Glutamine[143]
5	5a	Br^b, Zav^b	99.0	GPIa	G^{1648}	rs10471371	Glutamic acid[505]
	5b	Br^a, Zav^a, Hc^a	19.7		A^{1648}		Lysine[505]
6	6bw	Ca^a, Tu^a	0.7	GPIIIa	G^{1564}	rs13306487	Arginine[489]
					A^{1564}		Glutamine[489]
7	7bw	Mo^a	0.2	GPIIIa	C^{1267}		Proline[407]
					G^{1267}		Alanine[407]
8	8bw	Sr^a	<0.01	GPIIIa	T^{2004}		Arginine[636]
					C^{2004}		Cysteine[636]
9	9bw	Max^a	0.6	GPIIb	G^{2603}		Valine[837]
					A^{2603}		Methionine[837]
10	10bw	La^a	<1.6	GPIIIa	G^{281}		Arginine[62]
					A^{281}		Glutamine[62]
11	11bw	Gro^a	<0.25	GPIIIa	G^{1996}		Arginine[633]
					A^{1996}		Histidine[633]
12	12bw	Iy^a	0.4	GPIbβ	G^{141}		Glycine[15]
					A^{141}		Glutamic acid[15]
13	13bw	Sit^a	0.25	GPIa	C^{2531}		Threonine[799]
					T^{2531}		Methionine[799]
14	14bw	Oe^a	<0.17	GPIIIa	Δ AAG$^{1929-1931}$		Δ Lysine[611]
15	15a	Gov^b	74	CD109	C^{2108}	rs10455097	Serine[703]
	15b	Gov^a	81		A^{2108}		Tyrosine[703]
16	16bw	Duv^a	<1	GPIIIa	C^{517}		Threonine[140]
					T^{517}		Isoleucine[140]
17	17bw	Va^a	<0.4	GPIIIa	C^{622}		Threonine[195]
					T^{622}		Methionine[195]
18	18bw	Cab^a	<1	GPIa	G^{2235}		Glutamine[716]
					T^{2235}		Histidine[716]

(Continued)

TABLE 9.2 (Continued)

HPA System	Antigen	Alternative names	Phenotype frequency* (%)	Glycoprotein	SNP	SNP rs number	Amino acid change
19	19bw	Sta	<1	GPIIIa	A^{487} C^{487}		Lysine^{137} Glutamine^{137}
20	20bw	Kno	<1	GPIIb	C^{1949} T^{1949}		Threonine^{619} Methionine^{619}
21	21bw	Nos	<1	GPIIa	G^{1960} A^{1960}		Glutamic acid^{628} Lysine^{628}

* Frequencies based on studies in Caucasians.

SNP: single nucleotide polymorphism; rs: the international SNP reference number in the dbSNP database

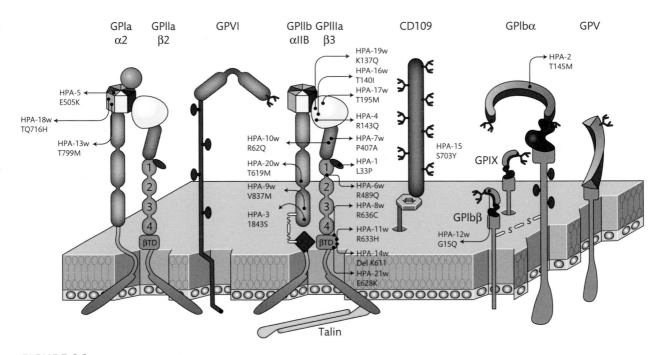

FIGURE 9.1

Representation of the platelet membrane and the glycoproteins (GP) on which the human platelet antigens (HPA) are localized. The major functional protein complexes (GPIa/IIa, GPVI, GPIIb/IIIa, CD109, and GPIbα/Ibβ/X/V) are depicted from left to right. The diagram also illustrates the transmembrane nature of these proteins and the interaction with the platelet cytoskeleton (represented by the protein talin) and which is responsible for platelet shape change that occurs in response to external stimuli such as von Willebrand factor and fibrinogen. The molecular basis of the HPAs are indicated by black dots, with the amino acid change in single letter code and by residue number in the expressed protein. (Adapted from Practical Transfusion Medicine Third Edition, 2009, Wiley-Blackwell.)

and are responsible for the stepwise process of platelet attachment to the damaged vessel wall. GPIb/IX/V is the major receptor for von Willebrand factor (vWF) and is implicated in the initial binding of platelets to damaged endothelium. The GPIbα-bound vWF interacts with collagen, facilitating the interaction of collagen with its signalling (GPVI) and attachment receptors (GPIa/IIa). GPVI related signalling leads to a change in the platelet integrins GPIIb/IIIa and GPIa/IIa, exposing the high affinity binding sites for fibrinogen and collagen respectively. The function of CD109 has not been fully elucidated. These proteins are represented pictorially in Figure 9.1.

Glanzmann's thrombasthenia and Bernard–Soulier syndrome are two rare and severe, autosomal recessive, platelet bleeding disorders caused by mutations in the genes encoding GPIIb and GPIIIa, or GPIbα, GPIbβ, and GPIX respectively, which result in either an absence, a numerical reduction, or functional impairment of these proteins.

The glycoprotein IIb/IIIa complex

The GPIIb/IIIa complex consists of two polypeptide chains. GPIIIa (CD61) is a 90 kDa glycoprotein consisting of three major domains: a large extracellular N-terminal region containing 28 disulphide bonds, a transmembrane domain, and a short cytoplasmic segment. GPIIb (CD41) is also a transmembrane protein consisting of an extracellular 116kDa heavy chain associated by a single disulphide bond with a 22kDa light chain. There are approximately 50–80,000 copies of GPIIb/IIIa per platelet. This complex requires Ca^{2+} ions for its function and upon platelet activation undergoes a conformational change that enables it to bind fibrinogen and fibronectin, vitronectin, and vWF.

The glycoprotein Ib/IX/V complex

The GPIb/IX/V complex (CD42) is involved in the initial stages of platelet adhesion via vWf to damaged subendothelium of the vessel wall under conditions of high shear stress. The vWf receptor is composed of four transmembrane components. Glycoprotein Ibα (CD42b) and GPIbβ (CD42c) are linked by a single disulphide bond and are associated with GPIX (CD42a) and GPV (CD42d). There are approximately 25,000 copies of GPIb/IX and 12,000 copies of GPV per platelet. The primary vWf binding site has been localized within GPIbα, but there is evidence that the other three components also contribute to receptor function.

The glycoprotein Ia/IIa complex

The GPIa/IIa (CD49/CD29) complex is another dimeric protein and is also found on activated T lymphocytes and several other cell types as well as platelets. The principal ligand of this heterodimer is collagen in exposed sub-endothelium. There are approximately 800–2,800 copies of GPIa/IIa per platelet.

Incidence of platelet alloantigens in different populations

There have been few comprehensive large-scale studies to assess the frequency of platelet alloantigens in different populations but there are a number of small-scale studies. Although incomplete, summarized data from these studies clearly show significant differences in the prevalence of some antigens between populations, for example the HPA-1 polymorphism is largely absent in populations of the Far East, while the HPA-4 polymorphism is largely absent in Caucasians but is present in Far Eastern populations. Consequently, it is important to take ethnicity into account when investigating clinical cases of suspected HPA alloimmunization.

Key points

Alloantigens on platelets are known as human platelet antigens (HPAs).

HPA typing

Until the early 1990s, HPA typing was performed by serology (phenotyping). This required the use of monospecific human antisera, which were relatively uncommon as the majority of immunized individuals produced HLA class I antibodies in addition to the HPA antibodies. The development of more advanced assays such as the MAIPA assay (Figure 9.2) that were able to elucidate complex mixtures of antibodies against different GPs permitted more extensive phenotyping, but antisera for many HPA specificities were unavailable or scarce.

Today, DNA-based typing techniques have largely replaced HPA phenotyping in most laboratories. A commonly used assay is the **PCR using sequence-specific primers (PCR-SSP)**,

Polymerase chain reaction with sequence specific primers (PCR-SSP)
The polymerase chain reaction using primers that recognize a DNA sequence encoding a unique heritable genetic characteristic—typically an SNP.

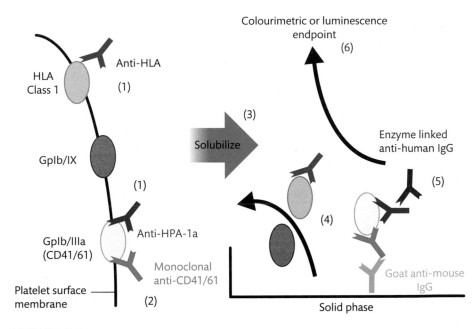

FIGURE 9.2

Monoclonal antibody-specific immobilization of platelet antigens (MAIPA) assay. This diagram demonstrates the detection of HPA-1a antibodies in the presence of HLA class I antibodies, a laboratory scenario that may not readily lead to the determination of HPA antibody specificity using a whole cell assay such as the platelet immunofluorescence test. The sequence of the assay is as follows: 1) Target (HPA typed) platelets are incubated with the test serum. HPA-1a antibodies will bind to HPA-1a (+) platelets but not to HPA-1a (–) platelets. 2) After washing, platelets are incubated with a platelet glycoprotein specific monoclonal antibody (anti-GPIIb/IIIa in this example). 3) After washing, the platelets are solubilized. 4) After centriguation, the resultant supernatant is added to a microtitre plate previously coated with goat antimouse IgG antibodies. 5) The solubilized complex of platelet glycoprotein, murine antibody, and human antibody of interest is captured by the immobilized goat anti-mouse antibodies on the microplate. 6) After washing the presence of human antibodies is visualized by the addition of enzyme linked anti-human antibodies.

which is a fast and reliable technique with minimal downstream handling (Cavanagh et al. 1997; Hurd & Lucas 2002). High-throughput HPA typing techniques with automated readout, such as Taqman assays, are now in routine use and have reduced the cost of large-scale typing. **Microarray techniques** for the simultaneous detection of numerous SNPs are emerging (Bugert et al. 2005) and are likely to become the routine typing method eventually.

Genotyping of foetal DNA from amniocytes or from chorionic villus biopsy samples is of clinical value in cases of HPA alloimmunization in pregnancies where there is a history of severe NAIT and the father is heterozygous for the implicated HPA. Non-invasive HPA genotyping assays based on the presence of trace amounts of foetal DNA in maternal plasma, as developed for red cell antigens and the prevention of haemolytic disease of the newborn (see Chapter 7), will reduce the risk to the foetus from invasive sampling procedures.

> **Microarray techniques**
> An assay system using labeled probes to simultaneously identify a range of different characteristics.

SELF-CHECK 9.2

What are the risks associated with amniocentesis or foetal blood sampling?

Platelet isoantigens, autoantigens, and hapten-induced antigens

In addition to the HPAs there are other antigens that can lead to the production of antibodies against platelets. GPIV is absent from the platelet membrane in 4% of Black Africans and 3–10% of Japanese. If these individuals are exposed to normal, GPIV-positive platelets as a consequence of pregnancy or transfusion they may produce GPIV isoantibodies. These antibodies may cause NAIT or platelet refractoriness, and may be responsible for non-haemolytic febrile transfusion reactions in multi-transfused recipients. Similarly, formation of isoantibodies can complicate the pregnancies and transfusion support of patients with Glanzmann's thrombasthenia and Bernard–Soulier syndrome.

The GPs carrying the HPAs are often the target of autoantibodies in autoimmune thrombocytopenia. Such autoantibodies bind to the platelets of all individuals regardless of their HPA type. Platelet autoimmunity is frequently associated with B cell malignancies and following haemopoietic stem cell transplantation during immune cell re-engraftment. The presence of platelet autoantibodies may also contribute to refractoriness to transfused platelets.

SELF-CHECK 9.3

How would you distinguish between platelet-specific allo- and autoantibodies in a transfused patient?

SELF-CHECK 9.4

What interventions might be used to reduce the impact of platelet autoantibodies in patients with platelet transfusion refractoriness?

Some drugs too small to elicit an immune response in their own right may bind to platelet GPs *in vivo* and act as a **hapten**. In some patients, the haptenized platelet GP can trigger the formation of antibodies that only bind to the GP in the presence of hapten. A classic example is quinine and its stereo-isomer quinidine. Typically, quinine-dependent antibodies are against either GPIIb/IIIa and/or GPIb/IX/V, although other GPs are sometimes the target. Many other drugs, particularly heparin and several antibiotics, have been associated with

> **Hapten**
> A substance that is unable to elicit an immune response by itself (usually because it is too small) but which can do so when combined with a larger molecule.

hapten-mediated thrombocytopenia. In haemato-oncology patients, who often receive a spectrum of drugs, unravelling the causes of persistent thrombocytopenia or poor responses to platelet transfusions can be complex because of the many possible causes of thrombocytopenia. If the thrombocytopenia is drug (hapten) mediated, withdrawal of the drug will result in rapid recovery of the platelet count.

9.3 Human neutrophil antigens (HNA)

Neutrophil membrane antigens are, compared to platelet antigens, often relatively poorly characterized. The antigens on the membrane of human **neutrophils** can, as with platelets, be divided into different categories. There are common antigens which have a wider distribution on other blood cells and tissues, for example I, Le^x, and sialyl-Le^x (CD15) blood group systems and HLA class I. There are 'shared' antigens which have a limited distribution amongst other cell types, for example the HNA-4a and HNA-5a polymorphisms associated with CD11/18. There are also a small number of truly neutrophil-specific antigens, for example HNA-1a, HNA-1b, and HNA-1c polymorphisms on FcγRIII (CD16). The current nomenclature for the HNA systems includes polymorphisms that are both cell-specific and 'shared' (Table 9.3).

Nomenclature

The human neutrophil antigen (HNA) system was published by Bux (1999) and includes both neutrophil-specific and more widely distributed antigens that may be present on other white cells and this is therefore a source of potential confusion. Other antigens which have not been incorporated into the HNA system, because of insufficient scientific information, continue to be referred to by the original acronym assigned at the time of discovery.

FcγRIIIb (CD16) and the HNA-1 system

The human FcγRIII (CD16) molecule is a member of the immunoglobulin superfamily which is distinct from other human Fc receptors for IgG (FcγR). FcγRIII exists in two non-allelic forms: FcγRIIIa and FcγRIIIb, encoded by separate genes. FcγRIIIb is linked to the neutrophil plasma membrane via a **glycosylphoshatidylinositol (GPI) anchor**, and has low affinity for IgG (Figure 9.3).

In immunoprecipitation and SDS-polyacrylamide gel electrophoresis studies, FcγRIIIb migrates as a broad band with a molecular weight between 50 kDa and 80 kDa. This variation in apparent molecular weight is the result of variations in glycosylation between FcγRIIIb^{HNA-1a} and FcγRIIIb^{HNA-1b} forms. At the DNA level, there are five nucleotide differences between the *FcγRIIIB^{HNA-1a}* and *FcγRIIIB^{HNA-1b}* genes but only four of these substitutions give rise to the changes in amino acids arginine/serine, asparagine/serine, aspartic acid/asparagines, and valine/isoleucine substitutions at positions 36, 65, 82, and 106, respectively, that define the difference between HNA-1a and -1b.

SELF-CHECK 9.5

What is meant by the term 'degeneracy of the genetic code'?

A single amino acid substitution alanine/asparagine at position 78 defines the HNA-1c polymorphism (see Figure 9.3). HNA-1a is the most immunogenic of the polymorphisms on neutrophil FcγRIIIb (CD16). Gene duplication appears to have led to the creation of HNA-1c,

---

Neutrophils

Together with eosinophils and basophils these circulating white cells are collectively known as granulocytes or polymorphonuclear cells. In normal healthy adults, neutrophils account for >90% of all granulocytes. Most laboratories do not attempt to separate these three cell types prior to antibody testing so any antibodies detected are more correctly called granulocyte-specific. Nonetheless, some HNA, i.e. HNA-1 and 2, have been shown to be truly neutrophil-specific in that they are expressed on neutrophils but not eosinophils or basophils.

Glycophosphotidylinositol (GPI) anchor

A chemical linkage between glycoproteins and the cell membrane which can be readily cleaved under certain conditions thereby releasing the glycoprotein from the cell surface.

TABLE 9.3 The human neutrophil antigen (HNA) systems.

HNA system	Antigen	Phenotype frequency* %	Glycoprotein/ CD classification	Nucleotide change	Amino acid change
1	1a	46	FcγRIIIb (CD16)	G^{108} C^{114} A^{197} G^{247} G^{319}	Arginine^{36} None Asparagine^{65} Aspartic acid^{82} Valine^{106}
	1b	88	FcγRIIIb (CD16)	C^{108} T^{114} G^{197} A^{247} A^{319}	Serine^{36} None Serine^{65} Asparagine^{82} Isoleucine^{106}
	1c	5	FcγRIIIb (CD16)	A^{266}	Aspartic acid^{78}
				C^{266}	Alanine^{78}
2	2	97	CD177	§	
3	3a	94.5	CTL2	G^{461}	Arginine^{154}
3	3a	35.9		A^{461}	Glutamine^{154}
4	4a	99.1	CD11b	G^{302}	Arginine^{61}
			CD11b	A^{302}	Histidine^{61}
5	5a	>99	CD11a	G^{2466}	Arginine^{766}
			CD11a	C^{2466}	Threonine^{766}

* Frequencies based on studies in Caucasians.
§ HNA-2 null phenotype is due to incorrect splicing resulting in mRNA strands containing introns with stop codons.

and consequently HNA-1c(+) individuals often have three rather than two FcγRIIIB genes (Koene et al. 1998). Normally there are between 100,000 and 200,000 copies of FcγRIIIb per neutrophil but HNA-1c(+) individuals frequently have increased expression of FcγRIIIb because of the additional gene. Large-scale studies of the incidence of the NHAs in different ethnic groups have not been performed but the available data indicates that the frequency of the HNA-1a antigen is more common in Japanese, Chinese, and Korean populations than in Caucasians.

The FcγRIIIb 'null' phenotype (~1:2,000 individuals) arises from an absence of the FcγRIIIb genes. The maternal deficiency of FcγRIIIb on neutrophils can cause immune neutropenia in the newborn due to maternal transfer of anti-FcγRIIIb isoantibodies (de Haas et al. 1995).

HNA-2 alloantigen

HNA-2 is localized on a 58–64 kD glycoprotein (CD177) expressed as a glycosylphosphatidylinositol-anchored membrane GP found both on the neutrophil surface membrane and

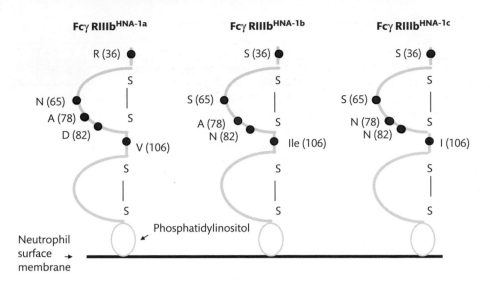

FIGURE 9.3

Representation of the amino acid substitutions resulting in the HNA-1a, -1b, -1c forms of FcγRIIIb. The positions of the amino acid substitutions arising from the allelic variation of the FcγRIIIb gene are depicted by black dots. Amino acids are given as one letter symbols. The single amino acid substitution which accounts for the difference between HNA-1b and HNA-1c are represented by a red dot. The intra-chain disulphide bonds create two domains which are closely related to the C-terminal heavy chain domains of IgG. Adapted from the illustration published by Salmon et al., (1996). The positions of the amino acids are noted according to the numbering system of Ravetch & Perussia (1989).

on secondary granules from 97% of the population. The percentage of neutrophils expressing HNA-2 varies between individuals, and HNA-2 alloantibodies typically give a bimodal fluorescence profile with granulocytes from HNA-2 positive donors (Figure 9.4). The HNA-2 status can be determined by phenotyping with polyclonal or monoclonal antibodies. There is no antithetical antigen to HNA-2.

FIGURE 9.4

Characteristic bi-modal binding pattern of HNA-2 antibodies to granulocytes. There is a population of cells expressing low levels of HNA-2 (on the left) and a population of cells expressing high levels of HNA-2 (on the right). The ratio and precise positions of the two peaks varies with individuals.

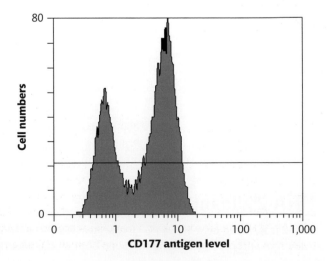

HNA-3 system

HNA-3a (previously known as 5^b) was originally described using antisera obtained from women immunized during pregnancy and was reported as being widely distributed on granulocytes, platelets, lymphocytes, kidney, spleen, and lymph node tissue. Biochemical techniques localized the HNA-3a antigen to a granulocyte glycoprotein with a molecular weight of 70–95 kDa. Recently, the molecular basis of this polymorphism was further localized to choline transporter like protein 2 (CTL2) and a single point mutation at amino acid 154 (HNA-3a encoded by arginine and HNA-3b encoded by glutamine) (Greinacher et al. 2010). The gene frequency of HNA-3a and HNA-3b has been reported as 0.792 and 0.207 respectively in the German population, with 64.1% of individuals as homozygous HNA-3a, 5.5% homozygous HNA-3b, and 30.4% heterozygous. Antibodies to HNA-3a have been associated with TRALI and in a case of neonatal alloimmune neutropenia (Haas et al. 2000). Antisera to HNA-3b (previously known as 5^a) have been described but the clinical significance of these antibodies is unknown.

HNA-4 and HNA-5

HNA-4a and HNA-5a are polymorphisms encoded by the genes for CD11b and CD11a respectively. CD11b and CD11a exist non-covalently with CD18 as heterodimeric proteins and belong to the integrin family of proteins. Alloantibody formation against the HNA-4a and 5a polymorphisms has been observed in transfusion recipients, and recently cases of neonatal alloimmune neutropenia due to HNA-4a and HNA-5a alloantibodies have also been described. HNA-4a has a calculated gene frequency of 0.906 and is expressed on granulocytes, monocytes, and a sub-population of T lymphocytes. The HNA-5a antigen is expressed on granulocytes, monocytes, T, and B lymphocytes in 91.8% of Dutch individuals.

Other antigens

There are a number of other incompletely described antigens reported to be located on granulocytes, for example LAN, SR, SL, 9a, ND, and NE.

Key points

Alloantigens on neutrophils and granulocytes are known as human neutrophil antigens (HNAs).

9.4 Antibody detection

Techniques for the detection of HPA and HNA antibodies have evolved from non-specific and insensitive tests, for example the platelet agglutination test, to non-specific and sensitive tests, for example the **platelet immunofluorescence test (PIFT)** and the **granulocyte immunofluorescence test (GIFT)**, and onwards to specific and sensitive assays that use purified or captured GPs, for example the MAIPA assay or **monoclonal antibody immobilization of granulocyte antigen (MAIGA) assay** and other solid-phase ELISA assays. A new generation of assays are currently being developed that may further enhance the detection of HPA and HNA antibodies. Assays that utilize recombinant antigen fragments bearing the major HPA (Stafford et al. 2008) may help streamline laboratory investigations and offer an

Platelet immunofluorescence test (PIFT)
A whole cell immunofluorescence assay capable of detecting platelet reactive antibodies.

Granulocyte immunofluorescence test (GIFT)
A whole cell immunofluorescence assay capable of detecting granulocyte reactive antibodies.

Monoclonal antibody immobilization of granulocyte antigens (MAIGA) assay
An ELISA assay which uses monoclonal antibodies against granulocyte antigens as the basis of detection and identification of granulocyte specific antibodies.

additional tool to further elucidate the presence of antibodies to rare HPA and define antibody specificity, while the application of surface-plasmon resonance (Socher et al. 2009) may provide a tool with which to detect low affinity antibodies which might be removed by multiple wash steps.

SELF-CHECK 9.6

What is the difference between antibody avidity and affinity?

Detection of HPA antibodies

Numerous techniques have been described for the detection of platelet antibodies. This text will describe in detail the two previously mentioned techniques, that is, PIFT and MAIPA assay, which have gained widespread use and have proven track records in quality assessment schemes. However, there are also alternative antigen capture and solid phase red cell adherence assays which are used by many laboratories.

It is generally accepted that reliance on a single technique is a sub-optimal investigation strategy for the detection of platelet specific antibodies and a combination of a whole cell assay with an antigen capture assay offers diagnostic advantages. Despite an inability to distinguish between platelet-specific and HLA antibodies, the PIFT with a flow cytometric endpoint remains widely used and one of the most sensitive assays available. The principles of the PIFT are described below.

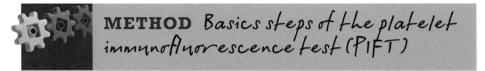

METHOD *Basics steps of the platelet immunofluorescence test (PIFT)*

The steps in the assay procedure include:

- Initial incubation of washed platelets with the serum sample being investigated
- Subsequent washing
- Addition of fluorescent labelled anti-human immunoglobulin
- Further washing

The endpoint of the assay can be determined manually using a fluorescence microscope or more usually a flow cytometer.

Typical results obtained by microscopy and by flow cytometry are shown in Figures 9.5 and 9.6 respectively.

(a) 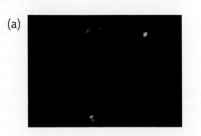   (b)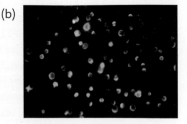

FIGURE 9.5
The results of microscopic analysis of the PIFT showing typical fluorescent staining with (a) negative control serum and (b) a strongly reactive HPA-1a antiserum.

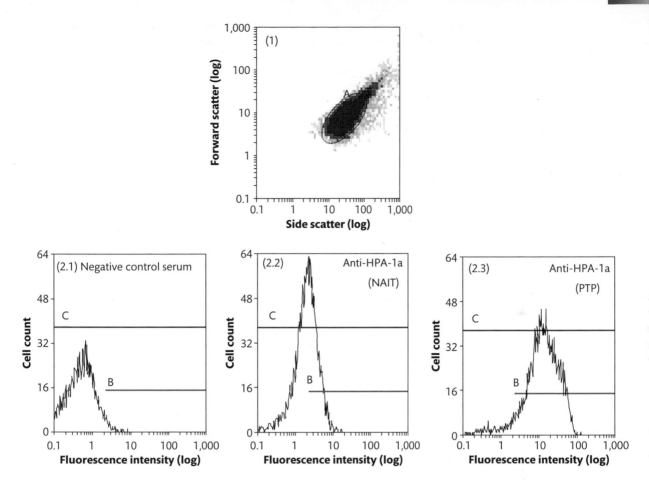

FIGURE 9.6

Typical results of flow cytometric analysis of the platelet immunofluorescence test (PIFT). A histogram plot of forward scatter (FS) and side scatter (SS) utilizes the ability of cells to scatter laser light on the basis of cell size and granularity. This type of plot can be used to define the population of cells (in this case platelets) for analysis (histogram 1). The identity of the cell population may be confirmed using a fluorescently labelled platelet glycoprotein-specific monoclonal antibody. The results of fluorescence binding for a negative control sample (histogram 2.1), a weak positive HPA-1a antiserum from a NAIT case (histogram 2.2) and a strong positive HPA-1a antiserum from a case of PTP (histogram 2.3). The results of the assay can be represented in different ways, either as the percentage of cells occurring above a certain threshold (typically >95% of a normal population) in region B or as the mean channel fluorescence values (from the X axis) obtained for region C.

 METHOD *Results of the platelet immunofluorescence test (PIFT)*

A histogram plot of forward scatter (FS) and side scatter (SS) is used to define the population of platelets for analysis (histogram 1) and this is often confirmed using a fluorescently labelled platelet glycoprotein-specific monoclonal antibody. The results of fluorescence binding for a negative control sample are shown in histogram 2.1; a weak positive HPA-1a antiserum from a NAIT case in histogram 2.2; and a strong positive HPA-1a antiserum from a case of PTP in histogram 2.3. The results of the assay can be represented in different ways, either as the percentage of cells occurring above a certain threshold (typically >95% of a normal population) in region B or as the mean channel fluorescence values obtained for region C.

However, assays based on the use of purified/captured GPs are now the cornerstone for the detection and identification of HPA antibodies. The MAIPA assay (Kiefel et al. 1987) captures specific GPs using monoclonal antibodies and can be used to analyse complex mixtures of platelet reactive antibodies in patient sera. The principle of this assay is shown in Figure 9.2.

METHOD *The procedure of the monoclonal antibody immobilization of platelet antigens (MAIPA) assay*

- Target platelets and the human serum sample to be investigated are incubated together (1).

- After washing to remove unbound antibodies, a murine monoclonal antibody directed against the glycoprotein being investigated, that is, GPIIb/IIIa is added. This step creates a trimolecular complex consisting of murine antibody, GpIIb/IIIa and the HPA-1a antibody (2).

- After washing to remove unbound murine monoclonal antibody, the platelets are solubilized using a non-ionic detergent and the lysate is centrifuged to remove any particulate material (3).

- The resultant supernatant is added to a microtitre well which has been previously coated with goat anti-mouse IgG antibodies (4).

- After further incubation, the trimolecular complex created in step (2) is captured to the solid phase by the goat anti-mouse antibody binding to the murine GpIIb/IIIa antibody.

- The other unbound platelet glycoproteins (e.g. GpIb/IX) and other bound antibodies, for example HLA class I antibodies bound to the appropriate antigen are removed from the microtitre well by washing.

- An enzyme linked goat anti-human IgG antibody is added to the microtitre well. After appropriate incubation and washing, an enzyme substrate is added and positive reactions are determined using a colorimetric or chemiluminescence endpoint (5).

The careful selection of reagents is critical to the performance of this assay, for example there must be no cross reactivity between the goat anti-mouse IgG antibody and human IgG antibodies or between the enzyme conjugated anti-human IgG antibody and either murine anti-GpIIb/IIIa antibodies or the goat anti-mouse IgG used to coat the solid phase. Equally, the selection of the glycoprotein specific antibodies in step (2) is critical as it must have an epitope binding site that does not compete with the binding site of the human antibodies we aim to detect.

The use of platelets expressing different HPA and different murine monoclonal antibodies, for example anti-GpIb/IX instead of anti-GpIIb/IIIa, makes it possible to routinely investigate and elucidate the presence of complex mixtures of platelet reactive antibodies in a way that is not possible with whole cell assays such as the PIFT.

The MAIPA assay requires considerable technical expertise in order to ensure maximum sensitivity and specificity, and selection of appropriate screening cells is critical, since the use of platelets heterozygous for the relevant antigen or from donors who have a low expression of particular antigens, for example HPA-15, may result in the failure to detect clinically significant alloantibodies. The combination of PIFT and MAIPA assay together with a panel of HPA typed platelets is currently the most reliable strategy for detecting and identifying platelet reactive antibodies.

Detection of HNA antibodies

The reliable detection and identification of neutrophil antibodies can be technically difficult. The main problems are the abundant expression of low affinity FcγR receptors for the constant domain of human IgG, which increases the binding of immunoglobulins to the cell surface and the requirement for fresh, typed donor neutrophils as panel cells, since neutrophils cannot be stored. Considerable technical expertise is required to investigate suspected cases of antibody mediated neutropenia and only a few laboratories worldwide undertake these investigations to a high standard.

Many techniques for neutrophil/granulocyte antibody detection have been evaluated over the years. Early assays such as the granulocyte cytotoxicity and agglutination tests had low specificity. The granulocyte immunofluorescence and granulocyte chemiluminescence tests have the advantage of good sensitivity but are not specific, that is, they cannot readily distinguish between granulocyte specific and HLA class I antibodies without further investigations. A combination of two techniques, including the granulocyte immunofluorescence test (GIFT), together with an HNA typed panel, is currently recommended as the optimal approach for antibody detection. For HNA systems expressed on CD16, CD177, and C11/18, MAIGA assays can be applied. The principles of the GIFT and the MAIGA assay are analogous to the equivalent platelet tests (PIFT and MAIPA) described earlier. An example of the forward scatter/side scatter histogram obtained with granulocytes and lymphocytes is shown in Figure 9.7. In contrast to the immunochemical assays commonly used in immunohaematology, the **granulocyte chemiluminescence test** is a biological assay (Lucas 1994). The assay measures the biochemical activity of human monocytes initiating the phagocytosis of opsonized (antibody coated) granulocytes (Figure 9.8a) and as such the results of this assay may provide a better correlation with clinical significance.

Granulocyte chemiluminescence test (GCLT)
A biological assay that utilizes human monocytes to detect granulocyte antibodies bound to the membrane surface.

 METHOD *The granulocyte chemiluminescence test (GCLT)*

Figure 9.8a shows the principle of the GCLT:

- Opsonized granulocytes (i.e. granulocytes coated with antibodies after incubation with test serum containing granulocyte reactive antibodies) are introduced to washed human monocytes. (The granulocytes are heat treated prior to opsonization to inactivate the phagocytic potential of these cells.)

- The FcR receptors on the monocytes interact with the Fc portion of the bound antibodies and via a process of trans-membrane signalling activate the biochemical processes in the monocyte to initiate phagocytosis.

- The biochemical pathways generate small amounts of light, which is amplified by an acceptor molecule (luminol) and the resultant increased signal is measured in a luminometer.

Figure 9.8b shows the kinetics of the interaction between opsonized granulocytes and human monocytes over 30–40 minutes. The three lines represent the light generated by inert serum (red line), and HNA-1a antibodies (blue line) and an HLA antiserum (green line):

- There is an initial lag phase as the monocytes initiate phagocytosis of opsonized granulocytes.

- The release of light peaks at 8–15 minutes depending on antibody class, antibody concentration, and antigen density.

- The reaction begins to subside as the biochemical reserves of the monocytes become exhausted.

FIGURE 9.7

Results of flow cytometric analysis of granulocytes and lymphocytes identified by forward scatter (FS) and side scatter (SS) characteristics as described previously for platelets (see legend of Figure 9.6). The cell population between the lymphocytes and granulocytes represents co-isolated monocytes.

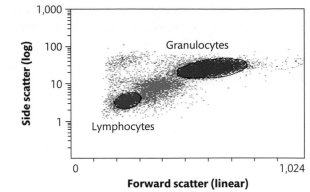

FIGURE 9.8

The granulocyte chemiluminescence test. Granulocytes incubated with antibody containing sera are washed and then introduced to isolated human monocytes. The monocytes recognize and are activated by the Fc portion of the bound antibodies to initiate phagocytosis. The monocytes produce small amounts of light which is amplified by the electron acceptor (luminol) and is measured in a luminometer (a type of spectrophotometer). The granulocytes are heat treated prior to incubation with the test sera to inactivate their own inherent phagocytic potential. (The enzymes which comprise the biochemical process of phagocytosis are temperature sensitive.)

(a) **Mechanism**

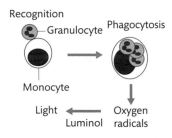

(b) **Kinetics**

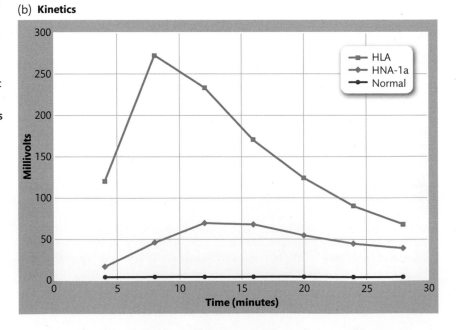

Typing for HNAs traditionally utilized monospecific alloantisera or more recently HNA-specific monoclonal antibodies, for example HNA-1a, -1b, and -2. Increased understanding of the molecular nature of HNA has enabled PCR based typing for HNA-1a, -1b, -1c, -3a, -3b -4a, -4b, -5a, and -5b and has opened the potential to develop recombinant HNAs, which may transform the serological investigation of granulocyte alloantibodies.

SELF-CHECK 9.7

What do you understand to be the major challenges in undertaking *in vitro* serological investigations with granulocytes?

SELF-CHECK 9.8

What would be the consequences of performing a sub-optimal number of washes in the PIFT or GIFT following incubation with patient serum?

Key points

Reliable detection and identification of HPA and HNA-specific antibodies requires the use of both whole-cell type assays such as the PIFT, GIFT, or GCLT and antigen-capture type assays such as the MAIPA and MAIGA assays, together with access to a HPA/HNA typed cell panel.

The detection of other platelet and granulocyte antibodies

The diagnostic value of detecting autoantibodies against platelets and neutrophils has been much debated because of the limited clinical benefit of these tests for many patients and, consequently, laboratory investigation is only indicated in certain clinical conditions. Detection of isoantibodies is of clinical importance in thrombasthenia patients and individuals with GPIV deficiency, whilst the identification of drug dependent antibodies can also have a profound effect on patient management.

SELF-CHECK 9.9

What are the main problems in the detection and identification of platelet and granulocyte antibodies?

9.5 Clinical significance of HPA alloantibodies

HPA alloantibodies are implicated in the following clinical conditions:

- Neonatal alloimmune thrombocytopenia
- Post-transfusion purpura (PTP)
- Platelet transfusion refractoriness
- Persistent post-bone marrow transplant thrombocytopenia

Unlike red cell and granulocyte immunohaematology, platelet antibodies with allospecificity have not been implicated in autoimmune thrombocytopenias.

SELF-CHECK 9.10

Give some examples of red cell antigens that are targets for autoantibodies.

Neonatal alloimmune thrombocytopenia (NAIT)

Neonatal alloimmune thrombocytopenia (NAIT) is by far the most important of the clinical conditions discussed in this chapter both in terms of the number of suspected cases referred for laboratory investigation and in terms of the impact upon transfusion service resources for HPA selected blood product support. Accordingly, more emphasis is given to this condition.

Neonatal alloimmune thrombocytopeniais the platelet equivalent of **haemolytic disease of the newborn (HDN)** and the first case was described in 1959. Neonatal alloimmune thrombocytopenia had been long suspected but laboratory confirmation had proved difficult because platelet antibody detection was technically more demanding than for red cell antibodies. Today, NAIT is a distinct clinical, but probably underdiagnosed, entity with an estimated incidence of severe thrombocytopenia due to maternal HPA antibodies of between 1 in 1,000 and 1,200 live births. Unlike HDN, about 30% NAIT cases occur in the first pregnancy.

Haemolytic disease of the newborn (HDN)
A disease associated with the foetomaternal transfer of red cell antibodies that cause haemolysis and red cell destruction in the infant (see Chapter 7).

Definition and pathophysiology

Neonatal alloimmune thrombocytopenia is usually due to maternal HPA alloimmunization caused by foetomaternal incompatibility for a foetal HPA inherited from the father but which is absent in the mother. Maternal IgG alloantibodies against the foetal HPA cross the placenta and bind to foetal platelets, thereby causing reduced platelet survival and thrombocytopenia. Severe thrombocytopenia in the term neonate, accompanied by haemorrhage, is generally caused by HPA-1a antibodies if the mother is Caucasian or Black African. Antibodies against antigens in the HPA-2 and HPA-4 systems are generally implicated in cases of Far Eastern ethnicity. In the latter group and in Black Africans, GPIV deficiency should also be considered. Anti-HPA-5b tends to cause mild thrombocytopenia, although on rare occasions intracranial cerebral haemorrhage (ICH) has been reported.

Neonatal alloimmune thrombocytopenia due to alloantibodies against the other HPAs is infrequent and HLA class I antibodies, present in 15–25% of multiparous women, are not thought to cause NAIT. Destruction of IgG-coated foetal platelets is assumed to take place in the spleen through interaction with mononuclear cells bearing Fcγ receptors for the constant domain of IgG. HPA-1a is known to be expressed on foetal platelets from 16 weeks' gestation, with placental transfer of IgG antibodies occurring from 14 weeks, so thrombocytopenia can occur early in pregnancy. Intracranial cerebral haemorrhage has been reported as early as 16 weeks' gestation.

Incidence

Prospective screening of pregnant Caucasian women has shown that about 1 in 1,200 neonates have severe thrombocytopenia (platelet count $<50 \times 10^9/l$) because of alloimmunization against HPA-1a (Williamson et al. 1998). However, the number of serologically confirmed, clinically referred cases suggests that NAIT is remains under-diagnosed. HPA-5b antibodies are frequently found in pregnant women, but they of less clinical significance than HPA-1a antibodies, possibly due to the low copy number of the GPIa/IIa complex on platelets (1–2,000 compared to 50–80,000 for GPIIb/IIIa).

Clinical features and differential diagnosis

There are many causes of neonatal thrombocytopenia, including bacterial or viral infections, premature delivery, intra-uterine growth retardation, inadequate megakaryopoiesis, inherited chromosomal abnormalities (particularly trisomy 21), and maternal autoimmune thrombocytopenia. In addition, platelet type von Willebrand's disease, in which there is a tendency for *in vitro* platelet aggregation, and a variety of technical problems, for example platelet clumping in EDTA, can also lead to falsely low platelet counts.

Typically, a full-term infant with NAIT presents with skin bleeding (purpura, petechiae and/ or ecchymoses), or more serious haemorrhage such as ICH, an isolated thrombocytopenia, but is otherwise healthy with a normal coagulation screen. Less commonly, ventriculomegaly, cerebral cysts, and hydrocephalus may be discovered *in utero* by routine ultrasound. Hydrops foetalis has also been reported in association with NAIT and this diagnosis should be considered if there are no other obvious reasons for the hydrops.

The precise incidence of ICH due to NAIT is unknown, but conservative estimates suggest that it is as low as 1 in 20,000 live births, which equates to approximately 35 cases per annum in the UK. Nearly 50% of severe ICHs occur *in utero*, usually between 30 and 35 weeks' gestation, but sometimes before 20 weeks. Severe NAIT (platelet count $<30 \times 10^9$/l) is a serious condition and appropriate management (see below) is essential to prevent ICH and the possibility of lifelong disability. Conversely, at the other end of the clinical spectrum, NAIT can be discovered incidentally when a blood count is performed for other reasons.

Laboratory investigations

The cause of severe thrombocytopenia in an otherwise healthy neonate should be determined with urgency and investigation for maternal HPA antibodies must be carried out by techniques with appropriate sensitivity and specificity. The use of the indirect PIFT and the MAIPA assay, together with a panel of HPA typed platelets is the current preferred option for many reference laboratories. In England, HPA antibodies are detected in approximately 15% of referrals of suspected NAIT. The most frequently detected specificities are anti-HPA-1a and anti-HPA-5b which are implicated in about 85% and 10% of confirmed cases of NAIT respectively. The ability of an HPA-1a negative mother to form anti-HPA-1a is partly controlled by the HLA DRB3*01:01 allele. HPA-1a negative women who are HLA DRB3*01:01-positive have a one in three chance of making HPA-1a compared to a frequency of 1 in 300 for DRB3*01:01 negative women. This highly significant association between an HLA class II type and the formation of HPA-1a alloantibodies has not been observed for any of the other antigens on platelets, red cells, or leucocytes.

Molecular typing of the parents and neonate for HPA-1, -2, -3, -5, and HPA-15 should be performed and the results reviewed in conjunction with the results of the antibody investigations. In patients of Far Eastern origin, HPA-4 typing should be undertaken and the platelets should also be investigated for GPIV expression.

Alloimmunization against low frequency HPAs, for example HPA-6bw, can cause NAIT and should be considered in referrals that have a negative antibody screen for the common HPA antibody specificities but a strong clinical history. Screening all suspected NAIT referrals for antibodies against low frequency HPAs is not cost effective and a recent study of more than 1,000 paternal DNA samples from NAIT referrals showed the presence of HPA-bw alleles in less than ten paternal samples. Investigations for alloimmunization against rare HPA-bw alleles should therefore be reserved for clinically severe cases of NAIT where there is a strong index of suspicion of NAIT and no alternative clinical diagnosis (Ghevaert et al. 2007). Genotyping of the paternal DNA sample for low frequency HPA is a cost-effective approach in this clinical setting.

Key points

Neonatal alloimmune thrombocytopenia is a common disorder and HPA-1a or HPA-5b antibodies are responsible for approximately 95% of Caucasian cases.

Neonatal management

A neonatal platelet count of $<100 \times 10^9/l$ should be confirmed and a blood film examined. The neonate should be carefully examined for skin or mucosal bleeding if a low platelet count is confirmed. If the platelet count is $<30 \times 10^9/l$ or if there are signs of bleeding, it is strongly recommended that the neonate is transfused with HPA-1a(-), 5b(-) platelets, as these will be compatible with the maternal HPA alloantibody in over 95% of NAIT cases. The transfusion of platelets that are HPA-1a(-), 5b(-) in NAIT caused by HPA-1a or HPA-5b antibodies results in a higher increment and more prolonged platelet survival than transfusion of random donor (HPA-1a positive) platelets (Allen et al. 2007). However, if HPA-1a(-), 5b(-) platelets are not immediately available and there is an urgent clinical need for transfusion then random ABO and RhD compatible donor platelets should be used in the first instance. Figure 9.9 illustrates the clinical advantage frequently observed as a result of using HPA-1a(-)5b(-) platelets to support infants with NAIT. Following the transfusion of platelets, a platelet count should be performed approximately one hour after the transfusion is completed, and at least daily thereafter until the platelet count has normalized. In a typical case, the platelet count should recover to normal within a week, although a more protracted recovery can occur. Intravenous immunoglobulin (IvIgG) is not recommended as first-line treatment as there is a delay of 24–48 hours before a satisfactory count is achieved, in contrast to the immediate effect of transfusing HPA-compatible donor platelets. A cerebral ultrasound scan of the baby should be considered if the platelet count is $<50 \times 10^9/l$, and is recommended when the platelet count is $<30 \times 10^9/l$.

Key points

Optimal post-natal treatment of NAIT is the transfusion of HPA-1a(-) and 5b(-) donor platelets.

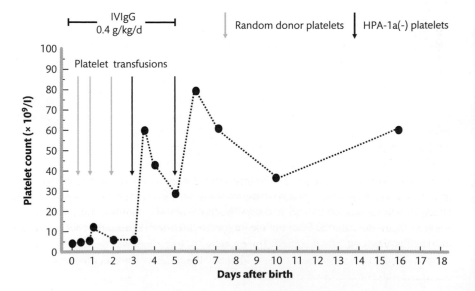

FIGURE 9.9

Neonatal platelet counts for an infant with NAIT due to HPA-1a antibodies. Initial treatment with random platelets and IvIgG did not produce a satisfactory platelet increment and only the use of HPA-1a(-) platelets resulted in the desired correction to the infant's platelet count.

Antenatal management

In a subsequent pregnancy of a mother with a previous pregnancy affected by NAIT, the pregnancy should be managed by an appropriately experienced foetal medicine team. The treatment strategy is based on the clinical history and outcome in previous pregnancies.

There are two main treatment options: high-dose IvIgG to the mother, or *in utero* platelet transfusion of the foetus, with the former being generally recognized as the safest, effective intervention to reduce the risk of ICH in the foetus. Maternal IVIgG (1 g or 0.5 g/kg body weight) is given at weekly intervals, usually commencing between 12 to 20 weeks of gestation, depending on the history of previous pregnancies. Early commencement of treatment is indicated in those cases where there is a history of antenatal ICH. A beneficial effect of IvIgG on the foetal platelet count occurs in approximately 70% of cases. Many treatment centres subsequently perform a foetal blood sampling (FBS) to ascertain the platelet count, usually after eight weeks' treatment with IvIgG. If a safe foetal platelet count has not been achieved at the time of sampling, the pregnancy may be managed by increasing the dose of IvIgG and/or adding corticosteroids (prednisolone, 0.5 mg/kg body weight) or switching to weekly foetal platelet transfusions. *In utero* platelet transfusions, carried out with FBS, carry a significant risk of foetal morbidity and mortality. This treatment should not be chosen as first-line treatment but as a rescue regime or in the management of pregnancies with a history of treatment failure on IvIgG. The intra-uterine transfusion of platelets has more complications compared to red cell transfusions for HDN, for example bradycardia, post-needle withdrawal cord bleeds, and the risk increases since this technically demanding procedure may need to be repeated on a weekly basis (see Figure 9.10).

Counselling

Couples with an index case of NAIT should be counselled about the risks of severe foetal/neonatal thrombocytopenia in a subsequent pregnancy and advice should be based on the

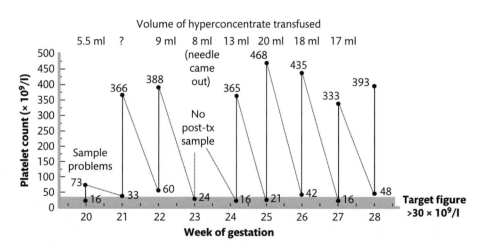

FIGURE 9.10

Third pregnancy of a mother with a history of NAIT due to HPA-1a antibodies. The first pregnancy was associated with intra-uterine death. The second pregnancy resulted in an infant with moderate thrombocytopenia. The foetal platelet counts during the third pregnancy are shown with IUT commencing at week 20 and continuing on a weekly basis until delivery by Caesarean section. The objective of treatment was to maintain the platelet count of the foetus above 30 × 10⁹/l and the target platelet count after transfusion after transfusion was >300 × 10⁹/l.

severity of disease in the infant(s) and the outcome of immunological investigations. The following should be taken into account:

- Thrombocytopenia in subsequent cases can be as severe or more severe.
- The best predictors of severe foetal thrombocytopenia in a future pregnancy are the occurrence of antenatal ICH and severe thrombocytopenia (platelet count $<30 \times 10^9/l$) in a previous pregnancy.
- Antibody specificity, titre, or the bioactivity of HPA-1a antibodies do not reliably correlate with the severity of NAIT, and are probably of little value in informing clinical management (Ghevaert et al. 2007b).
- The HPA zygosity of the partner.

SELF-CHECK 9.11

What is meant by the term zygosity?

Key points

Optimal antenatal treatment in women known to be HPA alloimmunized has yet to be determined but maternal IVIgG administration is generally preferred to intra-uterine transfusion of platelets.

HPA typed platelet donor panels

Establishing donor panels for foetal and neonatal platelet transfusion requires a major commitment from blood services and requires the use of high-throughput typing techniques. Although the frequency of HPA-1a negative individuals amongst Caucasians is 2.5%, potential donors for foetal/neonatal transfusions must also be negative for the mandatory microbiological tests, negative for antibodies against red cells, platelets and leucocytes, low titre anti-A and anti-B, and be cytomegalovirus (CMV) seronegative. Thus, in order to recruit one HPA-1a negative donor who is able to meet all of the above criteria approximately 1,500–2,000 donors will have to be typed for HPA-1a.

Therapeutic platelets should also be RhD compatible, as small amounts of red cells present in platelet concentrates may immunize RhD negative recipients. In order to recruit a single RhD negative, HPA-1a negative donor whose platelets will be suitable for a first foetal platelet transfusion, where the foetal/neonatal blood group is unknown, approximately 15,000–20,000 donors need to be typed. As a result of these logistical problems, the English Blood Service is the only organization to date to have made neonatal HPA-1a(-), 5b(-) platelets routinely available.

Post-transfusion purpura (PTP)

Post-transfusion purpura is an acute episode of thrombocytopenia occurring 5–12 days after whole blood, red cell concentrate, or platelet transfusion. Typically (95% of cases), it affects middle-aged or elderly women who have been alloimmunized against HPA-1a during an earlier pregnancy. The transfusion causes a secondary immune response which boosts HPA-1a antibody levels, although the mechanism of destruction of the patient's own HPA-1a(-) platelets remains unproven there is evidence to support the production of platelet autoantibodies during the strong secondary immune response. Post-transfusion purpura

Post-transfusion purpura (PTP)

An unexpected thrombocytopenia occurring 5–12 days after a blood transfusion that is associated with the presence of platelet-specific antibodies.

can occasionally affect men immunized by previous transfusion. An unusual case of this in which three different HPA antibody specificities were detected in addition to HLA antibodies (Lucas et al. 1997) provides a useful example of the ability of the MAIPA assay (see section 9.4) to elucidate complex mixtures of antibodies. Rarely, 'passive PTP' can occur immediately following infusion of plasma from a donor who has made HPA-1a antibodies following pregnancy.

SELF-CHECK 9.12

How might platelet autoantibodies be generated following blood transfusion in PTP?

Data reported by the **Serious Hazards Of Transfusion (SHOT)** scheme indicate that the incidence of PTP in the UK prior to universal leucodepletion is in the order of 1 in 0.5 million transfusions. The incidence has further reduced since leucodepletion by a factor of approximately 4 (Williamson et al. 2007).

Serious Hazards Of Transfusion (SHOT)
The UK haemovigilance scheme.

SELF-CHECK 9.13

What is leucodepletion?

SELF-CHECK 9.14

How could leucodepletion have reduced the incidence of PTP?

The onset of thrombocytopenia in PTP is usually rapid, with the platelet count falling from normal to below $10 \times 10^9/l$ within 24 hours or less of transfusion (Figure 9.11a). Haemorrhage is common, with widespread purpura (Figure 9b), bruising (Figure 9c), mucous membrane, gastrointestinal, and urinary tract bleeding. Post-transfusion purpura may be preceded by febrile non-haemolytic transfusion reactions. The natural history of PTP lasts between 7 and 28 days but early management is essential to reduce the risk of intracranial haemorrhage. High dose IVIgG over 2–5 days is the current treatment of choice, but platelet transfusions are not usually indicated unless the bleeding is severe. As the incidence of PTP is very rare, a diagnosis of heparin induced thrombocytopenia should be considered if the patient has received this drug.

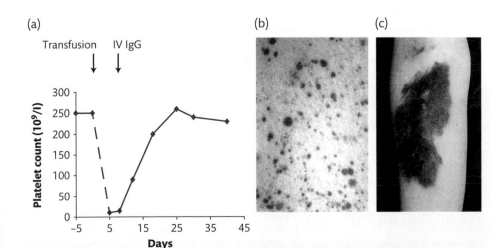

FIGURE 9.11

The main features of post-transfusion purpura (PTP). Figure 9.11a illustrates the typical crash in platelets following blood transfusion and the prompt recovery following IVIgG administration (usually within seven days). In the absence of IVIgG treatment the of the platelet count may take 1–2 months. Figures 9.11b and 9.11c illustrate typical manifestations of petechiae and ecchymoses associated with low platelets.

Recurrence of PTP following further transfusions has been reported but is unpredictable. In order to minimize the risk of recurrence, patients requiring further transfusions should receive HPA compatible red cells or platelets, but if these are not available, leucocyte depleted blood components are considered acceptable alternatives.

Platelet transfusion refractoriness

Platelet transfusion refractoriness
A suboptimal increase in circulating platelet count following platelet transfusion.

Platelet transfusion refractoriness may be defined as a failure to achieve a sustained increase in platelet count following a platelet transfusion. The current criteria for a successful platelet transfusion is an increase of $\geq 20 \times 10^9/l$ at 24 hours. Platelet transfusions are not normally given to adult patients unless the platelet count is $\leq 10 \times 10^9/l$ or there is a risk of haemorrhage.

In many cases, platelet refractoriness is due to 'non-immune' factors such as consumption due to coagulation problems, for example disseminated coagulation, or following surgery, concomitant bacterial infections, or increased sequestration of platelets as occurs in hypersplenism. When immunological destruction of platelets does occur it is usually due to the action of HLA class I antibodies. In such cases, satisfactory platelet increments can be obtained by providing HLA selected platelets. In a small proportion of patients, HLA selected platelets may not result in a satisfactory increment because of the presence of HPA antibodies. The incidence of HPA antibodies in refractory patients varies between 0–20% in different studies and the methodologies used to detect platelet antibodies. Typically, HPA antibodies occur together with HLA antibodies, although very occasionally (<1% of cases) only HPA antibodies are detected. The HPA specificities usually detected in this setting are HPA-1b, HPA-2b, and HPA-5b. Platelet autoantibodies, that is, with platelet glycoprotein rather than HPA specificity, can also occur in this context. Despite their low incidence, HPA antibodies, are often clinically significant and in HLA and HPA alloimmunized patients it may be necessary to select HPA compatible platelets in preference to HLA compatible platelets in order to achieve satisfactory increments and/or prevent/reduce haemorrhage.

HPA alloimmunization can also occur in the post bone marrow transplant setting and these may have an adverse impact on megakaryocyte engraftment and/or transfusion management in the recovery period (Lucas et al. 2010).

9.6 Clinical significance of HNA antibodies

HNA alloantibodies are implicated in the following clinical conditions:

- Neonatal alloimmune neutropenia
- Non-haemolytic febrile transfusion reactions (NHFTR)
- Transfusion-related acute lung injury (TRALI)
- Transfusion-related alloimmune neutropenia (TRAIN)
- Autoimmune neutropenia
- Persistent post-bone marrow transplant neutropenia

Neonatal alloimmune neutropenia (NAIN)

Neonatal alloimmune neutropenia (NAIN)
Neutropenia in a neonate (or foetus) caused by the maternal foetal transfer of granulocyte specific antibodies recognizing either HNAs or granulocyte glycoproteins inherited by the foetus from the father but absent in the mother.

Neonatal alloimmune neutropenia is the neutrophil equivalent of HDN but like NAIT can occur in the first pregnancy. Maternal alloimmunization against neutrophil-specific alloantigens on foetal/neonatal neutrophils is rare, with an estimated incidence of 0.1–0.2% of live births. Clinical presentation is primarily bacterial infection with an isolated neutropenia. Severe neutropenia in the newborn may require treatment with antibiotics and/or granulocyte colony stimulating factor (GCSF) to control bacterial infections and quickly achieve a normal neutrophil count. Left untreated, the neutropenia in some cases caused by HNA-1a and -1b antibodies has been reported to extend up to 28 weeks (Figure 9.12).

Non-haemolytic febrile transfusion reactions (FNHTR), transfusion-related acute lung injury (TRALI) and transfusion-related alloimmune neutropenia (TRAIN)

These three conditions are distinct entities but have some overlapping clinical characteristics. **Non-haemolytic, febrile transfusion reactions (NHFTRs)** are usually caused by bacterially contaminated blood products, particularly platelet concentrates, but can occasionally be associated with the presence of leucocyte (HLA, HPA, and HNA) alloantibodies in the recipient. In the UK, where there is universal leucocyte-depletion of blood products, investigations for bacterial contamination and IgA-deficiency should initially be carried out. The clinical management of NHFTRs, if pre-medication with anti-histamines and corticosteroids is not effective, is to alter product specification by using red cells or platelets with reduced plasma content. Serological investigations for platelet, HLA, and granulocyte antibodies are of limited clinical value as the diagnostic specificity of these tests for NHFTRs is low. Nonetheless, testing for HNA (and HPA/HLA) antibodies may be required in the rare cases in which a severe NHFTR cannot be otherwise explained and plasma-reduced components have proved ineffective.

Transfusion-related acute lung injury (TRALI) is a severe and sometimes life-threatening transfusion reaction that should by reported by the hospital to SHOT. The majority of cases are caused by donor leucocyte alloantibodies against alloantigens present on the patient's leucocytes, although patient alloantibodies have been involved in some cases. In most TRALI cases, HLA class I and II specific antibodies are implicated, but HNA antibodies, particularly HNA-1a and HNA-3a, have also been implicated as causal agents. Transfusion-related acute lung injury (TRALI) investigations are logistically complex but should initially include a screen for both HLA and HNA alloantibodies in samples from donors and, in a small number cases and if non-leucodepleted blood has been transfused, the patient. In some cases, a crossmatch between the donor's sera and the patient's granulocytes and lymphocytes may be required. The incidence of TRALI notified to SHOT has reduced in recent years (Chapman et al. 2009).

> **Non-haemolytic febrile transfusion reactions (NHFTRs)**
> An increase in temperature >1°C following a blood transfusion but which is not associated with red cell haemolysis.

> **Transfusion-related acute lung injury (TRALI)**
> Difficulty in breathing associated with *de novo* chest X-ray changes observed within six hours of transfusion that is not associated with transfusion overload or cardiac insufficiency.

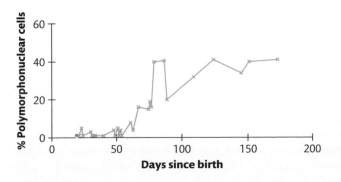

FIGURE 9.12
Sustained neutropenia in an infant affected by neonatal alloimmune neutropenia due to HNA-1b antibodies. There was a degree of compensation in the proportion of other white cells; the white cell count ranged between 9.8–13.0 × 10⁹/l during this period.

SELF-CHECK 9.15

What laboratory techniques would you use to investigate a suspected cases of TRALI?

Transfusion-related alloimmune neutropenia (TRAIN)
A transient neutropenia following infusion of a blood product due to the action of neutrophil-specific antibodies but which does not develop the symptoms of TRALI.

The first documented case of **transfusion-related alloimmune neutropenia (TRAIN)** occurred following the infusion of 80 ml of plasma-reduced blood after surgery on a four-week-old infant (Wallis et al. 2002). The plasma from the female blood donor was found to contain HNA-1b alloantibodies, and resulted in an absolute neutropenia in the infant, who typed as HNA-1a(+), 1b(+). The neutropenia was resolved after seven days after treating the infant with GCSF. The case is of interest since it demonstrates that, in some circumstances, infused passive HNA antibodies can trigger neutropenia rather than TRALI. This clinical entity has recently been confirmed by an additional case report.

Autoimmune neutropenia

Autoimmune neutropenia
An autoimmune disease in which the antibodies form target granulocytes. These antibodies can recognize HNAs, especially in children.

Autoimmune neutropenia is a rare condition which can occur as a transient, self-limiting autoimmunity in young children (typically presenting from 18 months to 4 years of age) (Bux et al. 1998) or in a chronic form in adults (Shastri & Logue 1993). The condition may be primary, that is, the sole presenting feature, or secondary to other conditions, for example rheumatoid arthritis, or systemic lupus erythematosus. The autoantibodies tend to target the FcγRIIIb (CD16), CD177, or CD11/18 molecules but can also be HNA specific, typically HNA-1a, especially in children. The most sensitive method for the detection of autoantibodies is to test the patient's neutrophils using the direct immunofluorescence test. However, a combination of severe neutropenia, difficulties of cell isolation, and the requirement for a fresh sample limit the applicability of this test, especially in children. Screening of a patient's serum sample with a panel of typed neutrophils in the indirect granulocyte immunofluorescence and granulocyte chemiluminescence or granulocyte agglutination tests provide a suitable alternative, and in some studies this approach has been found to be only slightly less sensitive than the direct test. The value in identifying these antibodies in children is that the condition is usually easily managed by use of antibiotics or GCSF and confirmation of antibodies avoids the need for expensive investigations for leukaemia and a bone marrow biopsy.

Persistent neutropenia after bone marrow transplantation

Antibody mediated neutropenia may be a serious complication of bone marrow transplantation. In this context, the neutrophil antibodies may be autoimmune and/or alloimmune in nature and laboratory investigation requires serological and typing studies to elucidate the nature of the antibodies involved. Granulocyte-specific antibodies in the post-bone marrow context can cause lineage specific delay in engraftment, which requires specific clinical management.

Other clinical consequences of HPA and HNA polymorphisms

Until recently, the importance of platelet and granulocyte polymorphisms was restricted to their ability to induce the formation of alloantibodies and thereby clinical conditions discussed earlier in this chapter. However, there is also evidence that certain platelet and granulocyte polymorphisms may affect cellular function and may be associated with increased risk of disease. On platelets, HPA-1b has been proposed as a risk factor in myocardial infarction and unstable angina. On granulocytes, the HNA-1a and -1b antigens can influence the function of the immunoglobulin FcγRIIIb receptor; granulocytes from HNA-1a individuals exhibit greater levels of phagocytosis than granulocytes from HNA-1b individuals.

CHAPTER SUMMARY

- Platelets and granulocytes have unique antigens (HPA and HNA respectively) on their surface.

- The advent of biochemical and molecular analysis of glycoproteins on platelets and granulocytes has enabled the elucidation of the HPA and HNA systems and provided investigative procedures for antigen typing and antibody detection.

- HPA and HNA give rise to immunological responses which typically result in either thrombocytopenias or neutropenias respectively, although, in some cases, more systemic pathology can also be initiated, for example TRALI.

- The clinical conditions caused by HPA and HNA antibodies are largely well-characterized but there remain areas of uncertainty, for example the clinical significance of some antibodies, the optimal antenatal management of NAIT, and the precise the mechanism and reasons for susceptibility to TRALI.

- The advent of biochemical and molecular analysis of glycoproteins on platelets and granulocytes has enabled the elucidation of the HPA and HNA systems and provided investigative procedures for antigen typing and antibody detection.

- Many of the techniques developed differ from those in use in red cell immunohaematology laboratories because of the unique biologic and antigenic characteristics of platelets and granulocytes.

- Advances in technology have led to improved treatment options for many of the clinical problems caused by immune responses to HPA and HNA, for example the provision of HPA selected platelets and use of IvIgG in NAIT, use of GCSF in the treatment of the more profound cases of NAIN and autoimmune neutropenia.

- The interplay between clinical observation, for example isolated cytopenias in a neonate or following transfusion, and development of technological advances in the laboratory have been crucial in improving the treatment of these conditions and increasing understanding of the immunopathology of these disorders.

- The link between antigens, immune response, and biological function of target molecules has had significance for the understanding of the basic biology of platelets and granulocytes.

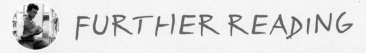

FURTHER READING

- **Bassler D, Greinacher A, Okascharoen C, *et al*. A systematic review and survey of the management of unexpected neonatal alloimmune thrombocytopenia.** *Transfusion*, **48 (2008), 92–8.**

An up-to-date survey of the management of unexpected thrombocytopenia in two countries.

- **Brand A. Alloimmune platelet refractoriness: incidence declines, unsolved problems persist.** *Transfusion*, 41 (2001), 724–6.

A review of the technical challenges in determining the cause of immunologically mediated platelet transfusion refractoriness.

- **Bux J & Sachs UJH. The pathogenesis of transfusion related acute lung injury (TRALI).** *Br J Haematol*, 36 (2007), 788–99.

A model of the pathogenesis of TRALI based on reported findings.

- **Kjeldsen-Kragh J, Killie, MK, Tomter G, et al. A screening and intervention program aimed to reduce mortality and serious morbidity associated with severe neonatal alloimmune thrombocytopenia.** *Blood*, 110 (2007), 833–9.

An alternative approach to antenatal management and prospective study of NAIT.

- **Lucas GF & Metcalfe P. Platelet and granulocyte polymorphisms.** *Transfusion Medicine*, 10 (2000), 157–74.

An earlier review containing some alternative diagrammatic representations of the key features of the platelet glycoproteins.

- **Murphy MF & Bussel JB. Advances in the management of alloimmune thrombocytopenia.** *Br J Haematol*, 136 (2007), 366–78.

An up-to-date review of the current treatment strategies in NAIT.

- **Ouwehand WH, Stafford P, Ghevaert C, et al. Platelet immunology, present and future.** *ISBT Science Series* 1 (2006), 96–102.

A review of the current key issues and advances in platelet immunology.

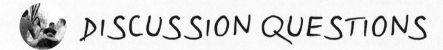 **DISCUSSION QUESTIONS**

9.1   There is an antenatal screening programme to identify women at risk of HDN. What would be the key elements for a screening programme to identify women at risk of having an infant due to HPA antibodies? Identify the limitations of such a strategy.

9.2   Identify strategies for reducing the incidence of TRALI.

Answers to the questions in this chapter are provided on the book's Online Resource Centre.

  Go to www.oxfordtextbooks.co.uk/orc/knight

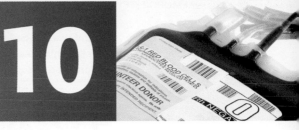

10

Haemopoietic Stem Cell Banking

Robert Walters

Learning objectives

After studying this chapter you should be able to:

- Understand the history and biology of haemopoietic stem cell (HSC) transplants.
- Describe the various sources and methods of stem cell collection.
- Understand the clinical and laboratory requirement involved in stem cell transplantation.
- Outline of the requirement standards of the various accreditation bodies.

Introduction

In the middle of the 1800s it was discovered that cells were the basic building blocks of life and that some cells had the ability to produce other cells. A number of attempts were made to fertilize mammalian eggs outside the body, but without success until the 1980s. In the early part of the twentieth century it was shown that some cells had the ability to generate blood cells—so-called *stem cells*. These cells are found mainly within the bone marrow but it was not until 1968 that the first bone marrow transplant was performed, successfully treating two siblings with a condition known as 'combined immunodeficiency'. Since then bone marrow transplants have been one of the main therapies to treat many haematological malignancies (e.g. leukaemias, myelomas) and other disorders such as immune deficiencies. In the UK some 65 new patients are diagnosed a day as having a haematological malignancy and each is a possible candidate for treatment with stem cells.

Some other notable events followed the initial bone marrow transplants within the field of stem cell research. In 1978 it was recognized that stem cells were quite numerous in human cord blood and techniques were later developed to use blood from the umbilical cord as a source of stem cells. In 1981 the first *in vitro* stem cell line was developed from mice, and in 1988 embryonic stem cell lines were created from a hamster. It was not until 1995 that the first embryonic stem cell line was derived from a primate and in 1997 a lamb was cloned from stem cells. In the same year it was demonstrated that leukaemic cells originated from *'affected' haemopoietic stem cells*; cells in which the DNA has been damaged, resulting in chaotic, abnormal cell division.

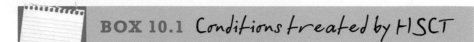

BOX 10.1 Conditions treated by HSCT

- Bone marrow failure, for example aplastic anaemia, congenital thrombocytopaenia.
- Leukaemia, for example acute myelogenous leukaemia (AML), acute lymphocytic leukaemia (ALL), and Hodgkin's and non-Hodgkin's lymphoma.
- Immunodeficiency, for example severe combined immunodeficiency disease (SCID).
- Congenital diseases, for example inherited metabolic disorders such as haemoglobinopathies, including sickle cell anaemia and beta-thalassaemia.
- Solid tumours, especially those that metastasize to bone where aggressive chemotherapy and or total body irradiation (TBI) follows solid tumour excision, such as breast, renal, ovarian, or testicular cancers.

10.1 Stem cells

Stem cells are special and have key features that separate them from other types of cell; they are unspecialized and renew themselves by dividing and are able, under specific conditions, to become cells with specialized jobs. Some regard them to be a bit like undergraduates—full of potential, not yet committed to any role but always thinking of reproducing themselves!

The potential use of stem cells in the treatment of diseases which affect millions of people around the world is virtually limitless and is an interesting branch of transplantation research. The potential of stem cells rests on their unique properties:

- *Self-renewal*: they can renew themselves almost indefinitely (proliferation).
- *Differentiation*: they have the ability to differentiate into cells with specialized characteristics and functions.
- *Unspecialized*: stem cells are largely unspecialized cells which then give rise to any number of specialized cells.

Stem cells are now thought to exist in most tissues, including the heart, skin, and even the CNS, where they contribute to repair damage. Research into understanding how these stem cells work should lead to innovative new therapies for regenerating, or treating diseased or damaged tissues and might replace the need for organ transplantation. The use of stem cell from human embryos that have far more of these cells than adult tissues and are also less resistant to expansion is very controversial. However, this chapter will deal with the established technologies using **haemopoietic** stem cells from bone marrow, cord blood, and peripheral blood.

Within the human body all haemopoietic blood cells, whether myeloid or lymphoid, are derived from a common **pluripotent** stem, or progenitor, cell (Figure 10.1) that is capable of self-renewal and progressive differentiation. When it becomes completely committed to a single cell type it loses the ability to self-renew and matures into fully differentiated

Haemopoietic
Blood cells produced in the bone marrow.

Pluripotent
Is the ability of the human stem cell to differentiate or become almost any cell in the body.

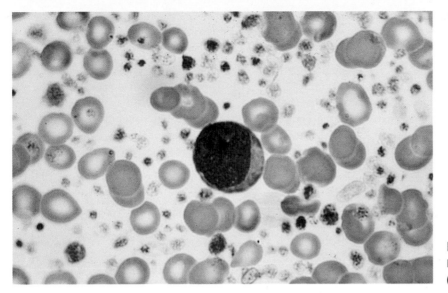

FIGURE 10.1
Pluripotent stem cell.
(© Nivaldo Medeiros.)

haemopoietic cell such as a granulocyte, monocyte, B or T cell (Figure 10.2). Haemopoietic progenitor cells (HPCs) are found in the largest numbers in bone marrow, also in increased numbers in umbilical cord blood, and in small numbers in the peripheral blood of adults.

To develop and differentiate *in vivo* HPCs require growth factors and a specific cellular environment. By giving potential stem cell donors some of these growth factors (e.g. granulocyte

(a) **(b)**

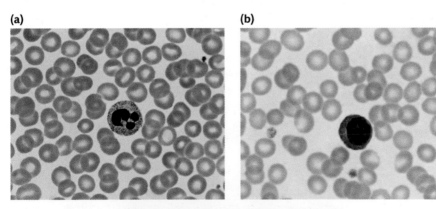

(c)

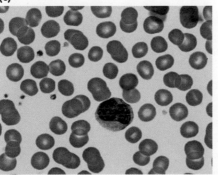

FIGURE 10.2
Leucocytes in peripheral blood. (a) Granulocyte, (b) lymphocyte, and (c) monocyte.

colony stimulating factor, GCSF) the number of HPCs in their circulation increases and they can be 'harvested' in sufficient numbers to be used in treating patients, as described in more detail below.

Morphologically, haemopoietic stem cells and progenitor cells appear under the microscope as either small lymphocytes or as blasts. The identification of stem cells is either by using a functional assay to count the number of colony forming units (CFUs) in a sample, or by surface marker analyses using a flow cytometer (Figure 10.3) to count the number of cells that have the surface marker CD34. The CD34 antigen is part of a family of *glycosylated type-1 transmembrane* single *chain glycoproteins*, expressed on virtually all haemopoietic precursor cells including **multipotent** stem cells.

Multipotent
Multipotent progenitor or stem cells can give rise to many but limited types of cell.

Key points

All haemopoietic blood cells such as a granulocytes, monocytes, or lymphocytes, are derived from a common pluripotent stem cell.

SELF-CHECK 10.1

What are haemopoietic stem cells?

10.2 Major histocompatibility complex and human lymphocyte antigens

The human major histocompatibility complex (MHC), which contains the genes for the *human lymphocyte antigens* (HLA) is the most polymorphic system of the human genome and is found on the short arm of chromosome 6. These polymorphic characteristics of these

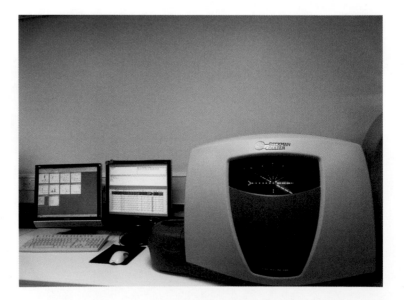

FIGURE 10.3
Flow cytometer. (Reproduced with kind permission from Specialist Haematology Laboratory, GSTS Pathology.)

antigens make them important in transplantation and HLA typing (identification of antigens or genes) is an essential step in selecting suitable donors for a bone marrow transplant.

The MHC or HLA comprises three major classes I, II, III. Class I genes are found furthest away from the centromere and are designated by capital letters, HLA-A, HLA-B etc, the best known and most significant in transplant are HLA-A, HLA-B, and HLA-C. Class II has five loci: DR, DQ, DP, DM, and DO, with DR, DQ, and DP being the most significant. Class III has a function which is very different from the other two classes and has its locus between the other two on chromosome 6. This locus is associated with complement, hormones, and intracellular peptide processing. See chapter 8 for more details of the HLA system.

Haemopoietic stem cell transplants present particular problems if recipient and donor are not closely HLA matched because the donor material will contain immunocompetent cells that will recognize antigens on the recipient cells (host) as foreign and mount an immunological attack. This is called graft versus host reaction (GvHR) and leads to **graft versus host disease** (GVHD) which can vary in severity from mild to severe and can cause death of the recipient.

Differences at HLA-A, HLA-B, or DRB1 loci increase the risk of acute GVHD but also decrease the post-transplant survival time, compared to a full match. There is a lower incidence of GVHD when cord blood is used even if there is an HLA mismatch; this is probably due to the immaturity and low number of immunocompetent T cells present. Mismatch of DQA, DPB1, or DPA has no significance, but matching at HLA-C, and possibly DQB1, can improve the outcome.

The best graft is from a monozygotic twin as they are genetically identical; next would be an HLA-matched sibling. Some 30% of patients will have an HLA-matched sibling, but for the remainder the only option is to perform a matched unrelated donor (MUD) transplant. It is recommended that patients and adult donors should be fully matched (8 out of 8 loci) for HLA-A, -B, -C, and -DBR1. Some centres now also include a match at DQB1. The matching required for cord blood units is less stringent, 6 out of 6, at HLA-A, -B, and DRB1. See Table 10.1.

> **Graft versus host disease (GVHD)**
> The most common cause of graft failure that is caused by donor immune cells, especially *T lymphocytes*, reacting against recipient tissue. The characteristic symptoms are the presence of a rash, diarrhoea, and abnormal liver function tests.

TABLE 10.1 HLA matching recommendations (National Marrow Donor Program USA).

HLA Locus	Tissue type patient	Match patient and donor
A	Yes, allele level	Yes
B	Yes, allele level	Yes
C	Yes, allele level	Yes
DRB1	Yes, allele level	Yes
DQB1	No*	No*
DRB3,4, 5	Desirable	No
DQA1	No	No
DPA1	No	No
DPB1	No	No

*Some centres match for DQB1.

Registries of HLA typed donors

There are more than 11 million HLA typed unrelated donors registered on international donor registries, with over 285,000 donors registered with the British Bone Marrow Registry (BBMR). Of these, 90% have been HLA typed for A, B, and DR and facilitate approximately 140 transplants annually. The largest and most successful UK registry is the Anthony Nolan Trust, with over 390,000 registered potential donors. In the UK there are over 60 transplant centres registered with the British Society for Bone Marrow Transplant (BSBMT), performing about 3,000 bone marrow or peripheral stem cell transplants annually. Of these, 35% are allografts and 65% autografts, mostly using peripheral blood rather than bone marrow derived stem cells.

Key points

Matching the potential donor and recipient for HLA is important to ensure a successful transplant.

10.3 Sources of haemopoietic stem cells

Stem cells can be harvested from:

- Bone marrow
- Peripheral blood
- Cord blood

Bone marrow stem cell donations

Bone marrow is the soft tissue found in the centre of the long bones and the sternum and it is here that blood cells of all lineages (red cells, white cells, and platelets) are produced from the haemopoietic stem cells. Once the cells have developed and matured in the bone marrow they then pass through the marrow-blood barrier and enter the peripheral circulation to carry out their specific functions.

Peripheral blood stem cells

There are a small number of haemopoietic stem cells in the normal peripheral circulation, but to collect sufficient numbers the donor has to be given a growth factor, for example GCSF (granulocyte-colony stimulating factor), to boost the number in their circulation. Regular counts are carried out to determine the number of CD34+ stem cells circulating by using a monoclonal anti-CD34 antibody by flow cytometry and when there are ten cells/cumm, or more, harvesting by *apheresis* can be undertaken.

Cord blood stem cells

The biggest advantage of using umbilical cord blood as a source of stem cells, as an alternative to bone marrow or peripheral blood, is the potentially unlimited numbers available, but the infrastructure to collect, process, store, and, when needed, recover them is not inconsiderable. The first transplant using cells from cord blood, took place in 1988. Since then cord blood banks have been set up in a number of countries and well in excess of 7,000 transplants with these cells have been performed worldwide.

Once the mother has consented and statutory tests for HIV, hepatitis, HLA type, etc. have been performed the cells are collected from the umbilical cord soon after delivery, then processed, stored frozen, and are then readily available for use. This is unlike the situation for bone marrow donation where once the need has been identified a 'compatible' donor has to be found, tested, and the marrow harvested—all of which takes time.

As the frequency of different HLA types varies geographically in the UK, collection of cord cells has been centred on areas with a high percentage of people from minority ethnic groups as these are generally underrepresented in the bone marrow registries. Therefore, when a stem cell transplant is needed for someone from one of these ethnic groups it is more likely that an HLA match will be found at a cord bank than from the bone marrow registry.

Cord blood immune cells are less mature than those of an adult and can be used with less risk of GVHD, even when only half of the HLA haplotypes match those of the recipient. Although the number of cells harvested from a cord is less than from a bone marrow or peripheral blood donation, they have been successfully used for both children and adults, but great care has to be taken with the collection, cryopreservation, and storage.

Key points

Haemopoietic stem cells can be obtained from bone marrow, peripheral blood, and cord blood.

SELF-CHECK 10.3

Why are cord stem cells better than adult stem cells?

Stem cell donations

Stem cell donations can be either:

- *Autologous*—the patient's own stem cells
- *Allogeneic*—donated by a family member or an unrelated donor
- *Syngeneic*—genetically identical or closely related

Autologous stem cells

The patient's own stem cells may be collected at any time during a period of disease remission and be stored frozen until high dose chemotherapy has been completed and the stem cells are required for marrow regeneration. The problem is that the patient's bone marrow and peripheral blood contains large numbers of malignant cells. Therefore, for the bone marrow to be of any benefit to the patient, the stem cell collection has to be carried out after the patient has gone into remission. Although there are no problems with graft versus host disease the patient's immune system will have been compromised by the chemotherapy treatment making the patient susceptible to infections.

Allogeneic stem cells

These are stem cells either collected from an HLA-matched live donor (a sibling or unrelated donor) or from stored cord blood preparations. Human lymphocyte antigen compatibility is required between recipient and donor as graft rejection is a real concern, although strong immunosuppressive drugs are used to diminish the immunological response and reduce the risk of rejection. The side effects of the chemotherapy (nausea, rashes, diarrhoea) will be the same for both autologous and allogeneic transplants.

Syngeneic stem cells

A patient receives stem cells from an identical twin. There are no biological or therapeutic problems with this method since they have the same major histocompatibility complexes (HLA type).

BOX 10.2 Apheresis

Stem cells are collected using a cell separator machine connected to the patient via a peripheral cannula. Blood is collected into the centrifuge bowl of the machine, where the mononuclear cells are separated from the red cell portion by centrifugation. The mononuclear cells are collected into a dedicated bag and the red cells are returned into the patient. Most cell separator machines require the use of two veins, one to withdraw and the second to return the blood—creating a continuous flow.

Donor leucocyte infusions (DLI) and graft versus tumour effect (GVT)

The aim of DLI is to induce a remission of the cancer by a process called *graft versus tumour effect* (GVT). DLI has been used after allogeneic transplantations for the treatment of recurrent malignancy. Its success varies depending on type of tumour, with the greatest success seen in CML (chronic myeloid leukaemia), although patients with relapsed acute leukaemia, chronic lymphocytic leukaemia, myelodysplasia, non-Hodgkin's lymphoma, Hodgkin's lymphoma, and multiple myeloma have also been treated successfully. Lymphocytes from the original HLA matched donor are collected and infused into the recipient to augment an anti-tumour immune response. Prior to DLI patients may require standard chemotherapy to reduce the number of malignant cells.

Key points

Stem cells collected, usually by apheresis, can be either autologous, allogeneic, or syngeneic.

10.4 Stem cell collection and processing

Patient conditioning

When stem cell therapy is used to treat a patient with a haematological malignancy or damaged immune system, their own malfunctioning cells need to be eliminated by chemotherapy and/or radiotherapy. Then, either their own previously harvested haemopoietic stem cells (autologous), or stem cells from another individual (allogeneic), are infused into the patient via a vein. The infused stem cells migrate to the bone marrow where they *engraft* and after a number of weeks they start producing cells that are released into the peripheral circulation.

Prior to infusion of stem cells, patients receive high dose chemotherapy and, in some cases in combination with radiotherapy; this is called conditioning. Eradication or suppression of the immune system is of great importance in recipients of allogeneic stem cells to prevent rejection of the foreign stem cells, so-called graft versus host disease (GVHD). There are a number of drugs used in the conditioning process, the most common is cyclophosphamide, which acts by damaging the DNA, thus interfering with cell replication. Other drugs such as busulphan, melphalan, and cytosine arabinoside are also used depending on the conditioning protocol. Total body irradiation (TBI) is used in patients with malignant diseases and is administered as a single dose or in smaller doses over several days.

BOX 10.3 *Effects of radiation*

As a result of the Chernobyl disaster a considerable number of people who had received a radiation dose of 500 rads died and only a few survived a dose greater than 800 rads.

Leukaemia patients who receive doses as high as 1,500 rads have been 'rescued' with bone marrow transplants.

The effect of chemotherapy on the bone marrow can be quite dramatic and even fatal. Chemotherapeutic drugs operate by destroying the fast growing malignant cells, but normal bone marrow cells are also very sensitive to these drugs, resulting in complete marrow destruction and marrow failure. Therefore, the patient's normal marrow function needs to be restored and this is done by transplanting stem cells.

Key points

Before a stem cell transplant a patient's own malfunctioning cells need to be eliminated by chemotherapy and/or radiotherapy.

Collection, manipulation, and storage of stem cells

All patients who may need to have their bone marrow or peripheral blood stem cells harvested will have been treated by a clinical haematologist or clinical oncologist and the question of transplantation will have been discussed. Prior to an autologous harvest a number of virological tests will be performed on the patient's blood (see below) to ascertain their viral status. It is essential that only material that is negative for these markers is stored in the same vessel to prevent contamination, albeit a very low risk.

The tests carried out on recipient and donor are:

- Anti-HIV-1
- Anti-HIV-2

- HIV-1-Ag
- Anti-HTLV
- HBsAg

Bone marrow harvest

Bone marrow harvest is an operating theatre, surgical procedure and uses a method developed by Thomas and Storb over a quarter of a century ago. The patient is anaesthetized and is laid face down on the theatre table and the bone marrow is aspirated from the posterior iliac crest (the top end of the femur) using a sterile bone marrow harvest needle (Figure 10.4). The aspirated marrow is placed into a 2-litre sterile blood collection bag containing ACD-A as anticoagulant. After 500 ml of marrow is collected, a 5 ml sample from the ACD-A/marrow mixture is removed aseptically and sent to the laboratory for a nucleated cell count so that a midway cell dose (indication of the number of nucleated cells collected) can be calculated. The midway cell dose will determine the final volume of bone marrow harvested. The NMDP (National Marrow Donor Program USA) uses a target dose of $2\text{--}4 \times 10^8$ nucleated cells/kg of patient or recipient body weight.

Once sufficient has been collected, the labelled collection bag is sent to the laboratory for concentration. This is done using an apheresis machine to remove the unwanted red cells and to concentrate the white blood cell population that includes the progenitor cells. The final concentrated material will then be manipulated, frozen, and stored (see below).

Peripheral blood stem cell harvest

To ensure sufficient stem cells are available to harvest, the donor is given GCSF, sometimes in conjunction with other drugs such as plerixafor, for a number of days and a WBC and CD34 count is carried out daily. When the CD34 count is >10/cumm then the stem cell harvest can proceed using an apheresis machine.

Apheresis equipment used can be single venous access or dual venous access). In either case, a large bore needle is inserted into one or both of the patient's *anticubital* veins. The collection system is a closed system and blood is collected into a bowl which is continually

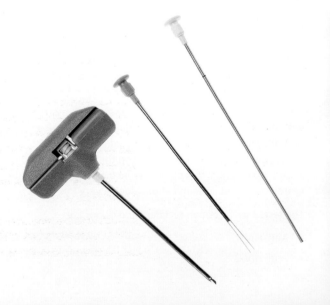

FIGURE 10.4
Bone marrow harvest needle. (© 2012
Angiotech Pharmaceuticals, Inc.
Reprinted with permission.)

centrifuging; the plasma is removed into a separate collection bag, the **buffy coat** (which is the concentrated WBC portion) into another bag, and then the remaining red cells and plasma are returned to the patient/donor. Most patients/donors are attached to the machine for up to six hours for sufficient stem cells to be collected. Once the collection has finished, the bag containing the buffy coat, and the plasma bag are labelled with the patient's name, hospital number, DoB, patient's weight, volume collected, and the date of collection. These are then sent to the laboratory for manipulation, CD34+ enumeration and colony forming units, CFUs. It is important to know the number of CD34 positive cells that have been collected. This is calculated:

Buffy coat WBC = A

A ÷ 100 × %CD34 = B

B × volume collected = C

C ÷ patient's wt kg = CD34 × 10^6/kg body weight

To determine the number of colony-forming units, a small amount of the nucleated cells from the buffy coat collected are incubated for 14 days in a semi-solid medium containing recombinant growth factors to stimulate specific cell growth and differentiation, in tissue culture conditions. Microscopic examination of the cells will reveal cell clusters (colonies) of the cells initially seeded that have responded to the growth factors. Different colony types GM (granulocyte-monocyte), E (erythroid), and MegK (megakaryocytic) are identified and counted. The assay indicates the presence of cells able to respond to the growth factors (CFS) present in the medium.

Manipulation

To store stem cells they have to be frozen and kept frozen. To prevent them being damaged during this process a cryoprotectant, such as glycerol or dimethyl sulphoxide (DMSO) is used (see Box 10.4). Manipulation of the cells is carried out in a laminar flow cabinet of grade A air quality situated within a clean room of grade B air quality to maintain sterility of the product that will be infused into a patient. Staff carrying out this procedure are required to wear sterile garments and follow the principles of good manufacturing practice (GMP) within this area.

Buffy coat the layer of WBC sitting on top of the red cell layer after centrifugation.

BOX 10.4 *Freezing cells*

When cells are frozen they are damaged, not directly by ice formation within the cell but by exposure to the high salt concentrations produced by freezing. *Cryoprotectants* act by penetrating the cell where they bind to water molecules in solution. The efflux of water is blocked from the cytoplasm during freezing which then prevents cellular dehydration or shrinkage and maintains a stable intracellular salt concentration and pH levels.

Glycerol is often used as cryoprotectant as it reduces the amount of ice forming, which restricts the increase in salinity that accompanies freezing.

Dimethyl sulphoxide (DMSO) also lessens the rise in salinity. It is used at lower concentrations than glycerol, and does not so readily enter the cell and can be added and removed, if necessary, much more easily than glycerol. For DMSO to be effective it is necessary for freezing to be rapid and to maintain a very low storage temperature, in liquid nitrogen for example.

A mixture of DMSO and plasma is added slowly to the cells via a plasma giving set with a three-way tap, mixing the bag continuously during the procedure. Once a final DMSO concentration of 8% has been achieved the plasma bag and giving set are removed from the three-way tap and a sterile cryocyte storage bag (specially designed to withstand low temperatures) is attached. A maximum of 100 ml of the plasma/cell mixture is added to the cryocyte bag using a 50 ml syringe to measure the amount.

Twenty-two ml of the plasma/cell mixture is retained, 10 ml being added to an aerobic blood culture bottle and another 10 ml added to an anaerobic culture bottle. The remaining 2 ml is aliquoted into three cryocyte bottles, frozen in the controlled rate freezer and stored in the liquid nitrogen phase. These aliquots are retained for retrospective testing if required.

The bags and aliquots are labelled with the patient's name, hospital number, date, volume, and a unique identifying number. The blood culture bottles are labelled and sent to the microbiology laboratory for culturing to ensure that the preparation is sterile.

Cryopreservation

A controlled rate freezer is used to freeze the cells with liquid nitrogen (Figure 10.5). A control unit (heating coil) that is attached to the freezing unit is placed in a Dewar of liquid nitrogen and secured. The freezing unit and heating coil are switched on and the required freezing programme entered into the unit. While the unit is coming to its start temperature, the bags and aliquots are placed in stainless steel holders and when the start temperature is reached they are placed within the unit and the freezing programme is allowed to run. At the end of the freezing cycle the bags and aliquots are removed and placed in the storage tank (Figure 10.6) until required. Stem cells can be stored in the *vapour phase of liquid nitrogen* indefinitely at a temperature of −150°C to −180°C.

Cord blood processing

Cord blood is collected into a bag from an umbilical vein soon after the cord has been cut and only takes about five minutes. The cord blood is then sent to the cord bank, where it

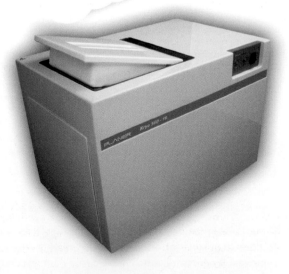

FIGURE 10.5
A controlled rate freezer. (© Planer.)

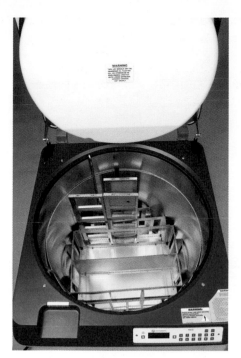

FIGURE 10.6
Liquid nitrogen storage tank.
(© Taylor Wharton.)

is processed using a 'slow sedimentation' technique to remove the red cells that are not required for the transplant. The volume is further reduced using a centrifugation method to separate the material into three blood components: plasma, buffy coat (the component needed) and buffy coat-depleted red cell concentration. The final volume of the buffy coat fraction will be about 30 ml and will be rich in progenitor and mononuclear cells. These latter cells are not removed because the patient may require support of more developed cells at the time of transplant to rebuild their immune system.

DMSO is added to the pellet as a cryoprotectant and the mixture is frozen using the rate control freezing method. After completing the freezing process the cord stem cell donations are stored in liquid nitrogen vapour at a temperature of $-150°C$ to $-180°C$.

Key points

Once stem cells have been collected they have to be stored at very low temperatures using a cryoprotectant.

Transportation

If the material for transplant is transported it should be in a specially designed container, such as a **Cryoshipper** (Figure 10.7). This is filled with liquid nitrogen that is absorbed into the inner lining of the shipper. The bags are checked before they are deposited in the shipper and a **ShipsLog™** (Figure 10.8) is attached to monitor the internal temperature of shipper during transportation.

Cryoshipper
A specially designed container used to transport material at a low temperature.

ShipsLog™
A temperature monitoring device attached to a cryoshipper to record the temperature.

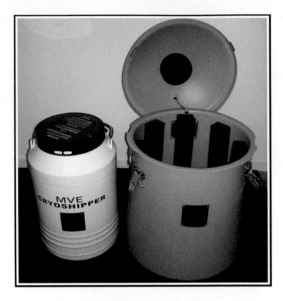

FIGURE 10.7
Cryoshipper for transporting
frozen cells with its outer
container. (© Planer.)

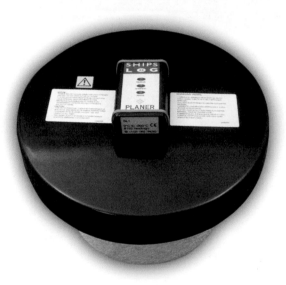

FIGURE 10.8
Cryoshipper with ShipsLog™
attached. (© Planer.)

10.5 **Reinfusion and engraftment**

When the clinical decision is made to infuse the stem cells, an authorized request has to be made to the stem cell laboratory for the material to be prepared. Transplant units work in different ways; in some units the stem cell material will be delivered to the ward and the ward staff will thaw out the material for reinfusion, while in other laboratories a staff member will accompany the material to the ward and will carry out the thawing procedure there.

The patient's demographic details are first checked by two staff members involved in the reinfusion of stored stem cell material, then the bag containing the required stem cells is placed in a water bath containing sterile saline at 37°C and allowed to thaw. This takes approximately five minutes, depending on the volume of material within the bag, and should be transfused within 20 minutes after thawing. A giving set is inserted into one of the ports on the bag and the other end attached to a three-way tap.

A 50 ml syringe is attached to one of the other ports on the three-way tap, the remaining port to a line inserted into one of the patient's veins. Some of the stem cell preparation is drawn into a 50 ml syringe and then slowly injected into the patient's vein. During the procedure the patient's blood pressure, temperature, and pulse are monitored as with any blood transfusion. (It is also possible to run in the material through a giving set as with any infusion of blood or saline.)

Engraftment takes place after the stem cells have been infused into the peripheral circulation, as they migrate to the bone marrow where they start to restore haemopoiesis. After a period of 10–14 days of severe **pancytopaenia** the first sign of engraftment will be the presence of neutrophils and monocytes in the blood, followed by an increase in the platelet count. Regular full blood counts (FBC) show any increase in white blood cell numbers, and an increase in the absolute numbers of circulating neutrophils and monocytes provide evidence of early engraftment.

> **Pancytopaenia**
> Low numbers of all blood cell lines (RBC, WBC, and platelets).

In patients undergoing autologous PBSCT the minimum number of stem cells which would be required for engraftment would be 2×10^6/CD34 + cells/kg. Increased stem cell dose can hasten neutrophil and platelet engraftment but there is little evidence that a dose of 5×10^6/CD34 + cells/kg is any more beneficial. The number of cells transplanted also plays an important role in the outcome in recipients of matched siblings and volunteer unrelated donor transplants.

Graft versus leukaemia effect (GVL)

It has been noted that during allogenic transplant the role of immunologically mediated GVL contributes in eradicating the patient's leukaemia. Graft versus leukaemia effect reduces the relapse rate in patients with severe GVHD but increases relapse rates when stem cells from identical twins have been used and reduces the ability of donor leucocyte infusions (DLI) to cure leukaemia in some patients.

Key points

Stem cells, infused into the peripheral circulation, migrate to the bone marrow where they engraft and start to produce normal cells.

10.6 Complications

Graft failure

Graft failure is defined as the failure to achieve a neutrophil count of $>0.5 \times 10^9$/l within 28 days of stem cell infusion. The most common cause is graft versus host disease (GVHD). The characteristic symptoms are the presence of a rash, diarrhoea, and abnormal liver function tests.

Graft versus host disease occurs in patients who have received allogeneic stem cell infusions and occurs near the time of engraftment in 40–70% of patients. This is caused by donor immune cells, especially T lymphocytes, reacting against recipient tissue. There are a number of risk factors that can be identified which increase the risk of GVHD; these include recipient age, HLA mismatch, and the use of female donors.

There are a number of methods that can be used as prophylaxis to try to prevent GVHD. Where there is a high degree of HLA mismatched, depletion of T cells from the donor stem cells can be achieved by using a monoclonal antibody-based technique using CD34 selection. The method is based on a monoclonal anti-CD34 antibody which is coupled to paramagnetic beads and added to the stem cell collection. The mixture of cells and antibody is incubated and washed, and then passed through a specially made set which magnetically removes the CD34+ cells allowing the T cell rich portion to pass through. Another form of prophylaxis is drug therapy in the form of cyclosporine and methotrexate. An alternative method is to give anti-T cell antibodies to the patient to remove the T cells by *in vivo* immunosuppression.

ABO incompatibility

Stem cells can be transplanted between a red cell antigen-disparate donor and recipient without an increase in GVHD or graft rejection. But if the recipient has ABO antibodies directed against donor red cells this *major incompatibility* can result in immediate haemolysis of red cells in the infused stem cell preparation. This can be minimized by reducing the red cell contamination of the stem cell preparation before reinfusion.

If the donor has been stimulated to produce red cell antibodies then viable lymphocytes in the stem cell material, once engrafted, can continue to produce these antibodies; this includes ABO antibodies. If these antibodies are incompatible with the recipient's red cells they might be haemolysed, but this is not normally noticed until about 14 days after the transplant (see Chapter 7 on immune red cell destruction).

Other complications

There are a number of other complications post allogeneic stem cell transplant, such as infections, including cytomegalovirus infections, fungal infections, and organ toxicity. Complications associated with autologous transplants are mainly related to immediate or delayed organ failure caused by conditioning regimes, or complications of **thrombocytopaenia** and **neutropaenia**.

In certain haematological **neoplastic** conditions (e.g. AML or ALL), malignant cells have been identified in the peripheral blood during mobilization and in leukophoresis products, although significantly lower than in bone marrow. This contamination is thought to influence disease recurrence, although it is not clear whether this is due to reinfusion of malignant cells or the inability of chemotherapy regimes to eradicate them.

Thrombocytopaenia
Low numbers of platelets.

Neutropaenia
Low numbers of neutrophil leucocytes.

Neoplastic
An abnormal growth of tissue.

Key points
Graft versus host disease is the main cause of graft failure.

SELF-CHECK 10.4

What are the main complications associated with haemopoietic stem cell transplants?

10.7 Health and safety, and statutory requirements

One of the main dangers in any stem cell bank is liquid nitrogen. Liquid nitrogen is colourless and odourless, but extremely cold, with a boiling point of −173°C. Contact with skin may result in cold burns and liquid contact with eyes can result in severe injury. Liquid nitrogen vapour can cause asphyxiation and therefore all areas where it is used must have 'low oxygen' monitors. All personnel handling liquid nitrogen should take appropriate personal protective measures, be properly trained, and have yearly competency assessments.

To guarantee the safety of the stored material the following should be in place:

- The storage facility is equipped with a backup electrical power generator.
- Each storage tank monitoring system has its own battery back-up.
- The temperature of the storage tanks is monitored 24/7, checked daily, and recorded.
- The flow of liquid nitrogen to the storage vessels should be automatically controlled.
- Laboratory is manned 24/7, 365 days per year.
- Each sample stored is given a unique bar code number, storage location in storage vessel, and the information stored on hardcopy and computer.

It is a statuary requirement that all transplant units in the UK are licensed by the Human Tissue Authority (HTA). The HTA has replaced the MHRA (Medicines and Healthcare products Regulatory Agency) as the licensing body and carries out site inspections every two years. All transplant procedures and processes must comply with the HTA standards as well as conform to the requirements of GMP. The objective of GMP is to ensure that products are consistently produced and controlled to particular quality standards. Each unit or laboratory must have a named designated individual (DI) and a licence holder. The DI is responsible for overseeing the whole procedure and processes and must make sure that all the HTA standards are met.

At the present time it is not a legal requirement for transplant centres to be accredited by JACIE (Joint Accreditation Committee-ISCT and EBMT) but the aim of JACIE is to promote high quality care and to ensure that the clinical, collection, and laboratory units work together to achieve excellent communication, effective common work practices, and increased guarantees for the patient.

NetCord-FACT (International Standards for Cord Blood Collection, Processing, Testing, Banking, Selection, and Release) produce the standards that apply to facilities and individuals performing the above activities in relation to cord blood.

Key points

In the UK, stem cell laboratories have to be licensed by the Human Tissue Authority and work to strict codes of practice.

10.8 The future of stem cell therapy

The potential use of stem cells for treating a whole range of diseases including degenerative disorders, is immense and research groups are working all over the world to develop stem cell treatments. Adult tissues are composed of fully differentiated cells but some have a very small number of stem cells that are capable of self-renewal and differentiation into a small range of tissues. The problem is getting to these cells and inducing them to increase in number without differentiating and then differentiating when required. Embryonic stem cells are more numerous and they seem to be capable of unlimited cell division and possibly being able to differentiate into any of the 220 cell types found in humans. This explains why so much research is being done with these cells but such research is controversial. However, it has been found that by re-programming normal adult cells, such as skin fibroblasts, into 'induced' pleuripotent stem cells (iPS); these have properties similar to embryonic stem cells and can give rise to multiple tissues. Such an approach might mean that embryos will not be needed and an individual's own fibroblasts could be re-programmed as required and specific graft material manufactured *ex vivo*. These developments are still in the early stages so there will be a continued need for donor derived HSCs for many years to come.

CASE STUDY 10.1 Peripheral blood stem cell harvest

A 50-year-old male suffering from multiple myeloma has received a number of cycles of intensive chemotherapy C-VAMP (cyclophosphamide, vincristine, Adriamycin®, and methykprenidolone) followed by an autologous stem cell harvest.

The patient was attached to the apheresis machine for six hours and 185 ml of material was collected, labelled, and sent to the laboratory. A total white blood cell count and a CD34 enumeration were carried out on this sample. The peripheral blood CD34 was 22 cell/cumm and the CD34 count of the collected material was 0.89%. The WBC count was 142 x 10^9/l. The patient's weight was 84 kg.

SELF-CHECK 10.5

What was the final CD34 count?

SELF-CHECK 10.6

Was it necessary for a further harvest to be carried out the next day?

CHAPTER SUMMARY

- The first bone marrow transplant took place in 1968 and haemopoietic stem cell transplantation is now widely practised.

- Typing for HLA (-A, -B, -DR) is an essential step in the selection of suitable donors for allogeneic transplants.

- Stem cells can be harvested from bone marrow, peripheral blood, or cord blood and can be *autologous* (the patient's own stem cells), *allogeneic* (donated by a family member or an unrelated donor), or *syngeneic* (genetically identical or closely related).

- Once collected, stem cells are processed, cryopreserved, and stored for use at a later date.

- The identification and enumeration of stem cells is by surface markers, such as CD34, and the use of growth factors sufficiently increases the number of circulating stem cells that can be harvested from a donor.

- The use of cord blood as a source of stem cells has increased the number of registered donors worldwide and the availability of material for transplantation has improved.

- The introduction of new chemotherapeutic drugs in the treatment of a number of neoplastic disorders have improved and the use of more sophisticated therapies has made certain complications of transplantation more manageable, for example GVHD.

- The advent of accreditation by MHRA and then by the HTA of all transplant activity in the UK has ensured that the requirements for GMP are rigorously applied and the safety of transplantation improved.

- The use of haemopoietic stem cells as a form of treatment for other non-haematological conditions may prove to be successful in the future. Many tissues can now be used as a source of stem cells, and with research and development stem cell therapy is becoming a growth area in healthcare provision.

FURTHER READING

- **Austin E, Guttridge M, Pamphilon D, & Watt SM. Blood services and regulatory bodies in stem cell transplanation.** *Vox Sanguinis*, 94 (2008), 18–32.

- **Bug G & Serve H. Stem cell and cord blood transplantation—state of the art.** *ISBT Science Series*, 5 (2010), 317–23.

- **McKenna DH & Brunstein CG. Umbilical cord blood: current status and future directions.** *Vox Sanguinis*, 100 (2011), 150–62.

- **NHS Blood and Transplant (NHSBT) Blood Matters is a regular publication with up-to-the-minute articles on all aspects of transfusion and transplantation: www.hospital.blood.co.uk/communication/blood_matters/index.asp.**

Answers to the questions in this chapter are provided on the book's Online Resource Centre.

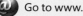 Go to www.oxfordtextbooks.co.uk/orc/knight

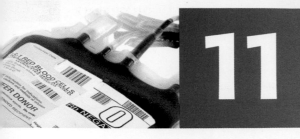

11

Tissue Banking

Richard Lomas

Learning objectives

After studying this chapter you should be able to:

- Describe the types of grafts that are currently used.
- Know what tissues are banked and how are they used.
- Outline how donors are selected, screened, and consent is obtained.
- Outline how tissues are procured from living and deceased donors.
- Outline how the collected tissue is processed.
- Outline how that tissue is preserved.
- Outline how tissues are stored and distributed.

Introduction

Tissue damage resulting from disease or trauma is a significant medical problem and many different ways have been tried to correct the damage, or to enable the patient to live with the problem. One of the earliest was the use of an artificial graft or a prosthesis, such as a metal plate to hold a fractured bone in place. But there are alternatives available. In other chapters, transplantation of cellular organs and stem cells have been considered and the need to HLA match the donor and recipient to prevent rejection of the transplanted organ. However, there are other tissues (e.g. bone) that can be used as grafts, whose effectiveness is not dependent on a good HLA match. This chapter describes how tissue grafts are used clinically, and discusses the process by which tissues grafts are collected and treated to improve their clinical efficacy, make them safer, and render them suitable for long-term storage.

11.1 **Types of graft**

There are many strategies for replacing or repairing damaged tissues, a significant one of which is the use of tissue grafts. There are three basic types of tissue graft:

- Xenografts (grafts prepared from animal tissue)
- Autografts (tissue grafted from another site on the patient's body)
- Allografts (tissue donated by another person, and the focus of this chapter)

Occasionally, biological grafts may be combined with prosthetic materials to form a composite, **bioprosthetic graft**. Prosthetic grafts (made from artificial materials) may also be used.

Autografts are universally agreed to be the gold standard for tissue grafting from a clinical performance viewpoint. The use of the patient's own tissue obviates any risk of disease transmission or immune rejection, and allows transplantation of a living graft, with the requisite biological and structural properties, to facilitate tissue repair and regeneration. For example, autograft obtained from the **iliac crest** is used in many bone grafting procedures, and autograft skin is essential for the repair of deep burns. Autografts do, however, have significant and insurmountable differences. First, any operation using autograft requires a secondary procedure to procure the graft, resulting in additional morbidity at the donor site. Second, the amount of tissue that can be safely taken for autografting is limited. Bone graft taken from the iliac crest may suffice for sinus reconstruction, but may be insufficient in volume for a spinal fusion, or hip revision, and a patient with 80% burns will not have sufficient undamaged skin available to graft the entire burnt area.

Prosthetic grafts address the deficiencies of autografts in that there are no restrictions on graft size or availability, but they also come with disadvantages. A general disadvantage with all grafts made of non-biological material is that they do not integrate well with the patient's own tissue, and are much more prone to infection than biological grafts. Prosthetic grafts placed in the cardiovascular system may also be **thrombogenic** and require the recipient to take prophylactic anticoagulants, with the attendant risk of side effects.

The principle advantages of using allografts is that as a biological material they do not have the drawbacks of prosthetic grafts, and also much better approximate the complex biomechanical properties of human tissue—it is generally better where possible to replace 'like with like'. They can also, to a limited degree, replicate the biological properties of an autograft. Whilst the cellular content of an allograft will be rejected if exposed to the recipient's immune system, grafts placed in immunocompromised areas such as the cornea or **articular cartilage** may retain the viability, and hence maintenance and reparative properties, of the donor cells. Even short-term retention of graft viability can be beneficial, for example in the case of *non-HLA matched* skin allografts which can temporarily engraft to a burn wound-bed, and promote regeneration of the recipient's own skin. The main drawback of allografts from a surgeon's viewpoint is the perceived risk of disease transmission from the graft to the recipient, originating either from the donor or from contamination acquired during procurement or preparation. If correct donor selection, testing, and tissue decontamination procedures are followed the risks of disease transmission are very low or negligible. However, allograft transmitted infections have been recorded and are a source of concern to clinicians.

Xenografts are prepared from animal material; the most commonly used in surgery are porcine (pig) heart valve grafts. Other types of xenograft include bovine and equine pericardium, commonly used in cardiac surgery, and bovine bone-derived grafts used in orthopaedic and maxillofacial surgery.

Bioprosthetic graft
A composite graft, comprising both prosthetic and biological materials.

Iliac crest
Part of the pelvic bone, often used as a source of bone autograft.

Thrombogenic
Material which causes blood to clot on contact.

Articular cartilage
Hard, smooth cartilage that lines bone in joint surfaces.

Key points

There are three types of graft available: xeno, auto, and allografts, plus prosthetic grafts. Although autografts are the most effective, allografts are becoming more widely used.

SELF-CHECK 11.1

What are the advantages and disadvantages of synthetic, auto, and allografts?

11.2 Which tissues are banked and how are they used?

Most tissue allografts are donated by deceased donors, although some tissues may be donated for grafting by living donors following surgical removal during routine operations. The clinical requirement for different types of allograft varies both temporally and geographically. As certain types of graft are shown to perform well or less well, requirements fluctuate accordingly. There are additionally geographical variations in allograft usage, which may result (for example) from a lack of suitable local banking services. Perhaps the most widely and commonly banked tissues are those of the musculoskeletal system. The repair of damaged bones with prosthetic grafts has been performed since prehistoric times, and there is a major demand for bone allografts in many surgical areas, principally orthopaedic (spine and joint surgery) and also in oral/maxilliofacial surgery. There are many different forms of bone allograft, ranging from massive **osteochondral grafts** used in trauma repair and following excision of large bone tumours, to fine, **morsellized bone grafts** used in joint and dental surgery. See Figure 11.1.

Osteochondral graft
A composite graft, comprising bone plus an intact articular cartilage surface.

Morsellized bone graft
Bone graft milled to granules or powders of different diameters.

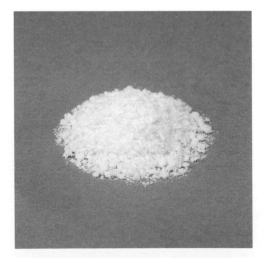

FIGURE 11.1
Morsellized cortico-cancellous bone graft.

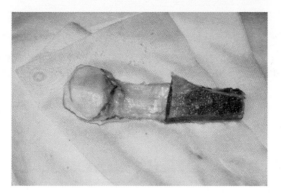

FIGURE 11.2
Patellar ligament graft, with patella bone and tibial bone block attached.

Tendon and ligament allografts are also commonly used, principally in knee surgery for the repair or ruptured or damaged **anterior cruciate ligaments**. There is also a growing use of more specialized musculoskeletal allografts, such as osteochondral grafts for the treatment of focal lesions of the joint surface, and allografts for repair of knee injuries. See Figure 11.2.

Skin allografts play a major role in the treatment of serious burn injuries. Whilst they do not permanently engraft they can be combined with small amounts of autograft, providing protection and cover to the wound-bed while the autograft induces the formation of new skin. Generally, a cadaveric skin graft comprises the epidermis and upper layer of the dermis. The allograft closely adheres to the recipient's wound-bed, covering exposed nerve endings and reducing pain and infection, whilst the presence of the intact epidermis reduces fluid and heat loss. There is also evidence that viable grafts are able to temporarily engraft to the recipient, further enhancing healing.

Other tissues that are banked include heart valves, blood vessels, pericardium, eye corneas and sclera, and amniotic membrane (used as a dressing in the treatment of eye and burn injuries). See Table 11.1.

> **Anterior cruciate ligament**
> A ligament located within the knee joint that plays a crucial role in stabilising the joint and a commonly damaged in sporting injuries.

TABLE 11.1 Types of tissue allograft used in different surgical specialities.

Surgical specialty	Types of graft used
Cardiac	Heart valves, vascular patches, pericardium
Orthopaedic (knee surgery)	Tendons, ligaments, meniscus, bone
Orthopaedic (hip)	Morsellized and structural bone
Orthopaedic (spine)	Morsellized and structural bone, demineralized bone matrix
Ophthalmology	Cornea, sclera, amnion
Burns	Skin, dermis
Plastic and reconstructive	Dermis
Oral and maxillofacial	Demineralized bone matrix
Vascular	Blood vessels

11.3 How are donors selected, screened, and consented?

The banking of tissues for therapeutic use is a multi-step process, the first stage of which is obtaining valid, informed consent for donation to take place. This section addresses the legal framework under which this consent must be obtained, and explains how this is accomplished by NHS Blood and Transplant Tissue Services (NHSBT-TS), the largest therapeutic tissue bank in the UK.

NHSBT-TS obtains tissues for therapeutic purposes and for ethically approved research projects. These may be obtained from living donors, where the tissue is removed following elective surgery (e.g. femoral heads donated following hip replacement), but most tissues are obtained from deceased donors.

It is crucial that when consent is obtained for tissue donation for any reason, be it for therapeutic or research purposes, it is both informed and valid. For the consent to be valid, it must be taken from the appropriate person in a manner that complies with legislative requirements. It also requires that the person giving consent is fully informed of all aspects of the donation process. Where the donor is deceased and consent is taken usually from bereaved relatives, there is a further challenge in ensuring that the process does not cause additional distress, whilst complying with legal and ethical requirements.

The primary legislation covering tissue donation is the Human Tissue Act. This was enacted in 2004, following well-publicized cases of organ retention following post-mortem examination without the knowledge or consent of relatives. Accordingly, the Human Tissue Act makes consent the fundamental guiding principle covering the use of donated tissue for any purpose, and provides for financial and custodial penalties for breaches of its requirements. It also established a regulatory body, the Human Tissue Authority (HTA), with a remit to license and inspect all establishments procuring and storing human tissue.

The HTA provides guidance and direction, through the publication of codes of practice, the first of which deals specifically with consent. This clarifies that the removal, storage, and use of relevant material from deceased donors, and the storage and use of relevant material from living donors requires consent. The HTA define the term 'relevant material' as 'material other than gametes, which consists of, or includes, human cells'. Certain tissues, such as hair and nail clippings, are not classified as relevant material and are not covered by the Act.

As already mentioned, for consent to be valid, it must be given by the appropriate person. With a living donor, this is generally the donor themselves. However, for deceased donors the situation is often more complex. The HTA defines a 'hierarchy of consent', specifying in order of relevance who can give consent in these cases. The highest priority is given to the wishes of the deceased themselves if expressed in life, for example through the organ donor register. If this was not done, then priority is given to the deceased's nominated representative, a person who was appointed in life by the deceased to make these decisions. If neither of these situations is the case, consent must be sought from a person who was in a 'qualifying relationship' with the deceased. This may be (in order of priority) a spouse or partner, blood relation, or friend.

It is also important for consent to be considered valid, that the person giving consent is fully informed with regard to all aspects of the donation process, including how, where, and when the donation will take place, how much tissue will be removed, and the purposes for which the tissue may be used. The scope of the consent must be defined as closely as it is practical to do; it is recognized that when tissue is donated for research purposes, a generic consent may be appropriate as the specific nature of the research for which the tissue may be used may not be known at the point of donation. However, where the tissue is donated for a specific purpose, such as a defined research project, or for transplantation, this information must be provided to the person giving consent.

The duration of the consent must also be specified; this may be enduring, that is, it remains in force unless it is specifically withdrawn, or time limited. The person giving consent may also withdraw it at any point before or after donation (providing that the tissue has not already been used), and it is important that they are informed of this right.

With the exception of anatomical examination or public display, where written consent is required, the Human Tissue Act does not specify the format in which consent should be recorded. Verbal consent, documented either by audio recording or in the patient's notes, is also valid. The Act recognizes that in itself, a signed consent document does not make the consent valid; it must be shown that all the information necessary for the person to give appropriate consent was given prior to the decision being made.

The procedure by which the NHS Blood and Transplant Tissue Services (NHSBT-TS) obtains consent for tissue donation was developed following consultation with a number of interested parties, including donor families and donor transplant co-ordinators, and has been ratified by the HTA. Indeed, during a recent inspection by the HTA the procedures in the National Referral Centre (NRC) were described as exemplary and are now used as an example of best practice in their *Code of Practice for Consent*.

Consent for tissue donation within NHSBT-TS is handled by a dedicated National Referral Centre (NRC), based in Liverpool. This unit is staffed by nurse practitioners (NPs) who are specially trained to assess the suitability of potential donors, and obtain valid consent for donation. The centralization of this service allows for rapid training of the NPs taking consent, quick dissemination of best practice, peer support for staff who need to undertake delicate and sensitive conversations with bereaved families on a regular basis, and also enables the application of lean working principles to maximize the efficiency of the unit.

Consent for tissue donation within the NRC is done by telephone, using a defined protocol. This is beneficial to donor families as it can be done at a pre-arranged time, in the surroundings of their own home with family members present for support. It also allows the option of donation to families of donors who have died outside a hospital environment. The NP must ensure that the conversation takes place in a quiet area without risk of disturbance, and a designated room is made available for this purpose. They then contact the donor family, and ensure that they are speaking to the appropriate person as defined in the hierarchy of consent. As the consent is verbal, the conversation is recorded to provide a record of the information that was provided by the NP, and what was agreed to by the person giving consent. The conversation requires that the NP provides appropriate information in order for the person giving consent to make an informed decision. This information includes:

- What the donor's expressed wishes in life were (if known). They establish this by checking if the donor is registered on the organ donor register prior to contacting the family.
- Which tissues may be donated.
- The timeframe under which donation will take place.
- How tissues are removed, and how the donor body is reconstructed afterwards.
- What is the clinical requirement for the donated tissues.
- How the donation process may affect the appearance of the donor.
- That viewing of the donor after donation is possible.
- That tissues may be stored in a tissue bank for a prolonged period of time before use.
- Sometimes, donated tissue is not suitable for transplantation; in these cases it may be used for ethically approved research, providing they so consent.
- That the donor's GP will be contacted to obtain medical history.
- That a blood sample will be taken to test for transmissible diseases, including HIV and hepatitis. If any of these test results may have significance for the health of other family members, they will be contacted and offered appropriate advice.
- Their right to withdraw consent at any time prior to use of the grafts, and an explanation of how to do so.

This is very much a two-way conversation, and the family are given the opportunity to ask questions and request further information about any aspects of the donation process. During the consent process, a detailed medical and behavioural history of the donor is also obtained from their family using a structured questionnaire to ascertain the medical suitability to donate. This is necessary to ensure the safety of the donated tissues. It must be considered that tissue grafts are in almost all cases used for 'life-enhancing', rather than 'life-saving' procedures; there are generally alternative treatments available (e.g. the use of inorganic bone substitutes in place of bone allografts, or the use of porcine heart valve grafts in place of allografts). The risk-benefit analysis for tissue allografts is therefore skewed more towards the risk side of the equation. Tissue donors are therefore, carefully selected to minimize the risk of either transmitting diseases from the donor to the recipient, or transplanting a tissue that may perform poorly. This selection process takes the form of physical testing, and a review of the donor's medical and behavioural history. The donor's relatives, and or friends are interviewed to elicit any lifestyle factors that may render the donor a higher risk for disease transmission, and the donor's GP and any other medical practitioners treating the donor are queried to obtain as accurate and complete a medical history as possible. Significant lifestyle factors that preclude donation are intravenous drug abuse, high risk sexual behaviour, and even the presence of recent tattoos. There are many medical conditions that either restrict or preclude tissue donation. Common reasons for total medical deferral include malignancy and sepsis, due to the potential risk of disease transmission. Other conditions may result in the deferral of tissues for physical reasons, for example the genetic condition **Marfan's syndrome** results in weakened connective tissue. Musculoskeletal and cardiovascular allografts would not be donated by a donor with Marfan's, but skin grafts would be acceptable. A comprehensive list of donor selection guidelines is maintained by the UK Blood and Tissue Transplantation Services, accessible online at: http://www.transfusionguidelines.org.

Marfan's syndrome
A genetic disorder, causing weakness of the connective tissue. A contraindication for donation of soft tissue allografts.

Screening of blood samples from potential tissue donors is also mandatory. Blood samples are screened for markers of a range of microbiological infections by using the same screening assays as used for testing blood donations. This screening includes the markers defined as mandatory, and any discretionary testing determined by the donor's medical or travel history, for example malaria and *T. cruzi*. All donors are screened for syphilis antibody, HBsAg, anti-HCV, anti-HIV, anti-HTLV, anti-HBc, and also by HCV-PCR, HIV-PCR, and HBV-PCR. The supplementation of routine serology testing with the new generation of nucleic acid tests serves to reduce the risk of false negative results, where a donor has only recently been exposed to a pathogen and not mounted sufficient immune response to trigger antibody tests. Nucleic acid testing is capable of detecting infection at a much earlier stage than the equivalent antibody test. However, serology screening still has the advantage of being able to detect a past exposure that may speak to lifestyle risks. This combination is especially important for testing of deceased tissue donors, where only a single blood sample can be taken at the time of donation. With donors of living tissue, it is possible to take a second blood sample at a time post donation to reduce the risk of these 'window period' infections. However, if PCR testing is used on the initial sample too, this is not now considered necessary.

A key limitation with serological testing is that it is only possible to test for diseases which are known about, and for which a validated test is available. It will take some time for the presence of novel transmissible diseases to become apparent, and even after a novel disease has been identified, it may be some time before a test is developed. A contemporary example of this problem is new variant Creutzfeldt–Jakob disease, which is known to be present in the donor population, especially in the UK. There is as yet no reliable blood test for this disease, and this screening must rely solely on assessment of a donor's medical history (did they show any clinical indications or dementia, etc.) and of any lifestyle risks (use of human growth hormone, etc.).

Assessment of donor safety is therefore a multi-step process, designed to investigate and identify any potential risks that might result from implantation of the tissue.

Key points

Before any tissue can be used, the donor, or in the case of a deceased donors, the nearest relatives, must have given consent; the donor's medical history must be reviewed and a sample of blood from the donor tested for the same microbiological markers as a blood donor.

SELF-CHECK 11.2

What is the role (in the UK) of the HTA?

11.4 How are tissues retrieved?

When a donor has been accepted for tissue donation, the next stage is to physically retrieve, or procure, the tissue from the donor. This is a very different procedure for deceased and living donors, and these will therefore be addressed in different sections. Irrespective of the type of donor, the overall objective of tissue procurement is to obtain the tissue to as high a standard as possible, minimizing or eliminating all risks to the tissue associated with the retrieval process.

With deceased donors, a key factor in ensuring the quality of the tissue grafts is the time post-mortem that the tissue is procured. Following death, the integrity of the intestinal walls deteriorates, and intestinal microflora begin to migrate throughout the body, contaminating other tissues. Additionally, autodegradation of all tissues commences as cells die and release

Warm ischaemia time
The time elapsing between death and a body being placed into a refrigerated environment.

lytic enzymes into the tissue. The rate of both these processes is critically dependent on temperature; therefore it is crucial that the **warm ischaemia time** is minimized and the body is cooled as soon as possible after death. The permitted time for post-mortem retrieval varies between different countries. However, generally a maximum post-mortem time of 48 hours is permitted, subject to an acceptable warm ischaemia time. The optimal time and place to procure tissues from deceased donors is in the operating theatre, immediately post-mortem. However, the availability of these facilities for tissue donation is limited, and is generally restricted to tissue grafts that can be obtained during routine organ procurement procedures, such as removal the heart for valve donation. In the UK, the large majority of tissue donations are performed in hospital mortuaries, or on rare occasions in funeral homes.

Retrieval of tissue in a mortuary, which is not designed for aseptic operations, is challenging. It is necessary to perform tissue retrievals once routine post-mortem examinations have been completed, to reduce the risk of cross contamination. It is crucial that prior to any retrieval activities commencing the donor is correctly identified. This involves checking the information given with the referral with information physically present on the donor, on a wrist band or toe tag. The cardinal rule here is that at least three points of identification (such as name, date of birth, address, or hospital number) must coincide. Once the retrieval team are satisfied that these requirements have been met, tissue retrieval can commence. Before any dissection activities take place, the donor is cleaned using surgical detergents, alcohol wipes, and sterile water. Any areas of the skin where incisions will be made, or where skin grafts will be retrieved from, are also shaved. The donor is then placed on a sterile field and the retrieval team will don sterile clothing to commence removal of tissues.

Generally, skin grafts (if consented for) will be retrieved first to prevent the skin becoming contaminated by internal body fluids following incisions to remove internal tissues. The areas of the body from where skin is retrieved are dictated both by aesthetic considerations and practicalities. Skin will not be retrieved from areas of the body that may be visible during an open casket funeral, such as the face, neck, hand, or lower arms. Additionally, given that the primary requirement for skin grafts is in burn surgery where large sheets of skin are required, skin is not retrieved from areas where this is not practical. In practice, skin grafts are retrieved from the back of the torso and the back and front of both legs. Skin is retrieved using an instrument called an *electric dermatome* that can be adjusted for cutting depth and width so that skin is taken in long strips of nominal thickness 0.3 mm. This results in a split skin allograft, which comprises the epidermis and the upper layer of the dermis—in practice the thickness of the skin varies considerably depending on the person performing the procurement, the donor, and the anatomical area it is being taken from. Care is taken to avoid taking skin grafts where the skin is excessively blemished (for example the presence of raised moles), and where the donor is tattooed. There is no clinical reason why tattooed skin is unsuitable for donation, but if the tattoo is considered to be identifiable to the donor it will be avoided. Following retrieval, the skin is transferred immediately to a cooled, buffered transport solution and transported to the tissue bank on wet ice. To prevent seeping of blood or other internal fluids from the body surface following retrieval, a dilute bleach solution is applied which seals the exposed dermis.

Other tissue grafts are located internally and must be retrieved by incision. If retrieving heart, pericardium, and thoracic aorta, the chest cavity must be exposed. This is accomplished by making an incision from the throat down to the bottom of the sternum. Care must be taken not to expose the abdominal cavity as this will significantly increase the risk of contamination. The skin is then retracted, and the ribcage cut away in an inverted 'V' shape. At this point, **costal cartilage** may be retrieved from the ribcage. With the ribcage removed, the pericardium can then be dissected away to expose the heart and great

Costal cartilage
Hyaline cartilage, located between the ribs. Utilized as a graft material in reconstructive surgery.

vessels (if required, the pericardium may be stored for subsequent banking). The heart is then removed, together with the associated ascending aorta, and pulmonary trunk and arteries. It is good practice to remove a significant length of these vessels, associated with the pulmonary and aortic valves, as it gives the surgeon more options when implanting the graft. Long vessel lengths (conduits) can also serve as grafts in their own right, or be opened up to create a vascular patch graft. Normally, the entirety of the heart is removed even though only the outflow valves are required. This allows the delicate valve dissection process to be performed under controlled conditions. Some tissue banks may remove the apex of the heart following procurement. This exposes the ventricles, and permits the heart to be flushed with sterile, buffered saline following procurement, as a means of reducing contamination. A further graft that may be procured from the chest cavity is the descending portion of the thoracic aorta. This is easily accessed following removal of the heart, but must be carefully procured so as to retain sufficient lengths of the branching **intercostal arteries** to permit the creation of stable **anastomoses** on implantation. The chest cavity can then be reconstructed using absorbent padding material to replace lost tissue mass and soak up fluids, followed by replacement of the ribcage and suturing of the initial incision.

Many other tissue grafts are obtained from the lower limbs, including bone (femur and proximal tibia), tendons and ligaments (patellar, Achilles, and hamstrings), **meniscal cartilage**, and femoral arteries. Bone grafts may also be obtained from other anatomical areas depending on clinical requirements. However, the leg bones offer a large mass of easily accessible **cortical** and **cancellous bone** that can be processed into a variety of different grafts, and permits straightforward reconstruction after donation.

When retrieving tendons and ligaments, the first step is to make a shallow incision to just below the level of the subcutaneous fat layer. The tendon/ligament connective tissue is located very close to this layer, and care must be taken not to damage it during the initial fibrocartiliase incision. The incision will be made to a generous length, to permit ease of access. Fine dissection is not required at this stage—during initial procurement the emphasis is on reducing the exposure of the tissues to environmental contamination, so excess connective tissue will be left attached to the graft. Where the tendon/ligament has a bone insertion point, a generous bone block is cut. In most cases, the whole length of the extensor mechanism will be exposed prior to dissection, although for hamstring tendons it may be possible to use tendon strippers to remove the tendon through a smaller incision.

Femoral arteries may also be procured from the legs. These can serve as lower limb bypass grafts, and may be obtained to a length of up to 30 cm, through an incision stretching from the groin to behind the knee. As with tendons, fine dissection is not performed in the mortuary, rather the whole vascular bundle containing the femoral vein (which may also be used as a graft) and sciatic nerve is retrieved for later fine dissection under controlled conditions. With careful dissection, the same incisions may be used for tendon, vascular, and bone graft retrieval.

For bone grafts, the whole femur is removed either as a single bone or cut into two or three separate sections. If meniscal cartilage grafts are being procured, the entire knee joint is dissected as an individual unit to permit later fine dissection. The distal femur, proximal tibia, and femoral head contain large quantities of good quality cancellous bone that may be used for structural grafting, and the femoral shaft is composed of thick cortical bone that may be used as strut or cylinder grafts, or dissected into more complex shapes. Again, fine dissection is not essential at this stage, the emphasis is on removing the grafts as quickly as possible, securely packaging them and getting them into a temperature controlled environment.

Intercostal arteries
Small arteries, branching of the thoracic aorta and supplying blood to the intercostal space.

Anastomosis
The connection of two structures, for example a blood vessel graft to a native blood vessel.

Meniscal cartilage
Crescent-shaped *fibrocartliage* structures within the knee joint, which distribute weight and reduce friction during movement.

Cortical bone
Hard, compact bone forming the external part of all bones and providing strength and stiffness to the skeleton.

Cancellous bone
Open "spongy" bone, mostly present in the ends of long bones.

Following retrieval of bone grafts, the legs are reconstructed. This may be done with anatomically formed prostheses, but may also be accomplished just as effectively with plastic or wooden rods and padding materials, prior to suturing of the incision sites. It is important that the prosthetic reconstruction is secure, so that the prostheses do not become dislodged when the donor is moved subsequently. When all retrieval activities have been completed, and the tissues safely packaged for transportation, the donor is cleaned and the cadaver restored to as normal appearance as possible. A toe tag is affixed to the cadaver to notify mortuary technicians and undertakers that tissue donation has taken place, and that they should take special care when moving the donor so as to avoid damaging incision sites and dislodging prostheses.

Once finished, the retrieval team return the donated tissues to the tissue bank as soon as possible. Water ice in an insulated container is ideal for this purpose, as it can be packed around the graft to quickly dissipate heat. The use of other cooling mechanisms, such as freezer packs, should be approached with caution as close association with the tissue may cause it to freeze, which will damage viable tissue grafts.

Key points

With deceased donors, it is important to ensure the quality of the tissues removed. This can be affected by the time post-mortem that the tissue is procured and the way it is removed so that contamination is minimized. A large number of different, useful tissues can be retrieved from one donor, including skin, heart and heart valves, bone, tendons, ligaments, and arteries.

Living donors

Tissue retrieved from living donors is generally classified as 'waste' material removed during surgical procedures, with very occasional exceptions (such as the donation of skin to treat a severely burned patient by relatives and friends). Another tissue that may be donated by living donors is the amniotic placental membrane following childbirth. The tissue most widely donated by living donors is bone, specifically the femoral head removed during hip replacement operations. In these cases, the articular cartilage on the surface of the bone has deteriorated, but the underlying bone is still usually of good quality. The femoral head provides a significant volume (up to 100 cm³) of cortico-cancellous bone that is of use to surgeons performing impaction grafting to replace lost bone stock during hip revision procedures. Bone removed during knee replacement operations has also been utilized for the same purpose in the past, but in practice is found to contain too high a proportion of cortical bone to be optimal for impaction grafting. Due to an ageing population, and the increasing incidence of hip replacement, this material is available in large quantities.

Obtaining tissue from living donors has many advantages from a tissue banking perspective. First, it must by necessity be retrieved in an operating theatre by surgeons rather than by the tissue bank staff. As the tissue is taken from living donors under aseptic conditions, the risk that it may be contaminated is greatly reduced, and a greater surety of safety with regard to transmissible viral diseases is possible as medical and behavioural history may be obtained directly from the donor themselves, and blood tests may be performed on fresh, good quality samples rather than post-mortem samples as is often the case with deceased donors.

Operationally, the tissue bank will set up a donation programme, usually with hospitals performing large numbers of hip replacements. This is a genuinely collaborative arrangement, as these hospitals will also have a need for the allograft to treat patients undergoing hip revisions and thus have a vested interest in the success of the programme. The hospital takes responsibility for screening and consenting patients, and retrieving the femoral heads, bacteriology testing samples, and blood samples using kits supplied by the tissue bank. The grafts and blood samples are then collected by the tissue bank who arrange for the blood and bacteriology samples to be tested by accredited laboratories, and store the grafts in quarantine until all the results are known. Depending on the surgeon's requirements, the grafts can then be issued as unprocessed, fresh frozen femoral heads, sterilized with gamma irradiation, or processed to remove donor marrow prior to issue—see below.

Donation of amniotic membrane is in principle a very similar process. The **amnion** is utilized as an ocular surface graft, and occasionally to treat burn wounds. It is donated by mothers undergoing elective Caesarian deliveries, whereby the placenta is removed surgically under aseptic conditions, exposing it to less risk of contamination than a vaginal delivery. The whole placenta is collected, and sent to the tissue bank for further processing.

Amnion
The innermost of the two membranes surrounding the placenta.

Key points

Tissues from living donors are regarded as being 'waste' material and as they are retrieved in the aseptic environment of an operating theatre this greatly reduces the risk of contamination.

SELF-CHECK 11.3

What steps are taken when retrieving tissues to reduce the risk of bacterial contamination?

11.5 Tissue processing and preservation

The major activity of a tissue bank is the processing of donated tissues. Whilst there are multiple ways in which tissue grafts can be processed, there are perhaps three core reasons why they are processed:

- To make them safer; for example by the use of decontamination protocols
- To make them more clinically effective; for example by the removal to donor cells to reduce immunogenicity and improve incorporation
- To make long-term storage (banking) possible; for example, the use of lyophilization or low temperature storage.

A fourth reason, which relates more to operational considerations, is to make tissues easier and cheaper to store and transport, for example a lyophilized graft can be stored and transported at ambient temperature, which reduces operating costs and the need for specialist low-temperature storage facilities.

The methods by which a graft can be processed depend on the properties of the graft that need to be retained. Whilst it may be desirable to sterilize a graft to increase safety, this is not practical where retention of donor cell viability is needed. This also affects the timescales under which a graft is processed. When grafts arrive at the tissue bank, they are still in quarantine, as much of the donor information required to release them for clinical use is not yet known. It is therefore best to hold them in quarantine until this information is obtained, to avoid the risk to both to personnel and the facility from handling tissue that may contain pathogens, and to avoid committing resources to processing grafts that may need to be discarded. This is achieved by deep freezing the grafts in their original packaging. However, this is not possible if tissue viability is an essential attribute for the graft, as deep freezing will render donor cells non-viable on thawing. Where this is required, as is the case with skin, heart valve, cardiovascular, and meniscus grafts, the tissue must be processed immediately on arrival at the tissue bank. Whilst individual protocols for different tissues may vary, the core methodology by which viable tissues are processed is broadly the same, comprising of dissection, decontamination by antibiotic cocktail, and cryopreservation. This methodology is discussed in detail by considering the procedures for banking the two most widely used viable grafts: skin and heart valves.

Skin

Toxic epidermal necrolysis
A serious life-threatening condition, usually caused by reaction to medication, resulting in the detachment of the epidermis from the dermis.

Necrotizing fasciitis
A serious infection of the skin and subcutaneous tissue, requiring aggressive debridement of infected tissue.

Skin grafts are utilized principally in the treatment of severe burn wounds, although they may be used to treat conditions with similar pathologies, such as **toxic epidermal necrolysis** and **necrotizing fasciitis**. There are conflicting opinions as to whether the grafts need to be utilized as viable grafts. As in many cases with tissue banking, good quality clinical data comparing different types of graft is scanty at best, and the bank is led by the requirements of individual surgeons. In the UK, it is the opinion of many burns surgeons that viable skin grafts, when applied to a wound bed from which all necrotic tissue has been excised, will temporarily 'take' to the wound, (the blood vessels in the graft anastomose to blood vessels in the wound bed) providing a blood supply to the graft and allowing the donor cells to assist the healing process. This is not a permanent engraftment, but is assisted by the fact that burns victims are naturally immunosuppressed. The graft will be rejected after a period of up to six weeks, but during this period it contributes actively to the healing of the wound.

The earliest method for the banking of skin was to place it in a refrigerator in a nutrient solution. This had the advantage of retaining cell viability, but only for a short period (up to two weeks) and was thus of limited practicality for tissue banking. The only feasible method for preserving viability long term is to cryopreserve the graft. The skin grafts are transported to the tissue bank in buffered, isotonic transport fluid which is essential to prevent acidification of the medium due to the metabolism of the donor cells. On arrival, the grafts are transferred to a decontamination solution, which comprises a range of broad spectrum antibacterial and anti-fungal antibiotics, prepared in a buffered nutrient medium. The use of antibiotics permits the selective targeting of microorganisms whilst minimizing damage to cells, and the use of a base buffered nutrient medium helps maintain cell viability during the incubation. The incubation may be performed at refrigerated, ambient, or normothermic temperatures, generally for a period of up to 24 hours with agitation. Prior to commencement of the decontamination, samples of tissue for microbiology testing are obtained ('pre-process' samples). It is necessary to test the tissue both pre- and post-process as residual antibiotics from the decontamination step may bind to the tissue and compromise post-process testing.

Following decontamination, the tissue is dissected and prepared for cryopreservation. All of these activities must be performed in a grade A environment within a grade B clean room. The strips of skin are laid flat, and trimmed so that the edges are flush. Any sections with perforations are discarded, as are any that are thought to be too fragile. Skin allografts do not require great mechanical strength, but must be able to withstand routine handling. The grafts are rinsed thoroughly to elute residual antibiotics from the decontamination step (although as mentioned previously some traces remain) and immersed in a cryoprotectant solution. This solution usually contains dimethylsulphoxide (DMSO) or glycerol dissolved in a buffered nutrient solution to a final concentration of 10–25%, depending on the bank. The grafts are incubated in the cryoprotectant solution for a short period to allow the cryoprotectant to fully permeate the skin; post-process microbiology samples are taken and the graft is spread onto a gauze or other supportive framework, and packaged. Given that the grafts will be stored cryopreserved at low (<–180°C) temperatures, appropriate packaging materials must be used; there are several plastic materials formulated for this purpose. When the grafts are sealed, using two layers of packaging, they can be removed from the clean room environment and cryopreserved. The grafts are maintained in a quarantine location pending satisfactory review of the processing paperwork, acceptable microbiology results, and release of the donor. They are then made available for issue.

METHOD *Principle of cryopreservation*

The principle of cryopreservation is to prevent the formation of large intracellular ice crystals during freezing through a combination of cryoprotectant impregnation and a controlled, slow rate of freezing. The controlled rate freezers are programmed to deliver a slow and steady cooling rate of –1°C per minute through application of nitrogen vapour and heating elements to dissipate the latent heat of crystallization, down to a temperature of –100°C. They are then removed, and placed into long-term storage in the vapour phase of liquid nitrogen at >–135°C. This temperature is below the glass transition temperature of the system, meaning that re-crystallization does not occur. Under these conditions, tissue can be stored effectively indefinitely without significant degradation.

Key points

Skin for transplant should ideally be a viable tissue. It is commonly used to treat burns, where it will temporarily 'take' to the wound, providing a blood supply to the graft and allowing the donor cells to assist the healing process, but is not a permanent engraftment and will in time be rejected.

Heart valves

Heart valve allografts are used principally for the repair of congenital defects in younger patients, and for the replacement of diseased or damaged valves in older patients. As with skin grafts, there are conflicting opinions as to whether the grafts need to be viable. In the early days of heart valve banking, the perceived wisdom was that donor cell viability was essential to the success of the graft as donor cells survived transplantation and contributed to the healing process. This lead to a preference for 'homovital' grafts, which had been stored refrigerated for a short period of time in nutrient medium. Current opinion is that donor cell viability is not essential (and may be disadvantageous due to provocation of cell mediated immune responses). Earlier data that suggested donor cells survived in the recipient for long periods has not been replicated, and evidence suggests that any viable donor cells present in the graft die very soon after transplantation. Therefore, the vast majority of heart valve banks today use cryopreservation to bank heart valves. The long-term storage afforded by cryopreservation permits thorough screening of the donor and the tissue prior to transplantation.

Hearts for valve donation may be obtained from deceased tissue donors during a traditional tissue retrieval, or in an operating theatre if organs are being donated. If a heart taken for transplantation proves unsuitable the valves can be used, or the heart is taken specifically for valve donation. Removal in an operating theatre is preferable as it permits organs to be taken in an aseptic environment immediately post-mortem. This is important as, perhaps more so than any other tissue, hearts are exposed to contamination from intestinal contents through the circulatory system or directly from the abdominal cavity. Where this is not possible, as in the case of tissue donors referred post-mortem, the heart is generally retrieved in a mortuary environment. Following retrieval, either in theatre or mortuary, the heart is transported to the tissue bank in a buffered, physiological transport solution on wet ice.

As the valve dissection is a delicate procedure that takes some time, the entire heart is retrieved rather than attempting valve dissection at retrieval. Adherent fatty tissue is removed from the heart and great vessels and the pulmonary and aortic valves dissected from the body of the heart. The mitral valve may also be banked; however, this is rarely required today. Every effort is made to retain as much vessel as possible, the ascending aorta and aortic arch in the case of the aortic valve, and the pulmonary trunk and pulmonary arteries in the case of the pulmonary valve. Following dissection, a thorough examination of the valve pathology is made. The internal walls of the valve vessels and coronary arteries are examined visually and with palpation for the presence of atheroma and calcification. Atheromatous plaques, which can cause calcification of vessel walls, are a common pathology associated with ageing, and lifestyle factors such as smoking and poor diet. Generally, any indication of calcification will render a valve unsuitable for transplantation, as will heavy atheroma; however, light atheroma would not preclude transplantation. A thorough examination is also made of the valve leaflets (cusps). These are checked for fibrosis (thickening of the leaflets which can reduce flexibility) and fenestrations (holes) which can cause the valves to leak. Any gross pathological abnormalities, for example bicuspid or quadricuspid valves, will also be noted and will generally contraindicate transplantation. The competency of the valves will be assessed by filling the lumen with physiological saline and checking for any leakage. Any observed pathology will be recorded, and valves may be rejected at this stage based on this. See Figure 11.3.

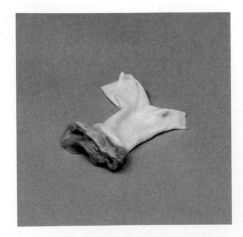

FIGURE 11.3
Pulmonary heart value graft.

The valves are then decontaminated with an antibiotic solution, with similar microbiological testing as described for skin grafts above. Following decontamination, the valves are measured. The annular diameters of the valve roots and any branching arteries are measured with *obturators*, and the length of the vessels associated with the valve recorded too. This is done post-decontamination as valves can contract post-mortem. They are then packaged utilizing packaging resistant to low temperatures and a cryoprotectant solution added. For heart valves, this is generally dimethylsulphoxide in a concentration of 10–20% (w/w), dissolved in a buffered physiological solution. This may contain nutrients and/or animal serum, depending on the individual protocol. A zwitterionic buffer such as HEPES is generally used as these remain effective at low temperatures. A secondary overwrap package is then added, and the valves cryopreserved as above. They may then be stored in quarantine pending completion of both donor and tissue related checks.

Key points

Cell viability of heart valves is not thought to be critical. The vast majority of heart valves used today are cryopreserved and this long-term storage allows thorough screening of the donor and the tissue prior to transplantation.

SELF-CHECK 11.4

What are the three main reasons for processing tissues? Briefly outline the two methods commonly used to preserve tissues.

Bone

For many types of tissue allograft, in particular musculoskeletal allografts, the presence of viable cells is not required and may in fact result in worse clinical performance. Typically, bone and tendon/ligament grafts are used as structural allografts, giving immediate mechanical support whilst providing a framework which is gradually reabsorbed and replaced by the recipient's cells. In this case, viable donor cells, or to a lesser extent cell remnants, are immunogenic and may provoke an immune response that weakens the graft material. In the interests of balance, it should be noted that it has also been suggested that this immunogenic response may enhance graft incorporation by provoking more rapid revascularization, but this is not based on sound clinical data. Most banking protocols for deceased donor bone therefore focus on removing the cellular elements whilst retaining the structural extracellular matrix.

Bone allografts can be deep frozen immediately following retrieval, as viability is not required. This enables all relevant information relating to the donor to be collated and checked before the tissue is processed, avoiding wasting resources processing tissue which may be unsuitable for clinical application. When the donation has been accepted, the tissue is processed. Following thawing, adherent soft tissue is dissected away from the bone. Depending on the type of graft required, the bone may then be cut using powered saws into a variety of shapes and sizes. These vary from large structural allografts, such as hemi pelvis, or distal or proximal femur, to fine powders composed of morsellized cortico-cancellous bone. Morsellized bone is prepared from larger chunks of bone that are mechanically ground. See Table 11.2.

TABLE 11.2 Bone products.

Role	Type of graft	Typical application
Structural	Hemi pelvis, cortical strut, femoral head	Replacement of large bone masses following trauma or tumour resection. Re-inforcement and replacement of bone weakened by artificial prostheses.
Space filling	Morsellized granules and powders of different sizes	Filling of large gaps in bone. Often impacted to form a solid support for prosthetic placement.
Osteoinductive	Demineralized bone matrix	Oral and maxillofacial repairs, spinal fusion.

The grafts are then cleaned, generally using a combination of chemical and physical processes. The overall objective of the cleaning process is to remove donor blood and marrow from the graft. A variety of different chemicals may be included in 'bone washing' protocols, including solvents and detergents to remove protein and lipid components, and active oxygen compounds that reduce bioburden and improve the cosmetic appearance of the graft. Physical processes, such as increased heat, negative and positive pressure, and centrifugation are often incorporated to improve the efficacy of the washing process. Many of the chemicals and physical treatments are also anti-microbial, and some bone washing protocols have been claimed to achieve sterilization of the graft in addition to marrow and blood depletion.

A more specialized type of processing is used to prepare a type of bone graft called demineralized bone matrix (DBM). This type of graft takes advantage of the fact that cortical bone contains small quantities of powerful **morphogens** called bone morphogenetic proteins (BMPs). These can actively induce the formation of new bone through initiating the 'osteogenic cascade', a sequence of events that involves the attraction of stem cells to the graft, induced differentiation of the stem cells into bone forming cells (osteoblasts), which then proceed to form new bone. This process is strikingly demonstrated in a mouse model, where subcutaneous implantation of DBM causes the formation of an ossicle of bone, replete with its own marrow cavity, independent of the skeletal system. Demineralized bone matrix is prepared by removing the mineral and lipid phases of bone with dilute acids and solvents, which leaves a collagenous matrix containing small amounts (in the order of picograms per gram) of BMPs. The process must be strictly controlled so as not to overexpose the BMPs to acid, which can damage them. Demineralized bone matrix is a unique type of bone graft in that its principal property is biological (active induction of bone formation) rather than biomechanical (passive support and provision of a framework for new bone generation).

Following completion of the processing protocols, the grafts must be preserved for long-term banking, and may also be sterilized. Preservation may be accomplished using either lyophilization or freezing, there being no requirement for the more sophisticated preservation protocols needed for viable grafts. Lyophilization (freeze drying) involves placing the grafts in a vacuum in the frozen state. Vapour is drawn off under the vacuum, and the graft dries at freezing temperatures, avoiding the possibility of damage occasioned by drying at higher temperatures. Lyophilized grafts may be stored and transported at room temperature, which permits for cheaper and less resource intensive storage infrastructure, and renders them more amenable for transport to, and local storage in, hospitals.

Morphogen
Molecule that influences undifferentiated cells to differentiate into specialised cells capable of making specific tissues.

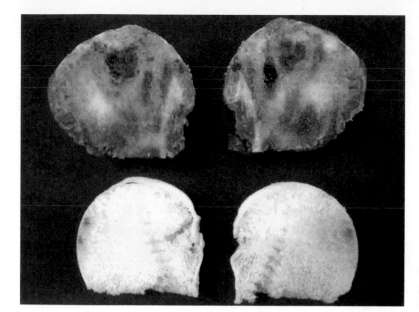

FIGURE 11.4
Cross sections of femoral head grafts before (above) and after (below) marrow depletion.

It is also common practice for bone allografts to be sterilized prior to issue. This is because (unlike with viable grafts) there is no need to retain cell viability and use of harsh sterilization processes is feasible. This adds to the overall safety of the graft. The most commonly used sterilization process is gamma irradiation, a relatively inexpensive, reliable, and controllable process which permits sterilization of the graft in its final packaging. It does, however, cause a dose dependent weakening of the bone structure, and should be employed with caution when applied to grafts which are intended to have a weight-bearing role. Where irradiation is utilized, it is good practice to minimize the required dosage by assessing the bioburden of the graft prior to sterilization. The harmful effects of irradiation may be ameliorated by the addition of radioprotectant chemicals to the graft prior to irradiation. Other protocols that may be used to sterilize bone grafts include chemical sterilization, with liquid chemicals, gases, or gas plasmas. Where chemical sterilization is employed, it is important that residual amounts of the sterilizing chemicals are eluted from the graft before it is implanted. Gas and gas plasma sterilization are only practical for lyophilized grafts. As has been previously mentioned, the chemical treatments applied during marrow and blood depletion may also be sufficient to sterilize the graft.

Tendons and ligaments

Tendons and ligaments may also be donated by deceased donors. Technically, a tendon joins muscle to muscle, or bone to muscle, whilst ligaments join bone to bone. Thus, certain types of tendon/ligament graft will have a bone block at one or either end. As with bone, tendon/ligament grafts may be stored frozen following retrieval pending completion of donor assessments. Processing of tendons is aimed at removing non-essential donor material whilst retaining the essential soft tissue matrix and any bone blocks. As the bone blocks contain the soft tissue insertion points, they need to be processed and banked as composite bone-tendon/ligament grafts. Processing generally commences with a dissection of the graft. In some cases, for example the patellar ligament, the graft may be retrieved as part of the larger knee joint, so the first step is to cut out the bone blocks with a powered saw. The bone blocks may also be dissected to defined sizes, with suture holes pre-drilled, to facilitate placement during transplantation. It is also necessary to remove any adherent muscle and fat. There are then a variety of protocols that may be used to clean the graft, and deplete donor cellular components. However, the soft tendon/ligament matrix is more vulnerable to damage than the hard, mineralized bone matrix, and care must be taken to ensure that the processing protocol does not damage this. Solvents and detergents are generally used in cleaning protocols. However, elevated temperatures (above 37°C) should be avoided as these can damage the soft tissue matrix. A further challenge with tendon/ligament grafts is sterilization. It may be possible to demonstrate that the washing protocol utilized achieves sterilization, but if not, the only widely used option for sterilization is gamma irradiation. This is problematic as the balance of evidence suggests that irradiation damages the structure of the soft tissue matrix, although this may be ameliorated by adjusting the dose applied, irradiating at low temperatures or using radioprotectant chemicals.

Key points

Bone and tendon/ligament grafts are generally used as structural allografts, giving immediate mechanical support whilst providing a framework which is gradually reabsorbed and replaced by the recipient's cells. As viability is not required, bone allografts can be deep frozen immediately following retrieval and processed only when all relevant information relating to the donor is collated and checked. Bone is made available as morsellized, structural bone, and demineralized bone matrix.

SELF-CHECK 11.5

How is bone processed and stored?

11.6 Storage and distribution

Therapeutic tissue banking is a relatively specialized field, and centralization of tissue banking activities permits concentration of expertise, and economies of scale afforded by banking multiple tissues in the same facility. In the main, tissue grafts are utilized in elective (planned) procedures, and it is not necessary for hospitals to hold local stocks for emergencies. There are some exceptions, for example major burn units require skin allografts to be close at hand, and some clinicians prefer to have grafts available locally on a 'just in case' basis, but generally the trend in recent years, encouraged by increasing regulation and inspection of tissue banks, has been towards centralized banking of tissues in regional or national facilities. One of the key aspects that differentiates tissue banking from organ donation and blood banking is that preserved tissues can be stored for long periods, and tissue banks therefore require large and well monitored storage facilities. A multi-tissue bank supplying a wide range of tissues will have facilities for ultra-low temperature storage (for cryopreserved grafts), frozen storage, and ambient temperature storage (for lyophilized grafts). These facilities must have sufficient (and ideally excess) capacity, be secure, reliable, and well monitored. Cryopreserved tissues are in most cases stored in liquid nitrogen cooled vessels, using vacuum insulated containers called Dewars. These allow tissue to be stored at temperatures below −180°C, well below that required to maintain cell viability. See Figure 11.5.

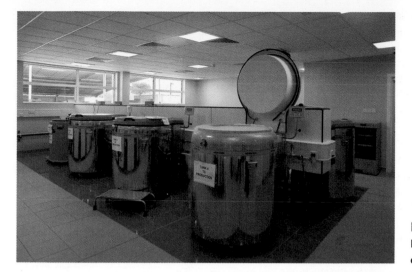

FIGURE 11.5
Large liquid nitrogen cooled storage vessels.

The use of liquid nitrogen gas requires the employment of strict safety protocols to deal with risks of cold burns and asphyxiation. Oxygen levels in the facility need to be continuously monitored, and powerful air extraction units included in case of a liquid nitrogen leak. Recently, advances in insulation technology have made possible the manufacture of mechanical freezers that can reliably maintain a temperature of −150°C, sufficient for the storage of cryopreserved tissues. These avoid the health and safety issues associated with liquid nitrogen. Non-viable tissues that have not been freeze dried are stored in mechanical freezers. The choice of storage temperature is dictated by the type of tissue, and the length of storage required—the colder the freezer, the longer the tissue may be stored for. Mechanical freezer storage facilities do not raise any specific health and safety issues, but it is important that sufficient air conditioning is provided, as the heat output from the compressors can raise the ambient air temperature to levels that are uncomfortable for staff, and at which the freezers may be unable to operate. Lyophilized grafts, by contrast, do not require any specialized storage facilities, only the requirement to maintain ambient temperature and humidity. The security of the facilities must also be considered; access to storage facilities should be restricted to designated individuals through the use of electronic or combination pass systems, and where possible individual Dewars, freezers, or cabinets containing tissue should be locked. Tissue banks may contain large amounts of tissue banked over a long period that cannot be easily or quickly replaced, so it is vitally important that temperature critical storage facilities are real-time monitored, with calibrated thermocouple probes linked to a data logging system and set to alarm at designated temperatures. Ideally, members of staff should be present in the facility and be able to respond to alarms immediately, and if not the alarms should be remotely monitored so that on-call personnel can respond quickly. Excess storage space should be available so that grafts affected by the failure of individual freezers, etc. can be rescued.

11.7 The future—regenerative medicine

As with any clinical science, tissue banking continues to develop and evolve. In its most basic form, tissue banking involves taking a tissue from a living or deceased donor, storing it for a period, then transplanting it into a recipient. We have discussed in this chapter many ways in which the tissue can be processed to make it safer and more clinically effective during the period between donation and transplantation, and one of the areas in which tissue banking has a key role is the emerging field of regenerative medicine, or tissue engineering, as it is also known.

The aim of the procedures discussed above is to replace a damaged tissue or organ with a graft that does not grow, but tissue engineering aims to regenerate and repair the damaged tissue. This is achieved by either adding a matrix into which cells can grow or by stimulating some of the remaining tissue to divide and regrow, or a combination of the two.

Regenerative medicine aims to bring together knowledge from the biological and biomechanical fields to create new solutions for the repair or replacement of diseased or damaged tissues. It is well established that the optimal type of tissue graft from a clinical performance standpoint is the autograft, although, as has been discussed, these come with problems of donor site morbidity and limited availability that cannot be overcome. The goal of regenerative medicine can be summarized concisely: to create tissue repair solutions with the advantages of autograft, but without the disadvantages. This requires that a tissue replacement be manufactured *ex vivo* (out of the body) and implanted.

The major components of a living tissue are cells and the extracellular matrix (ECM). The ECM portion of a graft may be derived from prosthetic materials, such as plastics or ceramics, processed biological components such as collagen gels, or animal or human tissue. The use of tissue for the ECM in the preparation of tissue engineered grafts has many advantages, principally the provision of appropriate mechanical properties and of a three-dimensional structure that facilitate colonization by the recipient's cells. If the objective is to replace a tissue, then the ideal replacement is a tissue. It may in fact not be necessary to add cells to the matrix *ex vivo*; if a tissue is processed to remove all donor cells and cell remnants the remaining ECM is minimally immunogenic, and can serve as a permanent graft. Acellular tissue matrices have shown a propensity in animal models and clinically to be integrated into the recipient's tissue and be recellularized *in vivo* by the recipient's own cells.

Examples of this include acellular dermis, which has been widely used clinically both as a direct dermal replacement in the treatment of burn injuries or chronic ulcers, and acellular heart valves, which have been used clinically for a number of years. In both cases, removal of donor cells enables the graft to integrate fully into the recipient as a replacement tissue, become recellularized *in vivo* with donor cells, and develop into a functional living tissue with the capacity to grow and self repair.

As with stem cell therapies, tissue regenerative research is expanding and new therapies are being tried clinically, giving hope to many who are suffering from degenerative diseases.

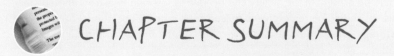

CHAPTER SUMMARY

- Diseases and injuries occasioning, or caused by, damaged tissues are a significant clinical and financial burden on the healthcare system.

- Allografts have a key role in treating these conditions, having attributes that cannot be replicated by prosthetic or other biological graft materials.

- Allografts can be donated by deceased or living donors. Appropriate and informed consent is a key legal requirement for donation to occur.

- Many different kinds of tissue may be banked, for example skin, heart valves, bone, tendons, and ligaments. The key difference between organ and tissue donation is that tissue grafts can be preserved for long periods.

- Allografts may be processed prior to being banked to make them safer and/or more clinically effective. Sometimes a compromise must be drawn between processes that improve safety, but may detract from clinical performance.

- They are different methods available for tissue preservation. The methodology chosen is informed by the need to preserve those qualities of the tissue important for clinical efficacy. Ultra-low temperature storage systems are required for storage of viable grafts.

- Tissue allografts can serve as excellent scaffolds for the generation of tissue engineered grafts that aim to regenerate and repair damaged tissue not just replace it.

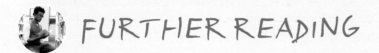

FURTHER READING

- **Galea G (ed.)** *Essentials of Tissue Banking*. **Springer, London, 2010.**

  A recent publication covering technical, medical, and scientific aspects of tissue banking.

- **Phillips GO (Series Editor).** *Advances in Tissue Banking*. **Volumes 1–7. World Scientific, Singapore, 1997–2004.**

  A series of books comprising invited review articles covering all aspects of tissue banking.

- *The Journal of Cell and Tissue Banking*.

  A quarterly journal, published since 2001, containing articles on all aspects of tissue banking.

- **UK Blood Transfusion Services.** *Guidelines for the Blood Transfusion Services in the UK*, **7th edition. The Stationery Office, London, 2007. Chapters 22 and 23.**

  UK Blood Service guidelines covering the selection of tissue donors, and the retrieval and processing of tissue grafts.

Answers to the questions in this chapter are provided on the book's Online Resource Centre.

 Go to www.oxfordtextbooks.co.uk/orc/knight

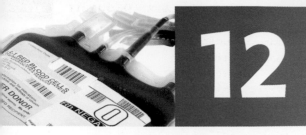

12

Quality Issues

John Barker and Joan Jones

Learning objectives

After studying this chapter you should be able to:

- Understand how the contributions of experts have shaped quality issues.
- Understand how the concepts of quality control, quality assurance, quality assessment, and good manufacturing practice (GMP) are related.
- Outline the basic ideals of GMP.
- Outline the GMP Standards required by the MHRA to conform with the Blood Safety and Quality Regulations (BSQR).
- Understand the requirements of the BSQR, Human Tissue Act, CPA (Clinical Pathology Accreditation), EFI (European Federation for Immunogenetics), JACIE (Joint Accreditation Committee-ISCT & EBMT), and their relationship to legislation.
- Describe what a quality management system (QMS) is and how it maintains and improves quality within blood transfusion and transplantation departments.
- Outline current haemovigilance systems in the UK.

Introduction

This chapter considers how blood transfusion and transplantation departments can satisfy the various standards and regulations that govern these disciplines, and guarantee the quality of the services they provide. It will also describe how a department can prove they are maintaining these standards to the regulatory bodies and demonstrate that they are improving the quality of the service. It will discuss quality assurance, quality assessment, quality management systems, and how the principles of GMP are an integral part of maintaining the system. The chapter also discusses **haemovigilance** and the current systems in place within the UK.

12.1 Evolution of quality

The move of *quality* to the top of organizational agendas has risen dramatically over the past 20 years. Much of the background stems from a number of industrial experts

Haemovigilance
Is defined as a set of surveillance procedures covering the whole transfusion chain (from the collection of blood and its components to the follow up of recipients) intended to collect and assess information on unexpected or undesirable effects resulting from the therapeutic use of labile blood components and to prevent their recurrence.

moulding managers' attitudes to quality within the workplace. Experts such as W Edwards Deming, Joseph Juran, and Philip Crosby have introduced concepts which although initially designed for consumer products, have spread into public services, such as the National Health Service. Many of the theories, such as Deming's 14 points and 'plan do check act' (PDCA) cycles, still hold true today, and although initially ignored by many industrialists they have become commonplace and the basis of quality management systems across the world. The concepts are designed to stop mistakes, introduce consistency, train staff, and improve processes, all virtues that blood transfusion and transplant professionals aspire too.

Traditionally all diagnostic laboratory tests have included *controls*, to ensure that the test has worked satisfactorily. With blood grouping, samples of known group are used as positive and negative controls, for example A and B cells for ABO grouping, K+ and K− cells for K typing.

In a test or assay where a numerical value is obtained, such as a haemoglobin estimation, there is an accepted level of experimental error and controls are used to ensure the accuracy and precision of that assay. In the late 1960s there were a number of pilot exercises to assess what variation there was between the same assay but performed by different laboratories. The value of such exercises was soon recognized and led to greater standardization of techniques and the introduction of more, and better, control materials. Initially schemes for haematology and transfusion these were run under the auspices of the British Committee for Standardization in Haematology (BCSH) but later they came under the umbrella of the UK National External Quality Assessment Scheme (NEQAS) as they remain today.

Over the years various *guidelines* have been developed, mainly by committees of BCSH, to help those working in the field of transfusion to develop them into *processes* and *procedures* that reflect the current state of technology and therapy. In clinical pathology laboratories, there was a marked improvement in the quality of the assays performed during the 1980s but there was growing concern about the management and staffing, both scientific and medical, of laboratories. The two major professional bodies involved in clinical laboratories, the Institute of Biomedical Science (IBMS) and the Royal College of Pathologists, cooperated in looking at ways in which these concerns might be addressed. In both Canada and Australia there were already standards written for clinical laboratories and inspection schemes in place. These were used as a basis for a UK scheme and after a number of pilots, Clinical Pathology Accreditation (UK) Ltd (CPA) was launched in January 1992. Although it was not mandatory that laboratories should be *accredited* under this professionally lead scheme, most soon saw its value, especially in the 'market place' atmosphere that was driving the NHS at that time. The diagnostic aspects of the blood centres' work, such as the reference laboratories, were accredited by CPA, but not the donor testing and component preparation as these had already been taken within the scope of the Medicines Inspectorate.

The original quality standards, such as BS 5750, were mainly concerned with the *product*; did it conform to the agreed specifications? But the later standards, the ISO 9000 series, also took account of the *process*, the steps taken to produce the product or result. Until 1988 all government run organizations, such as the NHS, had general immunity from prosecution for anything they did wrong or harm they did to patients. When it was proposed that this Crown privilege was to come to an end and blood was deemed to be a product within the scope of the Consumer Protection Act of 1987, the Blood Transfusion Services in the UK got together to produce some specifications for the blood components that they produced and agreed criteria for who could or could not give a blood donation. These were published in 1989 as the first edition of what came to be known as the Red Book—the *Guidelines for the Blood Transfusion Services in the UK*.

This first edition also contained a brief chapter on 'guidelines for a quality system for the collection and processing blood and blood products' that were in turn based on a British Standard 5750 for Quality Systems. This was the beginning of what some now describe as a quality culture, or the cynical as a quality industry, in the field of transfusion and transplantation.

The 1989 Red Book outlined for the first time details of what a bag of red cells, for example, should contain, and how many and how often such units should be tested to see if they complied with the standard. The main criterion for a unit of red cells was that the haematocrit or packed cell volume should be between 0.55 and 0.75, and that 1% of all units should be tested.

Many more and stricter standards then followed. To ensure products met these standards, quality monitoring laboratories were set up in blood (transfusion) centres to test the required number of units and to evaluate and validate any new processes introduced. The general quality standard BS 5750 became more rigorous as the ISO 9000 series was introduced, and to meet its requirements all aspects of the blood centres' activities came under the ever watchful eye of a new breed of employee, the quality manager and their new quality systems. These standards were for blood centres only and were not related to hospital blood banks. However, this soon changed with the introduction of the legally binding Blood Safety and Quality Regulations, 2005. The Human Tissues Act of 2004, brought transplant laboratories into the regulatory fold, with inspection and accreditation by the Human Tissues Authority. These are considered in more detail below.

The Department of Health has also produced a number of circulars aimed at improving transfusion practice across the country. The first circular known as *Better Blood Transfusion* (HSC 1998/224) was introduced following the recommendations of a symposium held by the UK Chief Medical Officer on evidence-based blood transfusion in 1998. These recommendations were designed to promote best practice by introducing local sets of rules based on national guidelines looking at the appropriate use of blood. The circular introduced the compulsory requirement for a hospital transfusion committee and the concept of transfusion practitioners in all trusts so that a multi-professional team could introduce and monitor these local guidelines. Other aspects looked at the training of staff, encouraging laboratories to become CPA accredited, the use of audit, and giving patients more information about transfusion. The circular has since been replaced by a number of new circulars, one in 2002, *HSC 2002/009 Better Blood Transfusion—Appropriate Use of Blood*, and one in 2007, *HSC 2007/001: Better Blood Transfusion—Safe and Appropriate Use of Blood*. All these recommendations are sent to the chief executive of NHS hospital trusts to be implemented by the transfusion laboratory within five years. The aims of the last circular were to:

- Build on the success of previous *Better Blood Transfusion* initiatives to further improve the safety and effectiveness of transfusion.
- Ensure that *Better Blood Transfusion* is an integral part of NHS care.
- As part of clinical governance responsibilities, make blood transfusion safer.
- Avoid the unnecessary use of blood and blood components (fresh frozen plasma and platelets) in medical and surgical practice.
- Avoid unnecessary blood transfusion in obstetric practice and minimize the risk of haemolytic disease of the newborn (HDN).
- Increase patient and public involvement in blood transfusion.

12.2 Quality management systems

Quality has always been a requirement within the blood transfusion department due to the serious consequences that an error may cause to a patient. Therefore, there is a need to prove that quality is an integral part of the daily work and departments are continually striving to improve the quality of the service they provide. This growth has been driven by legislation, such as the Blood Safety and Quality Regulations (BSQR) and has also been influenced by regulatory bodies such as the Medicines and Healthcare products Regulatory Agency (MHRA), and Clinical Pathology Accreditation (CPA), all requiring certifiable compliance and demonstrable improvements in quality. Other bodies such as the National Patient Safety Agency (NPSA) and the **Serious Hazards Of Transfusion** (SHOT) scheme are there to help us learn from our mistakes and prevent them from re-occurring. These are each dealt with in further details later in this chapter.

Blood transfusion is a key part of modern healthcare and it is the responsibility of the National Blood Services and hospital laboratories to provide an adequate supply of blood and components for all patients requiring transfusion. It is also vital that these products are safe, clinically effective, and of appropriate and consistent quality, so that patients are not put at risk. It is the responsibility of the management and staff at all levels to achieve these goals and make sure that the blood supply is 'fit for its intended use' and that it conforms to the required standard.

To achieve its quality objectives, laboratories must have well designed, structured, and organized quality in place that assures the user that the product or service provided is safe and efficient—a **quality management system**.

To accomplish this, the department must implement a **quality assurance** scheme that incorporates all the planned and systematic actions necessary to provide confidence that the product or service will satisfy the required standards. And to ensure that the laboratory is consistently producing a quality product or service the system needs standards that must be regulated by using good manufacturing practice (GMP) as part of this quality assurance programme. Good manufacturing practice provides a model on which to base a documented quality system and it describes the practical activities and controls which need to be in place so that the product or service achieves the appropriate standard.

Quality assurance

As stated above, quality management is a system to ensure both the accuracy and reproducibility of working practices are maintained and also to allow for improvement to be made. For consistency to be achieved, departments require protocols, called 'standard operating procedures' (SOP) that all staff can follow. An example of this could be how to perform a blood group test using manual techniques. Staff will be trained and their competency to follow these protocols assessed, before being allowed to perform the test unsupervised.

Serious Hazards Of Transfusion (SHOT)
The UK haemovigilance scheme.

Quality Management System (QMS)
Is a system of processes that ensures consistency and improvement of working practices, which in turn provides products and services that meet customer's requirements (e.g. a safe unit of blood).

Quality assurance
Is the prevention of quality problems through planned and systematic activities designed to detect, correct, and ensure that consistent quality is achieved. Good manufacturing process (GMP) is that part of the quality assurance system that assures that results and products are consistently produced, achieving the required standard and are 'fit for purpose'.

Quality control
Is any technique employed to achieve and maintain the quality of product, process, or result.

Internal quality control (IQC)
Is a set of procedures for continually assessing laboratory work and the results they produce to decide if they are good enough to be released.

External quality assessment (EQA)
Is a system of objectively checking the results of one laboratory with those from other, similar laboratories by the testing of undisclosed samples, thus ensuring that results are comparable wherever they are produced.

Statistical process control (SPC)
Is a method of quality control for a product or a process that relies on a system of analysis of an adequate sample size without the need to measure every product of the process.

The department will use a number of methods to assure themselves that the results they are reporting are accurate, and therefore safe. **Quality control** is essentially a way of assuring that the techniques used, and described by the SOPs, achieve and maintain the expected outcome.

A commonly used control is to test a number of samples with known blood groups in each batch of tests to make sure that the analyser is giving the expected result. These controls should also show up underlying trends in the assay by, for example, plotting OD data from an analyser, so that remedial action can be taken before a problem arises. This type of control is an example of **internal quality control (IQC)** that can be defined as a set of procedures for continually assessing each assay, and the results they produce, to decide if they are good enough to be released. This means that IQC has an immediate effect on the laboratory's activities and actually controls the output of the department. If the IQC fails then the results of a test, reagent, or process should not be released and an investigation should be initiated to find the cause of the problem and rectify it. Internal quality control is, therefore, controlling the day-to-day consistency of the laboratory's results and processes.

Another way of checking the quality of a department is to compare the results of the assays performed with other laboratories, thus monitoring the performance and effectiveness of their IQC measures. This inter-laboratory comparability is known as **external quality assessment (EQA)**. The various United Kingdom external quality assessment schemes help ensure that the results of investigations are reliable and comparable wherever they are produced. To achieve this, samples of known but undisclosed results are sent to laboratories who are members of the scheme. The department then tests the samples, using their normal procedures and processes, and returns the results to the scheme organizer. The results are then compared to the actual result and those from other laboratories so they can receive independent, objective, and impartial reports on their performance, enabling them to identify weakness and take appropriate action.

The UK Blood Services produce some three million units of blood and components every year, each one must be of a certain standard as laid down by the *Guidelines for the Blood Transfusion Service in the UK* (the Red Book). An example of this would be a standard level of Factor VIII in units of FFP so that users can expect that level of quality in each component. To maintain this quality, each service will perform quality monitoring tests and participate in the EQA scheme for each assay. However, it is not possible to test every product and therefore **statistical process control (SPC)** techniques are employed using data from usually 1% of components that are tested. This statistical method is used to observe the performance of the production process in order to predict significant deviations that may later result in a rejected product. An example of this is leucodepletion of whole blood, where 1% of all whole blood donations are tested to make sure that the volume of the donation is 470ml (±50 ml) in a minimum of 75% of tests, and that 99% of leucocyte depleted components have less than 5×10^6 leucocytes per unit. If this is not achieved then it identifies a problem somewhere in the process that must be investigated and corrected.

Statistical process control was pioneered by Walter Shewhart in the early 1920s. W Edwards Deming later applied SPC methods, in the USA during the Second World War, and successfully improved quality in the manufacture of munitions and other strategically important products. The power of SPC lies in its ability to look at a process, and variation within that process, to give a numerical value that can be used to assess the quality of the procedure and to allow the early detection of problems and thereby their prevention.

These three quality control mechanisms strengthen the quality assurance process, with IQC and SPC looking at the continuous process, and EQA assessing and comparing quality across laboratories. Once a department can establish that its procedures and processes are capable of meeting the expected quality another question now needs to be asked, 'Can we continue to do the job correctly?'

To answer this question we have to monitor the processes and the controls on them. This does not only mean the *detection* of quality problems but also how we can 'prevent' them from occurring; in other words can we *assure* quality.

Good manufacturing practice (GMP)

To obtain this quality objective a department needs to design and implement a QA system incorporating good manufacturing practice. Good manufacturing practice is that part of the quality assurance system that assures that results and products are consistently produced achieving the required standard and are 'fit for purpose'.

GMP is the basis of the UK *Rules and Guidance for Pharmaceutical Manufacturers and Distributors*, known as the 'Orange Book'. The basic requirements of GMP are:

- All processes are approved, documented, reviewed, and tested to produce the expected results to the appropriate quality.
- All critical steps and critical changes are validated.
- All necessary facilities for GMP are provided, including:
  - Appropriately qualified and trained staff to carry out procedures correctly
  - Adequate space and premises
  - Suitable equipment and services
  - Correct materials, containers, and labels
  - Approved procedures and processes

TABLE 12.1 Basic principles of good manufacturing practice.

1.	All processes are clearly defined and controlled. All critical processes are validated to ensure consistency and compliance with specifications.
2.	All processes are controlled, and any changes to the process are evaluated. Changes that have an impact on the quality of the blood/component are validated as necessary.
3.	Instructions and procedures are written in clear and unambiguous language.
4.	Operators are trained to carry out and document procedures.
5.	Records are made that demonstrate all the steps required by the defined procedures and instructions were in fact taken and that the quantity and quality of the blood/component was as expected. Deviations are investigated and documented.
6.	Records of testing and distribution that enable the complete history of an issued unit of blood to be traced are retained in a comprehensible and accessible form.
7.	The storage and distribution of blood minimizes any risk to their quality.
8.	A system is available for recalling any blood product.
9.	Complaints about products are examined, the causes of quality defects are investigated, and appropriate measures are taken with respect to the defective product and to prevent recurrence.

- There are suitable storage and transport facilities.
- Records for instrument and storage devices used in processes are recorded and any problems/deviations are recorded.
- A complete audit of the processes is required.
- A recall system of a product/result is required.
- Complaints and quality problems are corrected and changes introduced to stop them reoccurring.

A more comprehensive detailed breakdown of the chapters can be found in Table 12.2.

Within the Orange Book there are also various annexes that give additional information on procedural activities and validation processes for computerized systems and the use of ionizing radiation of blood components. The qualification and validation annex describes the principles of qualification and validation that are applicable to blood transfusion/transplantation laboratories to prove control of the critical aspects of particular operations. If there are any significant changes to the facilities, equipment, or the processes that may affect the quality of the product, then they must be validated prior to their introduction or reinstatement. A risk assessment approach should be used to determine the change in process to maintain the system in a validated state. In other words if you change any part of a process you must assess whether the system will give the same quality of result, this is known as *change control*.

Key points

Quality assurance in broad terms is the prevention of problems through planned and systematic activities (including documentation) so that the department can achieve control of its processes and achieve the consistent quality required by the patient.

SELF-CHECK 12.1

Can you name three differences between IQC and EQA?

12.3 Blood safety and quality regulations

Several years ago the European Commission (EC) agreed that for several reasons it would be worthwhile to 'set standards of quality and safety for the collection and testing of human blood and blood components. This would cover their processing, storage and distribution when intended for transfusion'. In effect the standard was to cover the whole process from donor to patient—from 'vein to vein'.

The main directive was 2002/98/EC—*Setting Standards of Quality and Safety for the Collection, Testing, Processing, Storage, and Distribution of Human Blood And Blood Components* (and amending Directive 2001/83/EC). It was supplemented by Technical Directive 2004/33/EC—Implementing Directive 2002/98/EC as regards certain technical requirements for blood and blood components.

TABLE 12.2 Details of GMP requirements.

1. Quality management	Requires: (a) Commitment and support of management (b) Quality policy defining the department's intentions in respect of quality (c) Quality manual which is a description of the quality system (d) Fully documented policies and procedures
2. Personnel	Requires: (a) Appropriate numbers of qualified and competent staff (b) Well-defined responsibilities (c) Personal development plan for every member of staff (d) Understanding of the requirements of health and safety
3. Premises and equipment	Requires: (a) Premises suitable for their intended use (b) Efficient workflow (c) Clean and temperature controlled (d) Equipment designed and maintained for its intended purpose (e) All changes must be controlled (f) Ensuring validated equipment, systems, and processes
4. Documentation	Requires: (a) Well-structured, easy to follow procedures (b) Controlled and reviewed on a regular basis (c) Fully audited amendments (d) Stored in a secure area
5. Service provision	Requires: (a) Work areas are secure (b) No unauthorized access (c) Documented procedures for all tasks (d) Traceability of all products from receipt to final fate (e) Inventory records
6. Quality control	Requires: (a) Internal quality control of all tests (b) Participation in external QC (c) Wrong results must be reviewed and actioned
7. Contract manufacture and analysis	Requires: (a) Scheduled equipment maintenance (b) Formal service level agreements with all contractors and users
8. Complaints and product recall	Requires: (a) Procedure for managing complaints (b) Procedure for recalling products not 'fit for purpose' (c) Investigation of complaints and recalls
9. Self-inspection	Requires: (a) Internal audits with all non-conformances addressed (b) Formal documentation of audit (c) Closure on all actions

Serious adverse reaction (SAR)

Is defined within the regulations as: 'An unintended response in a donor or in a patient that is associated with the collection or transfusion of blood or blood components that is fatal, life threatening, disabling, or incapacitating, or which results in, or prolongs, hospitalization or morbidity'.

Serious adverse event (SAE)

Is defined as: 'Any untoward occurrence associated with the collection, testing, processing, storage and distribution of blood or blood components that might lead to death or life-threatening, disabling, or incapacitating conditions for patients, or which results in, or prolongs hospitalization or morbidity'.

These two directives were transposed into UK law on 8 February 2005 as the Blood Safety and Quality Regulations (BSQR). Two further technical directives, on Haemovigilance and Quality Systems, were published and these were transposed into law in 2006.

The two directives, which became law in 2005, had an impact on all the UK blood services, but the impact was greater on the hospital blood banks as, for the first time, their activities came within legally binding regulations. It is the responsibility of the *competent authority*, currently the MHRA, to oversee compliance with BSQR by both the blood services and individual hospital blood transfusion laboratories. The latter are required to complete a *compliance report* every year for the MHRA, based on the principles of GMP, including being accredited by CPA.

The MHRA can inspect a laboratory if they feel, on review of their annual compliance report, that there might be a problem, or if a **serious adverse reaction** or **serious adverse event** has been reported that they deem might indicate some underlying problem. If an inspection is warranted the inspector will visit the department and perform an *audit* based on the GMP standards. All non-conformances identified at audit must be corrected within a specified timeframe before the department is deemed compliant. It is therefore essential that all personnel involved in blood transfusion understand the principles of GMP so that quality is built into the organization and the processes within it (see Figure 12.1). The MHRA also have the power to instigate a 'cease and desist' order or prosecute the 'responsible person' (nominally the chief executive) under criminal law if the standards are not met or information has been falsely submitted.

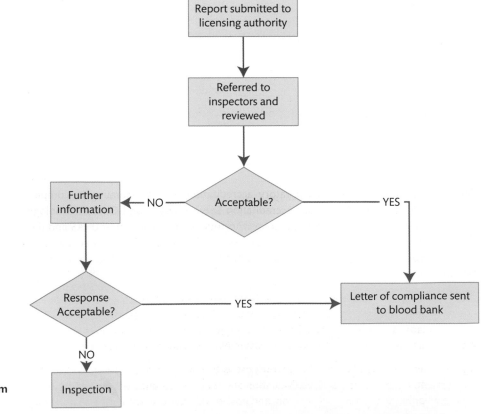

FIGURE 12.1
Annual compliance form review by MHRA.

12.4 The *In Vitro* Diagnostic Medical Devices Directive

One of the major elements of any laboratory assay is the reagent, or reagents, used. Over the years a number of countries developed their own criteria or standards for the commonly used reagents, such a blood grouping sera. With the advent of monoclonal antibodies there was a move away from grouping reagent produced in small batches from human sera, to producing large batches of monoclonal reagents by fewer manufacturers. Although these monoclonal reagents were more consistent batch to batch, and generally better than those from human sources, the differing standards made it difficult for one reagent to be sold in all countries. Within Europe some standards were agreed for the major reagents used in clinical tests, such as testing for HIV, hepatitis B and C, and for ABO and RhD blood grouping, and these became incorporated into the European *In Vitro* Diagnostic Medical Devices Directive (98/79/EC). The Directive was initially implemented into UK law by the In Vitro Diagnostic Medical Devices Regulations 2000, which have now been consolidated into the Medical Devices Regulations 2002.

The aim of the Directive was to deliver common regulatory requirements dealing specifically with the safety, quality, and performance of *in vitro* diagnostic medical devices (IVDs), and to ensure that IVDs do not compromise the health and safety of patients, users, and third parties, and attain the performance levels attributed to them by their manufacturer.

The Directive defines an IVD as:

Any medical device which is a reagent, reagent product, calibrator, control material, kit, instrument, apparatus, equipment, or system, whether used alone or in combination, intended by the manufacturer to be used *in vitro* for the examination of specimens, including blood and tissue donations, derived from the human body, solely or principally for the purpose of providing information.

The legislation mainly affects the manufacturers of reagents and other diagnostic devices, but users within Europe should ensure that any diagnostic device they use has the appropriate CE marking to show that it complies with these regulations.

12.5 Clinical laboratory accreditation

Within the UK there were two laboratory accreditation bodies, operating in complementary fields, the United Kingdom Accreditation Service (UKAS) and Clinical Pathology Accreditation (UK) Ltd (CPA). Clinical Pathology Accreditation is now part of UKAS and this has enhanced the development of accreditation policy, facilitation of the exchange of best practice and accreditation, and also has avoided the proliferation of accreditation standards for laboratories.

Clinical Pathology Accreditation focuses on the requirements for quality systems and *competence* as detailed in the *International Standards for Medical Laboratories*, ISO 15189-2007. These standards are for all clinical laboratories, not just blood transfusion laboratories, but help to ensure good quality systems are not just in place but are actually working.

Clinical Pathology Accreditation's stated purpose is to cover the organization and quality management, the resources, and the evaluation and quality assurance activities required to ensure that pre-examination, examination, and post-examination activities of the laboratory are conducted in such a manner that they meet the needs and requirements of the users. To asses that these objectives are being met laboratories are assessed, at present, on a four yearly cycle, with an additional surveillance visit every two years. These standards used when a laboratory is assessed cover the following areas:

- Organization and quality management systems
- Personnel
- Premises and environment
- Equipment, information systems, and materials
- The pre-examination phase
- Examination process
- The post-examination phase
- Evaluation and quality process

If on an assessment visit non-compliances are found, which is often the case, then the laboratory has to agree a timeframe in which to rectify the shortcomings. If these are not done, or the assessors feel that the laboratory has major failings then *they* are not accredited, or their previous accreditation is revoked.

12.6 The Blood Stocks Management Scheme

Another important aspect of quality is to ensure resources are used properly, and blood components, being a valuable resource, are no exception. The Blood Stocks Management Scheme (BSMS), was established to understand and improve blood inventory management across the blood supply chain and fits in with the *Better Blood Transfusion* objectives of avoiding unnecessary blood transfusion.

The BSMS is a partnership between hospitals and blood services, with an aim to maximize the use of donated blood by increasing the understanding of blood supply management. It was established in 2001 in England and now includes the blood services and hospitals in Wales, Northern Ireland, Scotland, and the Republic of Ireland. Central to the work of the BSMS is VANESA, a data management system where hospital and blood service data are collected, that now has a large bank of data on the blood supply chain and this has provided detailed knowledge of its various elements. Hospital participants can view real time data and charts and have the opportunity to benchmark performance against other users, for example those with similar blood usage. This has led to improvements in stock management. The BSMS provides inventory practice surveys and reports, publications, meetings, and training events, as part of its drive to improve stock management. More information about the work of the BSMS can be found at www.bloodstocks.co.uk.

Key points

Blood services and hospital transfusion laboratories now have to conform to certain legal regulations and these are enforced by a series of inspections. Clinical Pathology Accreditation assessments help laboratories maintain their quality systems in good order.

(a) What standards do CPA use for laboratory accreditation? (b) What standards are used by the MHRA to assess compliance to the BSQR?

12.7 Other legislation and regulatory bodies

The Human Tissue Act 2004

Following some highly publicized irregularities with the collection and use of hearts from children the Human Tissue Act was passed to regulate the removal, storage, use, and disposal of human bodies, organs, and tissues specifically for research, transplantation, education, and training. Laboratories involved in collecting and processing stem cells, bone marrow transplantation, or the retrieval of any human tissue are required to be licensed under this Act and are subject to inspection by the regulatory authority, the Human Tissue Authority.

Joint Accreditation Committee-ISCT and EBMT (JACIE)

This is a non-profit body established in 1998 to assess and accredit haemopoietic stem cell (HSC) transplantation. It aims to promote high quality patient care and laboratory performance and is an internationally recognized system of accreditation. It has established standards, conducts inspections, and accredits programmes to encourage organizations to meet these standards. This is a voluntary not legislative system to accreditation. Centres can demonstrate they have a QMS and will be issued with a certificate of accreditation.

European Federation for Immunogenetics (EFI)

EFI was formally founded in March 1985 with these aims:

- To advance the development of immunogenetics in Europe as a discipline of medicine and support research and training.

- To provide a forum for exchange of scientific information and to reinforce the skills and knowledge of young scientists and others working in the field.

- To create a formal organization of workers in the field of immunogenetics, histocompatibility testing, and transplantation.

- To elaborate recommendations for standardization of techniques, quality control, and criteria for accreditation and to support their implementation.

- To promote the organization and use of immunogenetic databases.

- To develop relations with similar organizations.

The EFI publish standards for histocompatibility testing, which provide a basis for the EFI accreditation process

12.8 Guidelines

As stated at the beginning of this chapter, the British Committee for Standards in Haematology (BCSH) develop and review many guidelines covering both laboratory and clinical aspects of transfusion medicine. These guidelines are accessed by following the link: www.bcshguidelines.

It is recommended that all laboratories comply with these guidelines and although it is not mandatory, regulating bodies are using these guidelines as standards that they expect a department to achieve.

12.9 Haemovigilance

In Chapter 6 we considered the two haemovigilance schemes that operate in the UK, SHOT and SABRE. The main aims of the SHOT scheme when it was launched in November 1996, were to improve the quality and safety of blood transfusions, and this was reinforced with the Blood Safety and Quality Regulations (BSQR); together they are a powerful tool in transfusion quality management systems.

From the cases referred to SHOT, which are analysed and reported annually, the four initial objectives of the scheme, listed below, have been realized and have had a positive impact on transfusion quality and safety in the UK.

The initial objectives of SHOT were:

- Improving safety of the transfusion process
- Informing policy within transfusion services
- Improving standards of hospital transfusion practice
- Aiding production of clinical guidelines for the use of blood components

More than a decade later these objectives are still relevant and the lessons learnt are also applicable to blood services outside the UK. The International Haemovigilance Network (IHN), with members from 28 countries, has the aim to develop and maintain a worldwide common structure with regards to safety of blood/blood products and haemovigilance of blood transfusion. The International Haemovigilance Network has established an international database so that in future comparisons can be made between the adverse events reported in various countries.

As said in Chapter 6, over the first decade of reporting, the trends observed by SHOT have demonstrated how an effective vigilance system can increase patient safety through a learning and improvement culture, rather than a punitive approach to errors, with the focus on safety and quality, monitoring, and audit. The number of events reported overall has risen, whilst the frequency of the most serious events, and the mortality directly related to transfusion, has fallen.

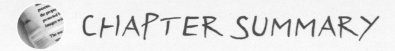

CHAPTER SUMMARY

- Over the past few decades methods have been introduced to improve the quality of blood transfusion/transplant departments by controlling and assuring that the blood, product, or result is of a high standard, fit for purpose, and is maintained at that level.

- As part of a planned quality assurance programme which is designed to detect, correct, and ensure that consistent quality is achieved, techniques such as internal quality control and statistical process control look at the continuous process, while EQA assesses and compares quality across laboratories.

- Statutory bodies like the MHRA inspect laboratories to determine conformance to legislation such as the BSQR. GMP is an important part of conforming to BSQR.

- All these processes combine to produce a QMS which helps provide products and services that meet the customers' requirements, for example a safe unit of blood to be transfused.

- The requirements of various expert committees, accrediting bodies, and legislation all help to improve the quality of the services provided by transfusion and transplant departments.

- Haemovigilance schemes, such as SHOT, use surveillance procedures to collect and assess information on unexpected or undesirable effects of blood and products to prevent their recurrence.

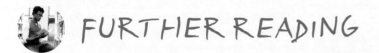

FURTHER READING

- Beckman N, Nightingale MJ, & Pamphilon D. Practical guidelines for applying statistical process control to blood component production. *Transfusion Medicine*, **19** (2009), 329–39.

- De Vries RRP, Faber J-C, & Strengers PFW. Haemovigilance: an effective tool for improving transfusion practice. *Vox Sanguinis*, **100** (2011), 60–7.

- BCSH Guidelines covering many aspects of blood banking and transfusion: www.bcshguidelines.com.

- Guidelines for the Blood Transfusion Services in the United Kingdom, other guidelines, useful information, and links: www.transfusion guidelines.org.uk.

- Blood Stocks Management Scheme reports: http://www.bloodstocks.co.uk.

- MHRA guidance for reporting incidents (SABRE): www.mhra.gov.uk/Safetyinformation/Reportingsafetyproblems/Blood/index.htm.

- Serious Hazards Of Transfusion (SHOT) annual reports: www.shotuk.org.

- International Haemovigilance Network (IHN) website: www.ihn-org.net.

Answers to the questions in this chapter are provided on the book's Online Resource Centre.

Go to www.oxfordtextbooks.co.uk/orc/knight

Glossary

Allele One of two or more alternative forms of a gene that arise by mutation and are found at the same place on a chromosome.

Alloantibodies Antibodies that react with an inherited antigenic characteristic that is lacking in the recipient.

Amnion The innermost of the two membranes surrounding the placenta.

Anastomosis The connection of two structures, for example a blood vessel graft to a native blood vessel.

Anterior cruciate ligament A ligament located within the knee joint that plays a crucial role in stabilizing the joint and is commonly damaged in sporting injuries.

Anticoagulant A substance which when it is added to the blood inhibits clotting.

Antisera Blood serum containing polyclonal antibodies.

Antithetical One of two or more alternative antigens.

Apheresis Collection of different blood cells using a machine.

Articular cartilage Hard, smooth cartilage that lines bone in joint surfaces.

Autoantibodies Antibodies directed against antigens on one's own cells, which can lead to an increased rate of cell destruction as in autoimmune haemolytic anaemia.

Autoimmune neutropenia An autoimmune disease in which the antibodies form target granulocytes. These antibodies can recognize HNAs, especially in children.

Batch pre-acceptance testing Tests performed to show batch of test kits/reagents received meets pre-defined criteria such as sensitivity and specificity and has not deteriorated during transportation.

Biallelic The two alternative alleles of a gene.

Bioprosthetic graft A composite graft, comprising both prosthetic and biological materials.

Biotin A water soluble B complex vitamin, necessary for the growth of cell, production of fatty acids, and metabolism of protein and fat. It is used in the laboratory because it interacts strongly with streptavidin. Thus molecules labelled with biotin can be detected with streptavidin conjugated to a reporter molecule.

Buffy coat The layer of WBC sitting on top of the red cell layer after centrifugation.

Cancellous bone Open 'spongy' bone, mostly present in the ends of long bones.

Cellular immunity That part of the immune system that is initiated by the recognition of a foreign protein or cell and leads to its removal or destruction by the interaction of complement, or cytokines produced by cytotoxic or killer T cells.

Clinically significant antibody An antibody capable of causing red cell destruction *in vivo*.

Codominant Allelic genes whose products are all expressed equally.

Codons Three base pairs that code for a particular amino acid.

Cold ischaemia time During transplantation this time begins when the organ is cooled with a cold perfusion solution after organs are harvested and ends after the tissue reaches physiological temperature during the implantation procedure.

Confidential unit exclusion This allows donors whose behaviour puts them at increased risk of acquiring HIV (or other TTI) who cannot avoid donating, to confidentially indicate that their blood should not be transfused.

Congenic Organisms produced as the result of specific inbreeding in an experimental setting so that they only differ in one gene locus.

Cortical bone Hard, compact bone forming the external part of all bones and providing strength and stiffness to the skeleton.

Costal cartilage Hyaline cartilage, located between the ribs. Utilized as a graft material in reconstructive surgery.

Cryoshipper A specially designed container used to transport material at a low temperature.

Cytosol The aqueous component of the cytoplasm in an intact cell.

Cytotoxic The ability to kill cells either by loss of membrane integrity, necrosis, or programmed cell death, apoptosis.

Differential centrifugation Subjecting a sample or donation of blood to accelerating force based on relative centrifugal force (or g force) and time to separate components according to size and density.

Drug-dependent antibodies Antibodies that react with a drug directly or with an antigenic structure created when the drug binds to a naturally occurring structure (referred to as haptenization).

Endosome A membrane bound intracellular compartment providing an environment for material to be sorted before degradation by the lysosome.

Extravascular lysis Immune mediated cell removal that takes place outside the circulation in the liver or spleen.

External quality assessment (EQA) Is a system of objectively checking the results of one laboratory with those from other, similar laboratories by the testing of undisclosed samples, thus ensuring that results are comparable wherever they are produced.

First field resolution This is how a low resolution HLA type is described because the numerals describing the HLA molecule are in the first field before the colon, for example HLA-DRB1*12.

Glycophosphotidylinositol (GPI) anchor A chemical linkage between glycoproteins and the cell membrane which can be readily cleaved under certain conditions thereby releasing the glycoprotein from the cell surface.

Graft versus host disease (GVHD) The most common cause of graft failure that is caused by donor immune cells, especially T lymphocytes, reacting against recipient tissue. The characteristic symptoms are the presence of a rash, diarrhoea, and abnormal liver function tests.

Granulocyte chemiluminescence test (GCLT) A biological assay that utilizes human monocytes to detect granulocyte antibodies bound to the membrane surface.

Granulocyte immunofluorescence test (GIFT) A whole cell immunofluorescence assay capable of detecting granulocyte reactive antibodies.

Haemolytic disease of the newborn (HDN) A disease associated with the foetomaternal transfer of red cell antibodies that cause haemolysis and red cell destruction in the infant.

Haemopoietic Blood cells produced in the bone marrow.

Haemovigilance Is defined as a set of surveillance procedures covering the whole transfusion chain (from the collection of blood and its components to the follow up of recipients) intended to collect and assess information on unexpected or undesirable effects resulting from the therapeutic use of labile blood components and to prevent their recurrence.

Haplotypes Linked genes, the alleles contributed from one or the other parent, in a blood group system that are passed on together.

Hapten A substance that is unable to elicit an immune response by itself (usually because it is too small) but which can do so when combined with a larger molecule.

Human neutrophil antigen (HNA) The term given to allelic forms of granulocyte glycoproteins that give rise to an alloimmune response.

Human platelet antigen (HPA) The term given to allelic forms of platelet glycoproteins that give rise to an alloimmune response.

Humoral immunity That part of the immune system that is initiated by the recognition of a foreign protein or cell and lead to its removal or destruction through the interaction of a specific antibody.

Hyperhaemolysis Characterized by marked reticulocytopenia (a significant decrease from the patient's usual absolute reticulocyte level), hyperbilirubinemla, and haemoglobinuria.

Iliac crest Part of the pelvic bone, often used as a source of bone autograft.

Immune response The body's ability to recognize and defend itself against substances that appear foreign and harmful such as bacteria and viruses.

Immunocompetent The ability to produce an immune response following a challenge with an antigen.

Immunodominant sugar residue The sugar residue that confers antigenicity on a carbohydrate antigen.

Immunogenic The likelihood that an antigen will stimulate an immunological response.

In utero Literally within the uterus.

Intercostal arteries Small arteries, branching off the thoracic aorta and supplying blood to the intercostal space.

Internal quality control (IQC) Is a set of procedures for continually assessing laboratory work and the results they produce to decide if they are good enough to be released.

Intracellular With in the cellular milieu.

Intra-membranous Within the cellular membrane.

Intravascular lysis Cells being lysed within the circulation by antibodies that activate the complement pathway, especially anti-A and anti-B.

Irradiation A process for inactivating donor lymphocytes using gamma (or X-ray) irradiation to prevent transfusion-associated graft versus host disease (TA-GVHD), a rare but potentially fatal consequence of blood transfusion.

Isoantibodies Antibodies that react with an antigen that is normally found in all individuals but which is lacking in the recipient.

Lectin A sugar-binding protein or glycoprotein of non-immune origin, which can agglutinate cells and/or precipitate glycoconjugates.

Leucodepletion A process for removal of white blood cells from blood components to less that 5×10^6 per unit through an in-line filter.

Linkage disequilibrium The tendency of certain alleles at different loci to occur on the same chromosome more often than expected by chance, for example HLA-A*01-B*08-DRB1*03:01 are in positive linkage disequilibrium as the observed frequency of this haplotype is greater than the expected frequency.

Marfan's syndrome A genetic disorder, causing weakness of the connective tissue. A contraindication for donation of soft tissue allografts.

Meniscal cartilage Crescent-shaped fibrocartliage structures within the knee joint, which distribute weight and reduce friction during movement.

Microarray techniques An assay system using labelled probes to simultaneously identify a range of different characteristics.

Mimotopes Short synthetic peptides that mimic natural epitopes of the individual blood group antigens that are being developed to be used in microarray antibody detection systems without the need for intact red cells.

Monoclonal antibody immobilization of granulocyte antigens (MAIGA) assay An ELISA assay which uses monoclonal antibodies against granulocyte antigens as the basis of detection and identification of granulocyte specific antibodies.

Monoclonal antibody immobilization of platelet antigens (MAIPA) assay An ELISA assay which uses monoclonal antibodies against platelet antigens as the basis of detection and identification of platelet specific antibodies.

Monoclonal antibody Produced from a single clone of cells.

Monoclonal Produced from one clone of cells.

Morphogen Molecule that influences undifferentiated cells to differentiate into specialized cells capable of making specific tissues.

Morsellized bone graft Bone graft milled to granules or powders of different diameters.

Multipotent Multipotent progenitor or stem cells can give rise to many but limited types of cell.

Necrotizing fasciitis A serious infection of the skin and subcutaneous tissue, requiring aggressive debridement of infected tissue.

Neonatal alloimmune neutropenia (NAIN) Neutropenia in a neonate (or foetus) caused by the maternal foetal transfer of granulocyte specific antibodies recognizing either HNAs or granulocyte glycoproteins inherited by the foetus from the father but absent in the mother.

Neonatal alloimmune thrombocytopenia (NAIT) Thrombocytopenia in a neonate (or foetus) caused by the maternal foetal transfer of platelet specific antibodies recognizing either HPAs or platelet glycoproteins inherited by the foetus from the father but absent in the mother.

Neoplastic An abnormal growth of tissue.

Neutropaenia Low numbers of neutrophil leucocytes.

Neutrophils Together with eosinophils and basophils these circulating white cells are collectively known as granulocytes or polymorphonuclear cells. In normal healthy adults, neutrophils account for >90% of all granulocytes. Most laboratories do not attempt to separate these three cell types prior to antibody testing so any antibodies detected are more correctly called granulocyte-specific. Nonetheless, some HNA, i.e. HNA-1 and 2, have been shown to be truly neutrophil-specific in that they are expressed on neutrophils but not eosinophils or basophils.

Non-haemolytic febrile transfusion reactions (NHFTRs) An increase in temperature ≥1°C following a blood transfusion but which is not associated with red cell haemolysis.

Null allele A mutant gene that does not function like the normal gene. Many null HLA alleles lack cell surface expression and cannot present peptides to the immune system.

Osteochondral graft A composite graft, comprising bone plus an intact articular cartilage surface.

Pancytopaenia Low numbers of all blood cell lines (RBC, WBC, and platelets).

Pathogen inactivation A process for removal of infectious agents in blood components/products through chemical or heat treatment and filtration.

Pathogen reduction Process for reducing or eliminating most infectious agents in blood components/products.

Phycoerythrin (PE) A red protein found in red algae and cyanobacteria. It is used as a fluorescent label for antibodies used in the laboratory for the detection of specific markers on cell surfaces, in the cytoplasm, or on DNA, by utilizing its ability to absorb blue green light and emit orange-yellow light (475 ± 10nm).

Platelet immunofluorescence test (PIFT) A whole cell immunofluorescence assay capable of detecting platelet reactive antibodies.

Platelet transfusion refractoriness A suboptimal increase in circulating platelet count following platelet transfusion.

Pluripotent Is the ability of the human stem cell to differentiate or become almost any cell in the body.

Polyclonal antibodies These are produced by more than one clone of cells.

Polymerase chain reaction (PCR) An enzyme reaction utilizing Taq polymerase to amplify the copy number and hence enable detection of a genetic characteristic.

Polymerase chain reaction with sequence specific primers (PCR-SSP) The polymerase chain reaction using primers that recognize a DNA sequence encoding a unique heritable genetic characteristic—typically an SNP.

Polymorphism The occurrence of more than one form of the antigen.

Post-transfusion purpura (PTP) An unexpected thrombocytopenia occurring 5–12 days after a blood transfusion that is associated with the presence of platelet-specific antibodies.

Proteasome An intracellular proteolytic complex that degrades cytosolic and nuclear proteins.

Public epitopes A region of an antigen shared by many different antigens that is recognized by antibodies, B cells, or T cells.

Quality assurance Is the prevention of quality problems through planned and systematic activities designed to detect, correct, and ensure that consistent quality is achieved. Good manufacturing process (GMP) is that part of the quality assurance system that assures that results and products are consistently produced, achieving the required standard, and are 'fit for purpose'.

Quality control Is any technique employed to achieve and maintain the quality of product, process, or result.

Quality management system (QMS) Is a system of processes that ensures consistency and improvement of working practices, which in turn provides products and services that meet customer's requirements (e.g. a safe unit of blood).

Second field resolution This is how a high resolution or allele level HLA type is described because the second field after the first colon is populated, for example HLA-DRB1*12:01.

Sensitivity This is the proportion of people who have a disease/infection (or products such as antibodies to it) which is correctly identified by a screening test.

Serious adverse event (SAE) Is defined as: 'Any untoward occurrence associated with the collection, testing, processing, storage and distribution of blood or blood components that might lead to death or life-threatening, disabling, or incapacitating conditions for patients, or which results in, or prolongs hospitalization or morbidity'.

Serious adverse reaction (SAR) Is defined within the regulations as: 'An unintended response in a donor or in a patient that is associated with the collection or transfusion of blood or blood components that is fatal, life threatening, disabling, or incapacitating, or which results in, or prolongs, hospitalization or morbidity'.

Serious Hazards Of Transfusion (SHOT) The UK haemovigilance scheme.

Serological crossreactivity This is where antibodies react with a public epitope shared by different HLA molecules. These HLA molecules that share a public epitope are often described as Cross Reactive Groups (CREG), for example anti-HLA-B7 antibodies can crossreact with a shared epitope on HLA-B42, B55, and B56.

ShipsLog™ A temperature monitoring device attached to a cryoshipper to record the temperature.

Single nucleotide polymorphism (SNP) A single nucleotide substitution in the DNA reading frame that encodes a particular inherited characteristic.

Specificity This is the proportion of people who are correctly identified by a screening test as negative for the disease/infection.

Statistical process control (SPC) Is a method of quality control for a product or a process that relies on a system of analysis of an adequate sample size without the need to measure every product of the process.

Streptavidin A bacterial protein purified from *Streptomyces avidinii* that has a high affinity for biotin.

Thrombocytopaenia Low numbers of platelets.

Thrombogenic Material which causes blood to clot on contact.

Toxic epidermal necrolysis A serious life-threatening condition, usually caused by reaction to medication, resulting in the detachment of the epidermis from the dermis.

Transfusion reactions This is a systemic response produced by the body to the infusion of blood or blood components/products. The adverse reaction may be to proteins in the blood or incompatible cellular components such as leucocytes, platelets, or erythrocytes.

Transfusion-related acute lung injury (TRALI) Difficulty in breathing associated with *de novo* chest X-ray changes observed within six hours of transfusion that is not associated with transfusion overload or cardiac insufficiency.

Transfusion-related alloimmune neutropenia (TRAIN) A transient neutropenia following infusion of a blood product due to the action of neutrophil-specific antibodies but which does not develop the symptoms of TRALI.

Validated Having documentary evidence to show that a system/equipment or process meets pre-defined requirements for its intended use.

Warm ischaemia time The time elapsing between death and a body being placed into a refrigerated environment.

Window period This is the period between the onset of the infection and the appearance of the detectable infectious agent or antibodies to it. For a virus, the window period is shorter for the detection of the viral RNA/DNA than antibodies which are produced later in the infection.

Abbreviations

2,3,DPG	2,3 diphosphoglycerate
ACD	acid citrate dextrose
AHG	anti-human globulin
AIDS	acquired immune deficiency syndrome
ALL	acute lymphoblastic leukaemia
AML	acute myeloid leukaemia
Anti-HBc	antibody to hepatitis B core antigen
Anti-HBe	antibody to hepatitis B e antigen
Anti-HBs	antibody to hepatitis B surface antigen
ATL	adult T cell leukaemia/lymphoma
ATR	acute transfusion reactions
BAT	bottom and top
BBMR	British Bone Marrow Register
BCSH	British Committee for Standards in Haematology
BM	bone marrow
BMP	bone morphogenetic protein
BPAT	batch pre-acceptance testing
BSBMT	British Society for Bone Marrow Transplant
BSE	bovine spongiform encephalitis
BSQR	Blood Safety and Quality Regulations
BTS	blood transfusion service
BWS	British Working Standard
CAD	compound adsorption device
CAPA	corrective and preventative actions
C-CAMP	cyclophosphamide, vincristine, adriamycin and methykprenidolone
CD	cluster distribution
CFS	colony stimulating factor
CFU	colony forming units
CH	chromosome
CHIKV	chikungunya virus
CLIA	chemiluminescence immunoassay
CML	chronic myeloid leukaemia
CMV	cytomegalovirus
CNS	central nervous system
CPA	Clinical Pathology Accreditation
CPD	citrate phosphate dextrose
CSP	cryosupernatant plasma
CPDA-1	citrate phosphate dextrose containing adenine

DBM	demineralized bone matrix
DI	designated individual
DLI	donor lymphocyte infusion
DMSO	dimethyl sulphoxide
DNA	deoxyribonucleic acid
dNTP	deoxynucleotide triphosphate
DoB	date of birth
E	erythroid
eBDS	enhanced bacterial detection system
ECM	extracellular matrix
EFI	European Federation for Immunogenetics
EIA	enzyme immunoassay
ELISA	enzyme linked immunosorbent assay
EQA	external quality assessment
FFP	fresh frozen plasma
FNHTR	febrile non-haemolytic transfusion reactions
FRALE	frangible anchor linker effector
FTA-abs	fluorescent treponemal antibody-absorbed
GCLT	granulocyte chemiluminescence test
GCSF	granulocyte colony stimulating factor
GIFT	granulocyte immunofluorescence test
GM	granulocyte-monocyte
GMP	good manufacturing practice
GP	glycoprotein
G.P.	general practitioner
GVHD	graft versus host disease
GVL	graft versus leukaemia
GVT	graft versus tumour
HAM	HTLV-I associated myelopathy
Hb	haemoglobin
HBc	hepatitis B core
HBcAg	hepatitis B core antigen
HBeAg	hepatitis B e antigen
HBsAg	hepatitis B surface antigen
HBV	hepatitis B virus
HCT	haemopoietic cell transplant
HCV	hepatitis C virus
HDN	haemolytic disease of the newborn

HEPES	4-(2-hydroxyethyl)-1-piperazineethanesulfonic acid	NHSBT-TS	National Health Service Blood and Transplant Tissue Services
HIV	human immunodeficiency virus	NIBSC	National Institute of Biological Standards and Control
HLA	human leucocyte antigens	NMDP	National Marrow Donor Program
HNA	human neutrophil antigens	NP	nurse practitioner
HPA	Health Protection Agency	NPSA	National Patient Safety Agency
HPA	human platelet antigens	NRC	National Referral Centre
HPC	haemopoietic progenitor cells	NTMRL	National Transfusion Microbiology Reference Laboratory
HSC	haemopoietic stem cells		
HTA	Human Tissue Authority	PBSC	peripheral blood stem cells
HTLV	human T cell lymphotropic virus	PCR	polymerase chain reaction
HTR	haemolytic transfusion reaction	PCR-SSP	polymerase chain reaction with site specific primers
IAT	indirect antiglobulin test		
IBCT	incorrect blood component transfused	PCT	photochemical technology
ICH	intra-cranial haemorrhage	PDCA	plan, do, check, act
ID	individual donation	PI	pathogen inactivation
IFA	indirect fluorescent antibody	PIFT	platelet immunofluorescence test
ISBT	International Society of Blood Transfusion	PR	pathogen reduction
ISCT	International Society for Cellular Therapy	PrPc	cellular form of prion protein
IQC	internal quality control	PrPsc	abnormal prion protein
IUT	intra-uterine transfusion	PTP	post-transfusion purpura
IVDD	*In Vitro* Diagnostics Device	QA	quality assurance
JACIE	Joint Accreditation Committee-ISCT and EBMT	QMS	quality management system
		RIBA	recombinant immunoblot assays
kg	kilograms	RNA	ribonucleic acid
MAIGA	monoclonal antibody immobilization of granulocyte antigens	RPR	rapid plasma reagin
		RT	reverse transcriptase
MAIPA	monoclonal antibody immobilization of platelet antigens	SABRE	serious adverse blood reactions and events
		SAE	serious adverse event
MB	methylene blue	SAG	saline, adenine, and glucose
MegK	megakaryocytic	SAG-M	saline, adenine, glucose, and mannitol
MHC	major histocompatibility complex	SAR	serious adverse reaction
MHRA	Medicines and Healthcare products Regulatory Agency	S/CO	sample optical density to cut-off ratio
		SEAC	Spongiform Encephalopathy Advisory Committee
MOP	metoxypsoralen		
MTU	multi-tube unit	SHOT	Serious Hazards Of Transfusion
NAIN	neonatal alloimmune neutropenia	SOP	standard operating procedure
NAIT	neonatal alloimmune thrombocytopenia	SPC	statistical process control
NAT	nucleic acid test	SPU	sample preparation unit
NEQAS	National External Quality Assessment Scheme	TA-GVHD	transfusion-associated graft versus host disease
		TBI	total body irradiation
NetCord-FACT	International Standards for Cord Blood Collection, Processing, Testing, Banking, Selection and Release	TMA	transcription mediated amplification
		TNBP	tri-(n-butyl)-phosphate
NHFTR	non-haemolytic febrile transfusion reactions	TPHA	*Treponema pallidum* haemagglutination assay

TPPA	*Treponema pallidum* particle assay
TRAIN	transfusion-related alloimmune neutropenia
TRALI	transfusion-related acute lung injury
TSP	tropical spastic parapheresis
TTI	transfusion-transmitted infection
URD	unrelated donor
vCJD	variant Creutzfeldt–Jakob disease

VDRL	Venereal Diseases Research Laboratory
vWF	von Willebrand factor
WBC	white blood cells
WHO	World Health Organization
WNV	West Nile virus
WP	window period

Index

A

A antigen 23, 25
A blood group 72, 127-8, 154
    transfused to O group 148
AB antigen 25
AB blood group 23, 126, 127, 154
Abbott PRISM test 94
ABO antibodies 25, 145
ABO antigens 23-4, 26, 43
ABO blood group 21-5, 22, 70, 114,
    120, 175, 189
   autoimmune haemolytic
      anaemias 154
   D grouping 124
   electronic issue 125
   emergency issue 125-6
   frequency of worldwide 24
   haemolysis post-
      transplantation 154, 155
   haemolytic disease of the newborn
      (HDN) 158, 159
   indirect antiglobulin test (IAT)
      crossmatch 122-3
   neonatal alloimmune
      thrombocytopenia 208
   platelets 127
ABO compatible plasma 146
ABO genotypes and phenotypes 24
ABO incompatibility 133, 138, 143-4,
    148, 155, 182, 232
ABO selection of red cells 120-1
acid citrate dextrose (ACD) 50
acquired immune deficiency syndrome
    (AIDS) 77, 78, 109
acupuncture 48, 75
acute normovolaemic haemodilution
    (ANH) 111-12
additional (discretionary) testing 81-4
adenosine 50
adenosine triphosphate (ATP) 50, 61
adverse effects 103, 105, 129-32,
    134-6
age of donor 46, 60
albumin 99
aliquots 125
alleles 168, 169, 190
allergic (urticarial) reactions 103, 130,
    133, 140
   see also anaphylactic reactions

allo-adsorption 153
alloanti-D 31-2
alloantibodies 145, 151, 153, 154, 188,
    206-10
   see also under human platelet antigens
allogenic blood components 107, 109
allogenic stem cells 225
allografts 222, 237, 238, 239, 244, 251
alloimmunization 105
amino acid substitutions 198
amnion 247
amniotic placental membrane 246-7
anaemia 101, 107, 114
   aplastic 41
   chronic normovolaemic 131
   haemolytic disease of the newborn
      (HDN) 155-6, 159
   normal physiological
      response to 99-100
   see also autoimmune haemolytic
      anaemias
anaphylactic reactions 132, 136
anastomosis 245
Anthony Nolan Trust 179, 222
anti-A 25, 70
anti-A/B 59, 121, 124
   haemolysis post-
      transplantation 154-5
   haemolytic disease of the newborn
      (HDN) 159
   high titre 72
   immediate spin crossmatch 123
   immune red cell destruction 143
   platelets 127
   polyclonal reagents 23
anti-B 25, 70
antibiotics 195, 213, 248, 251
antibody
   ABO, H and Lewis blood groups 25
   assay 73
   atypical 135
   clinically significant 145
   -dependent, cell-mediated
    cytotoxicity (ADCC) 176
   detection 199-205
    granulocyte
     chemiluminescence test
     (GCLT) 203-4
    human neutrophil antigens
     (HNA) antibodies 202-5

human platelet antigens
    (HPA) 200-2
monoclonal antibody
    immobilization of
    platelet antigens
    (MAIPA) assay 202
platelet immunofluorescence
    test (PIFT) 200, 201
Duffy blood group 40
   function 8-9
   incompatible transplants (AIT) 175
   isoantibodies 188
   Kell and Kx blood groups 38-9
   Kidd blood group 41-2
   Lewis blood group and secretor 27
   Lutheran blood group 36
   mediated red cell destruction 10-12
   MNS blood group 29
   naturally acquired 6
   polyclonal 4
   potency 146
   reactive but clinically
      insignificant 146-7
   screening 120-1, 124, 125
   structure 6-8
   see also alloantibodies; autoantibodies;
      immunoglobulins;
      in vitro detection of antigen-
      antibody reactions
anti-C 156-7, 158, 159
anti-C3 152-3
anti-CD3 therapy 173
anticoagulants 49, 50-1
anti-cytomegalovirus (CMV) 59
anti-D 35, 39, 70
   haemolytic disease of the newborn
      (HDN) 156-8, 158, 159
   immunoglobulin 106
   prophylaxis 157-8
   reagents 31-2
anti-E 147, 156, 158
anti-Fy^a 40, 158
antigens
   ABO, H, and Lewis blood
      groups 21-4
   antibody reactions 9-10
   assay 73
   Duffy blood group 39-40
   immune red cell destruction 143
   Kell and Kx blood groups 37-8